Cultural Competence *in* Caring *for* Muslim Patients

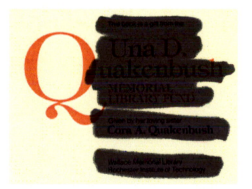

Dedicated to Adam Abu Isra Wa Asiyah Ibn Hussein Ibn Hassim Ibn Sahaduth Ibn Rosool Ibn Olee Al Mauritiusy, Yasmin Soraya, Reshad Hassan, Mariam, Isra Oya, Asiyah Maryam, Safian & Hassim.

The knowledge from which no benefit is derived is like a treasure from which no charity is bestowed in the way of the Lord.

—*Prophet Muhammad (✤[Peace be upon Him])*

Cultural Competence *in* Caring *for* Muslim Patients

Edited by

G. Hussein Rassool

palgrave
macmillan

First published 2014 by
PALGRAVE MACMILLAN

Palgrave Macmillan in the UK is an imprint of Macmillan Publishers Limited,
registered in England, company number 785998, of Houndmills, Basingstoke,
Hampshire RG21 6XS.

Palgrave Macmillan in the US is a division of St Martin's Press LLC,
175 Fifth Avenue, New York, NY 10010.

Palgrave Macmillan is the global academic imprint of the above companies
and has companies and representatives throughout the world.

Palgrave® and Macmillan® are registered trademarks in the United States,
the United Kingdom, Europe and other countries.

ISBN 978–1–137–35840–0

This book is printed on paper suitable for recycling and made from fully
managed and sustained forest sources. Logging, pulping and manufacturing
processes are expected to conform to the environmental regulations of the
country of origin.

A catalogue record for this book is available from the British Library.

A catalog record for this book is available from the Library of Congress.

Printed in China

Contents

Figures and Tables

Figures

Tables

List of Contributors

Dr G. Hussein Rassool, PhD MSc BA FRSPH ILTM Cert Ed. Cert Couns. Cert Supervision & Consultation
Professor and Executive Director, Sakina Counselling Centre; Director, Inter Cultural Therapy Centre; Academic Advisor, Doha Academy of Tertiary Studies. Formerly Professor of Addiction & Mental Health, University of São Paulo, Brazil; and Senior Lecturer, St George's University of London, UK. Florence Nightingale Foundation Scholar.

Dr Essmat Mohamed Gemaey, BN MSc DNs
Assistant Professor of Psychiatric and Mental Health Nursing, King Suad University, Riyadh, Saudi Arabia.

Dr Sandy Lovering, PHD RN DHSc CTN
Chief, Nursing Affairs, King Faisal Specialist Hospital & Research Centre (General Organization), Jeddah, Saudi Arabia.

Dr Sawsam Majali, PhD MSN BSc RN
Previously Head of Nursing Program, Dar Al Hekma College, Jeddah, Saudi Arabia. Currently, Director of the Queen Zein Al Sharaf Institute for Development, Amman.

Dr Chandbi Sange, PhD BSc RN
Research Nurse, Salford Royal Foundation, Manchester, United Kingdom.

Preface

The focus of the book is to offer a basic understanding of the tenets of Islam and the implications for the delivery of culturally appropriate and compassionate care to Muslim patients. As the population of Muslims increases in Northern and Western Europe, the Americas, Australasia and Oceania, it is reasonable to assume that many nurses and allied healthcare practitioners will more frequently encounter Muslim patients in the healthcare system. Therefore, the provision of a person-centred and holistic practice calls for promoting nurses' awareness of the ramifications of Islamic faith and belief, in their cultural competence in caring for Muslim patients.

This book is of particular relevance to non-Muslim and Muslim nurses and allied healthcare professionals, and for those wishing to gain increased insight into ways in which the Islamic faith is intertwined with the nursing and health care of Muslim patients. It also acts as a resource for those who have limited knowledge and contact with Muslims in their own context and social networks. Nursing approaches and care of patients with a diversity of culture and religion are both challenging and rewarding. The impact of this diversity means that nurses and allied healthcare professionals must learn to care in environments with different worldviews, language and communication styles, attitudes, and expectations. The ICN Code of Ethics for Nurses (International Council of Nurses, 2006) contains the following statement:

> Inherent in nursing is a respect for human rights including cultural rights, the right to life and choice, to dignity and to be treated with respect. Nursing care is respectful of and unrestricted by considerations of age, colour, creed, culture, disability or illness, gender, sexual orientation, nationality, politics, race or social status. In providing care, the nurse promotes an environment in which the human rights, values, customs and spiritual beliefs of the individual, family and community are respected.

Muslim patients are a heterogeneous group with varying values, attitudes and customs that affect their patterns of health and illness. To meet this nursing challenge, it is essential that nurses and allied healthcare professionals operate from a solid foundation of knowledge, skills and attitude based on a set of standards for cultural competence in nursing practice. The Expert

Panel on Global Nursing and Health (2010) stated that to be adequately prepared for cultural competence in nursing practice, 'nurses shall gain an understanding of the perspectives, traditions, values, practices, and family systems of culturally diverse individuals, families, communities and populations for whom they care, as well as knowledge of the complex variables that affect the achievement of health and well-being'. This awareness will enhance the qualities of caring, competence and professionalism. It is within the context of understanding the culture, beliefs and traditions, and the display of cultural competence, that individualised holistic care becomes attainable.

In a clear, reader-friendly format, the chapters address issues related to the identity and religious beliefs of Muslims; caring as an act of spirituality; spiritual/religious orientation; the ethical dimension in caring; understanding the Muslim family system; perception of health and illness; health behaviours and concerns; health considerations during fasting and pilgrimage (*Hajj*); food practices; cultural and religious factors in mental health; addictive behaviours; reproductive and developmental issues; rites de passage – birth and death rituals; organ transplantation and end-of-life decisions. Reflective activities and case studies have been provided throughout the book to illustrate the contemporary nature of caring for Muslim patients and to integrate theory and clinical application.

The essence of this book is based on the following notions:

- The fundamental principle of Islam as a religion is based on the Oneness of God.
- The tenets of Islam are the Noble Qur'aan and Hadith.
- Muslims believe that cure comes solely from Allah (God).
- Seeking treatment for ill health does not conflict with seeking help from Allah.
- Central to Islamic teachings are the connections between knowledge, health, holism, the environment and the 'Oneness of Allah', the unity of God in all spheres of life, death and the hereafter.
- Health is a state of complete physical, psychological, social and spiritual well-being.
- Islam takes a holistic approach to health. Physical, emotional and spiritual health cannot be separated.
- The importance of meeting spiritual needs comes before physical needs.
- Islam places great emphasis on both the physical and the spiritual, cleanliness and purification, a well-balanced diet combined with physical activity and exercise.

- Emerging cultural competence in nursing is aiming to make healthcare services more responsive to the needs of Muslim patients.
- There is wide consensus amongst Muslim scholars that psychiatric or psychological disorders are legitimate medical conditions – that is, distinct from illnesses of a supernatural nature.
- Organ and blood donation and organ transplantation are consistent with Islamic belief.
- The family are partners in the care of the patient, and make decisions on the patient's care with the healthcare team.
- Application of the Crescent of Care model places the patient and family at the centre of caring action, in the provision of psychosocial, interpersonal, cultural, clinical and spiritual care.
- Caring, in the Islamic context, is an act of shared spirituality between nurses and patients, where the nature of the shared spirituality is fluid, depending on the patient's spiritual needs.
- It is a sign of respect that Muslims utter or repeat the words 'Peace Be Upon Him' (PBUH) after hearing (or writing) the name of the Prophet Muhammad (PBUH).

References

Expert Panel on Global Nursing and Health (2010). Standards of Practice for Culturally Competent Nursing Care Executive Summary, available at www.tcns.org/files/Standards_of_Practice_for_Culturally_Compt_Nsg_Care-Revised.pdf, date accessed 21 April 2013.

International Council of Nurses [ICN] (2006) *The ICN Code of Ethics for Nurses* (Geneva, Switzerland: ICN).

Acknowledgements

Bismillah Ar Rahman Ar Raheem

All Praise is due to Allah, and may the peace and blessings of Allah be upon our Prophet Muhammad (PBUH) his family and his companions.

I would like to thank Kate Ahl for her valuable and constructive suggestions during the planning and development of the manuscript. Thanks also to Kate Llewellyn, at Palgrave Macmillan Higher Education, for her support in the final stage of the publication of this book. I am also particularly grateful to all the contributors who showed great patience, perseverance and commitment in making the book a reality. I am particularly grateful to Akbar Ally Hossenally, BA (Shariah) Islamic University of Madina, Saudi Arabia, for reviewing the issues of Islamic jurisprudence. I would like to acknowledge the contributions made by my teachers who enabled me, through my own reflective practices, to follow the path.

I am thankful to my beloved parents who taught me the value of education. My special thanks also to Mariam for her unconditional support and encouragement to pursue my interests. I owe my gratitude to Adam Abu Isra Wa Asiyah Ibn Hussein Ibn Hassim Ibn Sahaduth Ibn Rosool Al Mauritiusy for his unconditional love and for showing an interest in my work; and special thanks to Yasmin Soraya, Reshad Hassan, Isra Oya and Asiyah Maryam for their love and support and for being here.

Finally, whatever benefits and correctness you find within this book are out of the Grace of Allah, Alone, and whatever mistakes you find are mine alone. I pray to Allah to forgive me for any unintentional shortcomings regarding the contents of this book and to make this humble effort helpful and fruitful to any interested parties. 'Whatever of good befalls you, it is from Allah; and whatever of ill befalls you, it is from yourself' (An-Nisā' [The Women] 4:79).

The authors and publishers would also like to thank: Dr Sawsam Majali, previously Head of Nursing Program, Dar Al Hekma College, Jeddah, Saudi Arabia, currently Director of the Queen Zein Al Sharaf Institute for Development, Amman, for permission to use his case study in Chapter 5; WHO Regional Office for the Eastern Mediterranean (EMRO) for permission to reproduce

Table 7.1: 'The Amman Declaration of Health Promotion', originally published in *Health Promotion through Islamic Lifestyles: The Amman Declaration* 5 © 1996; Transcultural Nursing for the case study in Chapter 7 originally from Fernandez and Fernandez (1999) Transcultural Nursing: Basic Concepts and Case studies (online) www.culturediversity.org © 1999; Radcliffe Publishing for permission to reproduce Figure 8.1: 'Crescent of Care Nursing Model', published in 'The Crescent of Care: a nursing model to guide the care of Arab Muslim patients', by S. Lovering, in *Diversity and Equality in Health Care* 9, 3 © 2012; Dr Chowdhury and ESP Bioscience for permission to reproduce the case study in Reflective Activity 9.2, originally published in 'Severe hypoglycaemia in a Muslim patient fasting during Ramadan', by T.A. Chowdhury, in *Diabetic Hypoglycemia* 4, 2, 11–13 © 2011; Community in Action for Tables 10.1, 10.3 and 10.4 from the *Ramadan Health Guide* © 2007, reproduced under the Open Government Licence v2.0; the Islamic Medical Association of North America for Table 16.1, from IMANA Ethics Committee, 'Islamic Medical Ethics: the IMANA Perspective'; and S. Attar for Table 17.1, from 'Information for Health Care Providers when Dealing with a Muslim Patient'.

PART
1

Background and Context

Muslims and the Islamic Faith: an Overview

1

G. Hussein Rassool

Learning Outcomes:

- State the difference between Islam and Muslim.
- Discuss the fundamentals of Islam as a religion.
- Examine the relationship between Islam and Judeo-Christian religion.
- Have an awareness and understanding of the pillars of Islam.
- Have an awareness of Muslims' religio-cultural practices.

Reflective Activity 1.1

State whether the following statements are true or false. Give reasons for your answers.

	True	False
1 Islam is an Arabic term, which, when translated literally, means 'surrender' or 'submission'.		
2 Arabs make up most of the Muslim population worldwide.		
3 A Muslim is a person who submits to the will of God.		
4 Islam is a new-age religion of the 20th century.		
5 Islam is a monotheistic religion, involving the belief in the one God.		
6 The Qur'aan was written by Muhammad and copied from Christian and Jewish sources.		
7 Muslims do not believe in Jesus or other Prophets.		

	True	False
8 The Kaa'ba (Black Cubicle in Makkah) is the place of worship which God commanded Abraham and Ishmael to build over four thousand years ago.		
9 Performing all five prayers is not compulsory for Muslims.		
10 The 'Five Pillars' of Islam are the foundation of Muslim life.		
11 Islam oppresses women.		
12 Muslim beliefs and practices are based on the Qur'aan and Sunnah.		
13 Islam is intolerant of other faiths.		
14 Muslims are violent, terrorist extremists.		

Introduction

Islam is an Arabic term, which translated literally means 'surrender' or 'submission'. The same Arabic root word gives us *'Salaam alaykum'* ('Peace be with you'), the universal Muslim greeting. In a religious context, it means complete submission to the will of Almighty God (Allah) in heart, soul and deeds. 'Muslim' refers to a person who engages in the act of submission, acceptance, or surrender. Therefore a Muslim is a person who submits to the will of God, or a person who is a follower of Islam. 'Allah' is the Arabic name for God, which is used by Arab Muslims and Christians alike. Islam, as a way of life, is the second largest religion in the world, with over 1 billion (1,000 million) followers from a vast range of races, nationalities and cultures across the globe, united by their common Islamic faith. It is considered one of the Abrahamic, monotheistic faiths, along with Judaism and Christianity. This chapter will enable the reader to have a basic understanding of the principles of the Islamic faith and the Muslim community.

The Muslim world

Nearly a quarter of the world's population today is Muslim and the total Muslim population, with over 1.62 billion followers worldwide, could reach 2.2 billion in 2030 (Pew Forum on Religion and Public Life, 2011). If current trends continue, 79 countries will have a million or more Muslim inhabitants in 2030, up from 72 countries today. The seven countries projected to rise above 1 million Muslims by 2030 are: Belgium, Canada, Congo, Djibouti, Guinea Bissau, the Netherlands, and Togo (Pew Forum on Religion and Public

Life, 2011). Although Islam is often associated with the Arab world and the Middle East, fewer than 18% of Muslims are Arabs. While Asia has the largest number of Muslims compared with other continents, it is second to Africa in terms of the percentage of Muslims with respect to the total population. Accordingly, the percentage of Muslims in Africa is 43.3% with a total Muslim population of 447 million, which constitutes 27% of the world Muslim population. It is thought that a majority of the world's Muslims (about 60%) will continue to live in the Asia-Pacific region, while about 20% will live in the Middle East and North Africa, as is the case today. However, Pakistan is expected to surpass Indonesia as the country with the largest Muslim population. The portion of the world's Muslims living in sub-Saharan Africa is projected to rise, and in 20 years, for example, more Muslims are likely to live in Nigeria than in Egypt. Although there are Muslim minorities in almost every area, including Latin America and Australia, Muslims are also found in India, China, the Balkans, and Russia.

In 2010, it was estimated that more than 44 million Muslims were living in Europe, excluding Turkey (Pew Forum on Religion and Public Life, 2011). In Western and Northern European countries, the proportions of Muslims were: 6 per cent in Belgium, 7.5 per cent in France, 5.5 per cent in the Netherlands, 2.3 per cent in Spain, 5.7 per cent in Switzerland, 5 per cent in Germany, and 4.6 per cent in the United Kingdom (Pew Forum on Religion and Public Life, 2011, 124). In some countries, such as Bosnia and Herzegovina, Macedonia, or the Russian Federation, the Muslim population has been established for centuries. In Albania, Kosovo and Turkey, Muslims represent the majority of the population. Muslims are expected to constitute a growing share of the total population in Europe and the Americas.

There is great diversity in the ethnic composition of Muslim migrants in Western and Northern Europe. The presence of different groups of Muslims in specific countries varies depending on a wide range of factors including post-decolonisation migration patterns, a history of European labour markets, and refugee flows (Amnesty International, 2012). For example, the biggest groups of Muslims in France are originally from Algeria, Morocco, Tunisia, and sub-Saharan Africa, while in Belgium and the Netherlands the majority are of Moroccan and Turkish origin. A considerable share of Muslims living in Switzerland came from former Yugoslavia, whereas the biggest groups of Muslims in Catalonia (Spain) are originally from Algeria, Mali, Morocco, Pakistan, and Senegal. Muslims from Iran and Iraq are relatively numerous in Sweden, Norway, and Denmark, if compared with other European countries (Amnesty International, 2012).

The United Kingdom (UK) has a long history of contact with Muslims, with links forged from the Middle Ages onwards (Muslim Council of Britain, 2002). An example is the Yemeni community of South Shields, which began at the end of the nineteenth century when Yemenis working as stokers on steamships moved ashore and set up boarding houses in the dock area. During the 1960s, significant numbers of Muslims from South-East Asia (Bangladeshi, Pakistani or Indian origin) and some East African Asians came to the UK to take up employment. Permanent communities formed and at least 50% of the current population were born in the UK. Significant communities with links to Turkey, Cyprus, Iran, Iraq, Afghanistan, Somalia, and the Balkans also exist. However, in the UK, only a small percentage came originally from Northern Africa. The top countries of origin for Muslim immigrants to the United States (US) in 2009 were Pakistan and Bangladesh. About two-thirds of the Muslims in the US today (64.5%) are foreign-born, first-generation immigrants, while slightly more than a third (35.5%) were born in the United States. By 2030, however, more than four-in-ten of the Muslims in the US (44.9%) are expected to be native born (Pew Forum on Religion and Public Life, 2011).

Background to Islam

Islam is not a new religion, as it was the religion of all the Prophets. The religion of Islam is finally complete because Prophet Muhammad (Peace Be Upon Him) is the seal of all the Prophets and the last to convey the religion of Allah to mankind. Allah stated in the Noble Qur'aan (interpretation of the meaning):

☐ *This day I have perfected your religion for you, completed My Favor upon you, and have chosen for you Islam as your religion.* (Al-Mā'idah [The Table Spread]) 5:3)

Prior to Islam, the beliefs of the tribes of Arabia involved the worship of stones, stars, caves and trees. Around AD 610, Prophet Muhammad began to receive visions and revelations from the Angel Gabriel, proclaiming that 'God is one' and that the Prophet is the 'messenger of God'. He began preaching in Makkah where he met with considerable resistance. This was because Prophet Muhammad's message threatened not only popular polytheism, but the political, social and economic powers of the local tribes. The Kaa'ba (Black Cubicle in Makkah) is the place of worship which God commanded Abraham and Ishmael to build over four thousand years ago. The building was constructed of stone on what many believe was the original site of a sanctuary established by the Prophet Adam. God commanded Abraham to summon all mankind to visit this place, and when pilgrims go there today, in millions during the *Hajj* pilgrimage, they say *'At Thy service, O Lord'*, in response to Abraham's summons. Muslims pray in the direction of the Kaa'ba but do not worship the

Kaa'ba. To escape prosecution Prophet Muhammad migrated to Yathrib, today known as Madinah, and his escape is referred to as a turning point in Islam. The *'Hijira'* (migration) marks the beginning of the Islamic calendar. In AD 630, Prophet Muhammad and his followers took over Makkah without resistance. By the time Prophet Muhammad died in 632, Islam had already reached large portions of Asia, Africa and parts of Europe. Today, Islam is regarded as the world's fastest growing religion.

How other religions interlink to Islam

Islam is not a new religion but is the continuation of the religion of our patriarch Abraham, focusing on monotheistic belief. The basic beliefs of Muslims fall into six main categories, which are known as the 'Articles of Faith'. Muslims believe in One, Unique, Incomparable God; in the Angels created by Him; in the Prophets through whom His revelations were brought to humanity; in the Day of Judgement and individual accountability for actions; in God's complete authority over human destiny; and in life after death. Muslims believe in a chain of Prophets starting with Adam and including Noah, Abraham, Ishmael, Isaac, Jacob, Joseph, Job, Moses, Aaron, David, Solomon, Elias, Jonah, John the Baptist, and Jesus. However, God's final message to man, a reconfirmation of the eternal message and a summing-up of all that has gone before, was revealed to the Prophet Muhammad through Gabriel (Islamic Affairs Department, 1989).

Judaism and Christianity have similarities to Islam. For example, Christianity and Judaism, like Islam, believe in the 'oneness' of God, and go back to the Prophet and Patriarch Abraham, from whose sons the prophets are directly descended (Morgan, 2010). In fact, the Noble Qur'aan states that 'Abraham was not a Jew nor a Christian, but he was a *Hanif* (he was true in Faith) and bowed his will to Allah's (which is Islam), and he associated no partners with Allah' (Āli `Imrān [The Family of Ali] 3:67). The Prophet Muhammad is descended from the eldest son of Moses, Ishmael, and Jesus is a descendant of Isaac. Muslims believe that all the Prophets that came before Muhammad preached the same religion of Islam, and the belief in the One, Unique, Incomparable God. Islam has, at its core, a simple message that applies to all human beings. Islam tolerates other beliefs as it is one function of Islamic law to protect the privileged status of minorities, and this is why non-Muslim places of worship have flourished all over the Islamic world. History provides many examples of Muslim tolerance towards other faiths. Islamic law also permits non-Muslim minorities to set up their own courts, which implement family laws drawn up by the minorities themselves. In fact, the Constitution of Madinah (*Ṣaḥīfat al-Madīnah*), the earliest known written constitution in the world, concerns the rights and responsibilities of the Muslim, Jewish, and other Arabic and tribal communities of Madinah during the war between that city and its neighbours. To this effect, it instituted a number of rights and responsibilities for the Muslim, Jewish, and pagan communities of Madinah. The Muslims were brought within the fold of one community – the 'Ummah'.

The Prophet and Messenger

No one knows exactly when the Prophet Muhammad was born, but the most cited year is AD 570, on a Monday in the City of Makkah, to Abdullah and Amina. The Prophet's father died a few months before Muhammad was born, and six years later, his mother died. The grandfather of the Prophet, Abd al-Muttalib, took over his care, but unfortunately after two years he died too. Prophet Muhammad was taken under the care of his uncle, Abu Talib, where he grew up to be a young and successful merchant. Prophet Muhammad was unlettered and had led a very uneventful life before he began to receive revelations from Allah and announced his mission to the world at the age of forty. The life of Prophet Muhammad is full of countless examples that show his status as a role model for Muslim societies and individuals. This is characterised by an exceptional morality, good habits, noble and gentle feelings and superior skills. Any individual can find truths in Prophet Muhammad's life that constitute an example for them to follow (ICSFP, 2010). The following are examples of what non-Muslim scholars have said about Prophet Muhammad:

> Philosopher, orator, apostle, legislator, warrior, conqueror of ideas, restorer of rational dogmas, of a cult without images, the founder of twenty terrestrial empires and of one spiritual empire that is Muhammad. As regards all standards by which human greatness may be measured, we may well ask, is there any man greater than he? (Lamartine, 1854).

According to Bosworth (1874),

> He was Caesar and Pope in one; but he was Pope without Pope's pretensions, Caesar without the legions of Caesar: without a standing army, without a bodyguard, without a palace, without a fixed revenue; if ever any man had the right to say that he ruled by the right divine, it was Mohammad, for he had all the power without its instruments and without its supports.

Napoleon Bonaparte (1914) said:

> I hope the time is not far off when I shall be able to unite all the wise and educated men of all the countries and establish a uniform regime based on the

principles of Qur'aan which alone are true and which alone can lead men to happiness.

George Bernard Shaw (1936), Irish playwright and a co-founder of the London School of Economics, stated that:

> I believe that if a man like him were to assume the dictatorship of the modern world he would succeed in solving its problems in a way that would bring it the much needed peace and happiness: I have prophesied about the faith of Muhammad that it would be acceptable to the Europe of tomorrow as it is beginning to be acceptable to the Europe of today. (Sir George Bernard Shaw, cited in *The Genuine Islam*, vol. 1, no. 8, 1936).

Thomas Carlyle (1920), Scottish philosopher, satirical writer, essayist, historian and teacher during the Victorian era, stated that:

> The lies (Western slander) which well-meaning zeal has heaped round this man (Muhammad) are disgraceful to ourselves only... How one man single-handedly, could weld warring tribes and wandering Bedouins into a most powerful and civilized nation in less than two decades... A silent great soul, one of that who cannot but be earnest. He was to kindle the world; the world's Maker had ordered so.

M.K. Gandhi (1927), pre-eminent leader of Indian nationalism in British-ruled India, stated that:

> I became more than ever convinced that it was not the sword that won a place for Islam in those days in the scheme of life. It was the rigid simplicity, the utter self-effacement of the prophet, the scrupulous regard for his pledges, his intense devotion to his friends and followers, his intrepidity, his fearlessness, his absolute trust in God and his own mission. These, and not the sword carried everything before them and surmounted every trouble.

Michael H. Hart (1992), in his book entitled *The 100: A Ranking of the Most Influential Persons in History*, stated that:

> My choice of Muhammad to lead the list of the world's most influential persons may surprise some readers and may be questioned by others, but he was the only man in history who was supremely successful on both the religious and secular level.

However, Prophet Muhammad's status as a role model is an issue based on the Holy Qur'aan and the Sunnah (the practices and examples of the Prophet).

The fundamentals of Islam as a religion: the Oneness of God

Muslims follow a strict monotheism with one creator, who is just, omnipotent and merciful 'Allah'. The term 'Allah' shows no plural or gender, unlike the term 'God', which may take the plural sense 'Gods' and feminine form 'Goddesses'. This is the most important fundamental teaching of Islam: the Oneness of God, which is termed '*Tawheed/shahadah*' and the first pillar of Islam:

☐ *I testify that there is no true God but Allah Almighty, who is one (and the only one) and there is no associate with Him; and I testify that Muhammad (peace and blessings of Allah be upon him), is His messenger.*

The oneness of God is noted throughout the Qur'aan, and is the fundamental belief of Islam. God is described in the Qur'aan (interpretation of the meaning):

☐ *Say (O Muhammad): "He is Allah, (the) One." Allah-us-Samad (The Self-Sufficient Master, Whom all creatures need, He neither eats nor drinks). He begets not, nor was He begotten; And there is none co-equal or comparable unto Him.* (Al-'Ikhlāṣ [The Sincerity] 112:1–4)

The Noble Qur'aan

The Qur'aan, the last revealed Word of God, is the prime source of every Muslim's faith and practice. The Qur'aan is a record of the exact words revealed by God through the Angel Gabriel to the Prophet Muhammad. It was memorised by Prophet Muhammad and then dictated to his Companions, and written down by scribes, who crosschecked it during his lifetime. There are 114 chapters in the Qur'aan, which is written in classical Arabic. All the chapters except one begin with the sentence *Bismillah ir Rahman ir Raheem*, 'In the name of Allah, the Entirely Merciful, the Especially Merciful.' The longest chapter of the Qur'aan is Surah Baqarah (The Cow) with 286 verses, and the shortest is Surah Al-Kawthar (Abundance), which has 3 verses. Translations of the Qur'aan exist in over 40 native language. Not one word of its 114 chapters has been changed over the centuries, and Verse 15:9 states that God will personally protect and guard the Qur'aan from corruption. The Qur'aan deals with subjects that concern us including: wisdom, doctrine, worship, and law, but its basic theme is the relationship between God and His creatures. At the same time, it provides guidelines for a just society, proper human conduct and an equitable economic system. Other sacred sources include the Sunnah, the practices and examples of the Prophet, which is the second authority for Muslims. A Hadith is a reliably transmitted report of what the Prophet said, did, or approved. Belief in the Sunnah is part of the Islamic faith.

Beliefs and the pillars of Islam (fundamentals of Islam)

Islamic practices and behaviours are not only related to divine revelations but as a theology, generate particular social practices in culture, manners, food, and language. According to Ahmed (1999), Islam is sociology and a philosophy of life. Islam means submission, and has a moral code as well as a civil law with a unifying ethical framework. It creates a monotheistic culture, the aim of which is for one to create peace in one's self, family, and society by actively submitting to and implementing the will of God (Gordon, 2002).

The duties of Muslims are known as the five pillars of Islam, and are the model framework that all Muslims around the world will follow in relation to their daily activities, lifestyle, and practices.

- Recite the shahadah (have faith in Allah) termed *Imaan*: '*There is no true God but Allah, and Muhammad is his Messenger.*'
- Perform prayers five times a day, known as salaat: all five prayers contain verses of the Qur'aan, and all Muslims will face towards the Kaa'ba in Makkah to perform prayers. Prayer, according to the Prophet, is the borderline between a believer and a non-believer; it is a relationship between the performer and God.
- *Zakat* is one of the most important principles of Islam. It holds that all things belong to God, and all humans are trustees of such wealth. *Zakat* literally means 'to increase' or 'to cleanse'. In Islamic law (*shari'ah*), *zakat* means that fixed portion of wealth that an owner has to give annually to poor and needy Muslims as prescribed in the Qur'aan and Hadith.
- Fast during the Holy month of Ramadan: all Muslims are obliged to fast in the month of Ramadan, known as 'the month of Endurance and Sympathy'. The month of Ramadan marks the historical event of '*Laylat-ul-Qadr*', as the Night of Power when the Qur'aan was revealed.
- Perform the pilgrimage referred to as *Hajj*: *Hajj* is the largest annual gathering of Muslims from across the globe, in the Holy city of Makkah. *Hajj* symbolises devotion to Allah and obedience to his commands.

These are the five fundamentals and the framework of Muslim life. Muslims are by the Islamic law required to care for and nurture all of Allah's creations, and cause no harm to others. These common practices and shared beliefs help to explain why, to many Muslims, the principles of Islam seem both clear and universal (Pew Forum on Religion and Public Life, 2012).

Cultural and religious practices

The concepts of 'religion' and 'culture' are practically synonymous in many parts of the world and there is no clear differentiation between the two terms. Culture has been defined as 'the system of shared beliefs, values, customs, behaviours, and artifacts that the members of society use to cope with their world and with one another, and that are transmitted from generation to generation through learning' (cited in Culture and Religion). Whereas religion, like culture itself, consists of systematic patterns of beliefs, values, and behaviour, acquired by people as members of their society (Religion and Culture). Our culture, which is dynamic, shapes our worldview as it influences all of our behaviours and interactions. Religion is a component under the umbrella of culture because it is the religious beliefs that are often the sources of moral strength and a basis for the cohesion of the cultural groups. The belief system of the religion shapes the culture in relation to the habits, customs, traditions, superstitions, tribal or ethnic codes of conduct, hopes and fears of the group or community. Religions can play a significant role in some cultures and not in others. It has been stated that there is no homogeneity among religions as there are differences of interpretation of principles and meanings (Religion and Culture).

Islam can be regarded as a religio-cultural phenomenon whereby the behaviours of the believers are shaped by religious values and practices rather than cultural practices. Muslims from different parts of the world will have varying cultures even though they share the same religious values and practices. However, their behaviours are often shaped by cultural practices which may not be in concordance with basic religious practices. According to Saidi (2008), many of the countries that are commonly called 'Islamic countries', which in reality are merely 'Muslim-majority countries', use an amalgam of Islamic and pre-Islamic/non-Islamic practices and some of those countries have remained patriarchal. Some of the cultural (or pre-Islamic) practices performed by Muslims are given an Islamic dimension although these practices are not Islamic. Generally, religious or Islamic practices include all the practices that have roots in the Qur'aan and Sunnah (traditions).

Islamic/Muslim religio-cultural practices

The Muslim culture is based on Islamic teachings from the Qur'aan and the Sunnah and is embedded in the common belief that there is no God but Allah and that Muhammad is His Messenger. 'Islamic culture' is a term used to describe all cultural practices common to many Muslims around the world with a foundation of modesty (*hayaa*) and simplicity. Ibrahim (2009) stated that some things that Muslims do almost subconsciously are actually mandated, or encouraged, and come from the Qur'aan and Hadith. For example:

- Women wearing the hijab and conforming to other Islamic dress standards.
- Greeting other Muslims with '*As-Salaamu Alay-kum*'. This greeting is standard amongst all Muslims the world over.
- Saying *Bismillah* (in the name of Allah) before doing just about anything.
- Saying *Inshallah* (if Allah wills) when speaking of future events.
- Saying *Alhamdulillah* (praise is entirely and only for Allah) in all situations.
- Men growing beards and trimming the moustache.
- Using the right hand to eat with and the left hand for the bathroom.
- Using a stick for cleaning teeth (*Miswak*).
- Shaking hands when greeting someone.

Muslims are known to have larger families than the white majority as the foundation of Islamic culture is the family (IPCI, 1989), which includes grandparents, cousins, siblings, children, neighbours and the community. The extended family is the fundamental component within Muslim culture that determines acts, practices and behaviours (IPCI, 1989). The peace and security offered by a stable family unit is greatly valued, and seen as essential for the spiritual growth of its members. Caring for one's elderly parents in this most difficult time of their lives is considered an honour and blessing, and an opportunity for great spiritual growth. Mothers are particularly honoured: the Prophet taught that 'Paradise lies at the feet of mothers.' Children are treasured. Therefore, a harmonious social order is created by the existence of extended families. Islam sees a woman, whether single or married, as an individual in her own right, with the right to own and dispose of her property and earnings. Islam is both a religion and a complete way of life.

For Muslims, Islamic practices dominate every aspect of the individual's life and behaviour. In the Noble Qur'aan, human beings are taught that they were created in order to worship God, and on that basis, all true worship is God-consciousness. Since the teachings of Islam encompass all aspects of life and ethics, God-consciousness is encouraged in all human affairs (Masters et al., 2007). There are injunctions and commandments which concern virtually all facets of one's person, one's family and civil society. These include such matters as diet, clothing, personal hygiene, interpersonal relations, business ethics, responsibilities towards parents, spouse and children, marriage, divorce, inheritance, civil and criminal law, fighting in defence of Islam, and relations with non-Muslims (Masters et al., 2007). Muslim beliefs and practices are based on the following issues:

- Welfare and Society. The society is responsible for the welfare of an individual – community obligation (*fard al-kifaya*),
- Morals and manners. Muslims are forbidden from: dishonesty, theft, murder, suicide, bribery, forgery, usury, gambling, lottery, consumption of alcohol or pork, backbiting, gossiping, slandering, hoarding, destruction of property, cruelty to animals, adultery, fornication, and public nudity.
- Modesty in dress and behaviour. Muslims should wear decent and dignified dress. Men should cover their body from their navel to their knees, and women should cover their entire body except for their face and hands.
- Care of children and the elderly. Caring for one's children or parents is considered an honour and a blessing.
- Racism and prejudice. Muslims believe that they should not discriminate against anyone for any reason, since we are part of a larger brotherhood of humanity. The Prophet proclaimed, in his last sermon, that no Arab is superior over a non-Arab, and no white person is superior over a black.
- Dietary rules. Islamic dietary laws provide direction on what is to be considered *halal* (lawful) and *haram* (unlawful). Food hygiene is part of the Islamic dietary law.
- Marriage. Islam is a strong advocate of marriage and considers it a moral safeguard as well as a social building block. Furthermore, marriage is the only valid or *halal* way to indulge in intimacy between a man and a woman.
- Relations with non-Muslims. Our relationship with the people of other faiths should only be avoided when it becomes harmful for Muslims. There is no reason why Muslims should not cooperate with non-Muslims with regard to establishing truth and combating falsehood, to support the oppressed and ward off danger for mankind, such as cooperating to fight pollution or to protect the environment, or to combat epidemic diseases and so on (Sheikh Muhammad Salih Al-Munajjid).
- The 'Five Pillars' of Islam are the foundation of Muslim life. A testament of faith, prayer, giving alms to the needy (*zakat*), fasting during the month of Ramadan, and undertaking a pilgrimage to Makkah once in a lifetime for those who are able; these parameters essentially define what it means to be a Muslim.

Conclusion

This chapter has considered and summarised the Muslim way of life, Islam, as a religion and a way of life. In the Muslim world, there is an increasing recognition of the need to distinguish between cultural traditions, which may have nothing to do with Islam, and the true teachings of Islam. The cultural fabric of the Muslim community according to Raza (1991) reveals an intricate web, including social, economic, and healthcare areas. Islam as a religion has a major influence on the way in which Muslims view and understand their lives, their being and purpose. Cultural practices of Muslim communities are strong and very closely linked to their religious beliefs, so that separating the two can prove difficult, if not impossible. Some Muslims vary a lot in their day-to-day practices and these are simply local customs taken as Islamic culture. The lack of adherence to Islamic practices arises when people confuse cultural practices with religion.

Reflective Activity 1.2

- What is the nature of the Muslim population in your local community?
- Are the Muslim population in your local community ethnically diverse?
- How familiar are you with the healthcare needs of the Muslim community in your area?
- What are the key health needs or concerns for the Muslim community?
- Are there any health disparities between the Muslim community and the general population?
- Identify some of the socio-economic factors impacting on the health of the Muslim community.
- In relation to psychological health, are there differences between the Muslim community and the general population?
- Are there differences in healthy behaviours and unhealthy behaviours amongst the different Muslim communities?
- Are there wide variations in the use of the health services among this religious group?
- What healthcare services are being provided to the Muslim community in your locality?
- How accessible are these services (for example, hours, location, language capacity)?
- Is there an interpreting service for those whose mother tongue is not English?
- What are the problems faced by the Muslim community in accessing health and social care services?

- What outreach efforts are made to educate the Muslim community about access to the services provided?
- Have you or your local healthcare providers been prepared on cultural competence in working with Muslim patients?
- Reflect on how you can learn more about the Muslim community?
- Have you identified your learning needs regarding cultural competence in working with Muslim patients?

References

Ahmed, A.S. (1999) *Islam Today: A Short Introduction to the Muslim World* (London: IBS Tauris).

Amnesty International (2012) *Choice and Prejudice: Discrimination against Muslims in Europe* (London: Amnesty International).

Bosworth, S. (1874) *Mohammad and Mohammadanism* (London), p. 92.

Carlyle T. (1920) *Heroes and Hero-worship* (New York: Encyclopedia Americana).

Culture and Religion, www.cultureandreligion.com/, date accessed 27 July 2013.

Gandhi, M.K. (1927) *Young India* (New York: Viking Press).

Gordon, M.S. (2002) *Understanding Islam: Origins, Beliefs, Practices, Holy Texts, Sacred Places* (London: Duncan Baird).

Hart, M.H. (1992) *The 100: A Ranking of the Most Influential Persons in History* (New York: Hart Publishing Company), p. 33.

Ibrahim, A. (2009) *Muslim Culture*, http://islamiclearningmaterials.com/muslim-culture/, date accessed 27 July 2013.

ICSFP – International Committee for the Support of the Final Prophet (2010) *The Importance of Prophet Muhammad and His Status as a Role Model*, www.icsfp.com/en/contents.aspx?aid=6880, date accessed 27 July 2013.

IPCI (1989) *Understanding Islam and the Muslims* (Birmingham: IPCI), pp. 23–5.

Islamic Affairs Department (1989) *Understanding Islam and the Muslims*, The Embassy of Saudi Arabia, Washington DC, Consultants (Cambridge: The Islamic Texts Society).

Lamartine, Alphonse de (1854) *Histoire de la Turquie* (Paris), Vol. II, pp. 276–7.

Masters, D., Kaka, I. and Squires, AbdurRahman R. (2007) *The Islamic Way of Life*, www.islam-truth.com/Islamic_Life.htm, date accessed 30 July 2013.

Morgan, C.W. (2010) *This Dynamic World* (Bloomington, IN: Author House).

Muslim Council of Britain (2002) *The Quest for Sanity* (London: The Muslim Council of Britain).

Napoleon Bonaparte, quoted in Christian Cherfils (1914) *Bonaparte et Islam* (Paris).

Pew Forum on Religion and Public Life (2011) *The Future of the Global Muslim Population. Projections for 2010–2030*, http://pewresearch.org/pubs/1872/muslim-population-projections-worldwide-fast-growth, date accessed 27 July 2013.

Pew Forum on Religion and Public Life (2012) *The World's Muslims: Unity and Diversity*, www.pewforum.org/Muslim/the-worlds-muslims-unity-and-diversity-executive-summary.aspx, date accessed 27 July 2013.

Raza, M.S. (1991) *Islam in Britain, Past, Present and Future* (Leicester: Volcano Press).

Religion and Culture, http://web.mesacc.edu/dept/d10/asb/religion/index.html, date accessed 1 February 2013.

Saidi, T. (2008) *Islam and Culture: Don't Mix them Up*, www.minnpost.com/community-voices/2008/02/islam-and-culture-dont-mix-them, date accessed 1 February 2013.

Shaw, G.B (1936) cited in *The Genuine Islam* 1, 8.

Sheikh Muhammad Salih Al-Munajjid. Principles and guidelines for Muslims' relations with non-Muslims, http://islamqa.info/en/ref/26721, date accessed 2 February 2013.

2 Nursing, Healing and the Spiritual Dimension: an Islamic Perspective

G. Hussein Rassool

Learning Outcomes:

- Identify the relationship between religion and spirituality in the Muslim context.
- Discuss the relationship between caring and spiritual dimension.
- Identify some of the features of caring from an Islamic Perspective.
- List the 'Islamic Code of Ethics'.
- Define what is cultural competence.
- Identify the components of a culturally competent healthcare setting.

Reflective Activity 2.1

State whether the following statements are true or false. Give reasons for your answers.

	True	False
1 In the Western world, religion as a concept is perceived as not being interchangeable with spirituality.		
2 Spirituality plays a major role in the motivation to deliver a high quality nursing care.		
3 There is widespread misunderstanding of the concept and practice of Islam within the context of health care and nursing practice.		

	True	False
4 Change in any aspect of an individual's life brings change to every aspect of his existence.		
5 Holism is the interconnectedness of body and mind only.		
6 In Islam, there is a distinction between religion and spirituality.		
7 In Islam, caring is expressed at the level of action only.		
8 Everyone has the right to freedom of religion.		
9 In Islam, caring is expressed at three different levels: intention, thought and action.		
10 There are injunctions in the provision of care for Muslim and non-Muslim patients with HIV/AIDS or substance misuse.		
11 Many aspects of caring in Islamic nursing today include the attributes of empathy, kindness, patience and human touch.		
12 It is worth remembering that the Muslim population around the globe is a homogeneous entity.		
13 Anti-discriminatory practices and equality are laid down in Islam and they are regarded as fundamental expectations and requirements of Muslims; in the healthcare system this applies be they patients or nurses.		

'Bismillah Ir'Rahman Ir'Rahim'

In the name of Allah, the Entirely Merciful, the Especially Merciful. Muslims frequently recite the above phrase in their daily lives, in health and sickness, as an invocation for any virtuous or permissible acts. There is widespread mis-understanding of Islamic beliefs and practices and a failure to recognise that Islamic faith is intertwined with the health care of Muslim patients. Thus the nursing approach, with a Eurocentric orientation, is devoid of provision of a holistic and person-centred care in meeting the needs of Muslim patients. The focus of this chapter is to provide an examination of spirituality and holism, Islamic health practices, health behaviours, code of ethics, and the framework of Islamic perspectives on caring and spirituality.

Holism, spirituality and religion

The biopsychosocial approach takes into consideration an individual's physical, psychological, sociological and spiritual needs so that patients are treated as whole human beings rather than only their symptoms or their diagnostic labelling being addressed. Holistic nursing is the interrelationship of body, mind and soul as a unified total and is not just the sum of the patient's body parts. Holistic nursing is defined as 'all nursing practice that has healing the whole person as its goal' (American Holistic Nurses' Association, 1998). Change in any aspect of an individual's life brings change to every aspect of his or her existence and differentiates the quality of the whole person (Erickson, 2007). The practice of holistic nursing requires nurses to recognise the interconnectedness of body, mind, and soul and to integrate the spiritual dimension within the framework of the process of nursing.

Spirituality is acknowledged as being a basic human need and a universal human right. The right to express our spirituality in our lifestyle and behaviours applies to everyone and is enshrined in European and UK law, based on the Universal Declaration of Human Rights. Article 18 of the Universal Declaration of Human Rights states that: 'Everyone has the right to freedom of religion; this right includes freedom to change his religion or belief, and freedom, either alone or in community with others and in public or private, to manifest his religion or belief in teaching, practice, worship and observance.'

Spirituality has different meanings and this depends on the context in which the concept is used. Individuals may express their spirituality in varied ways. It may be their religion or faith; meaning and direction in their life; their worldview; or a belief in a higher being. Spiritual need is defined as 'Any factor that is necessary (requisite, indispensable) to support the spiritual strengths of a person or to diminish the spiritual deficits' (Simsen, 1985). However, the psychosocial and spiritual needs of a patient are much less tangible than physical needs and are sometimes overlooked. It has been stated that 'Spiritual needs, if expressed outside of a religious framework, are very likely to be unnoticed' (Hutchinson, 1997). So if we are to identify the spiritual needs and provide spiritual care, it is necessary to have some understanding of the nature of the spiritual dimension of Muslim patients.

Religion, as a concept, is perceived by some in the Western hemisphere as not being interchangeable with spirituality. In this context, the concept of spirituality has a broader meaning than religion and encompasses philosophical ideas about life, its meaning and purpose (Dyson et al., 1997). In most secular societies, it is acknowledged that not every individual who seeks self-awareness, self-empowerment and self-actualisation pursues a particular religious belief (Rassool, 2000). However, spirituality is often seen as broader than religion. Accordingly, spiritual needs may or may not be expressed within a religious framework. Some spiritual beliefs are particular to an individual, whereas the beliefs attached to a religion are shared by large groups of people who follow established teaching (www.mentalhealth.org.uk). In the Islamic context, there is no spirituality without religious thoughts and practices, and the religion of Islam provides the spiritual path for salvation and a way of life. Muslims embrace the acceptance of the Divine, and they seek 'meaning, purpose and happiness' in worldly life and the hereafter. This is achieved through the belief in the 'Oneness of Allah' (*Tawheed*), without any partner, and the understanding and application of Qur'aanic practices, and in the guidance of the Holy Prophet (Rassool, 2000). *Tawheed* means ' "unification' and is used in reference to Allah. According to Philips (1994), *Tawheed* is the very foundation of Islam on which all the other pillars and principles depend. It is the belief that Allah is One, without partner, One without similitude in His essence and attributes and One without rival in His divinity and in worship. These form the fundamental basis of *Tawheed*. In this framework, Allah's unity must be maintained spiritually, intellectually and practically in all facets of human life.

Caring and spiritual dimension: an Islamic perspective

Spiritual care is important for all people, not only those who express a religious belief, as spirituality is a fundamental need that goes beyond religious affiliation. Central to Islamic teachings are the connections between knowledge, health, holism, the environment and the 'Oneness of Allah', the unity of God in all spheres of life, death and the hereafter (Rassool, 2000). Inherent in Islamic principles is the holistic framework that embodies the physical, psychosocial, environmental and spiritual dimensions of caring. Thus, caring is an attribute of Islam. Hence, it would seem totally alien for Muslim patients to receive care without its spiritual entity (Rassool, 2000). The Qur'aan wants the faithful to be caring and compassionate. Allah says in the Qur'aan (interpretation of the meaning):

> ☐ *and to parents do good, and to relatives, orphans, the needy, the near neighbour, the neighbour farther away, the companion at your side, the traveller . . .* (An-Nisā' [The Women] 4:36)

The spiritual dimension of caring from an Islamic perspective is embedded in the act of 'doing good' (*Maaruf*) or evading 'wrong doing' (*Munkar*). In Islam, caring is expressed at three different levels: intention, thought and action. Underlying the intention and verbal expression of caring is the understanding of what, when, who to care for and why (Salleh, 1994a). At the action level is the question of how, and this is related to knowledge, skills and resources (accountability and responsibility are embedded with the process and outcome of caring). In a Hadith, Allah's Apostle said: 'Each of you is a guardian and is charged with a responsibility, and each of you shall be held accountable for those who have been placed under your care' (Bukhari [a]). Whilst Islam clearly opposes alcoholism, gambling, sexual promiscuity or lifestyle issues, it does not prohibit Muslim nurses and other healthcare professionals from caring for both Muslim and non-Muslim patients. There are no injunctions in the provision of care for Muslim and non-Muslim patients with HIV/AIDS or substance misuse. In a Hadith, the Prophet said: 'The merciful are shown mercy by the All-Merciful. Show mercy to those on earth, and God will show mercy to you' (Tirmidhî and Abu-Dawud). Caring, under Islamic ideology and practice, does not look to the belief of the sufferer, or his or her ethnic group, or social status, or wealth. Hence, it cares for and treats non-Muslims the same as their Muslim counterparts (Rassool, 2000).

Islamic code of ethics

An Islamic code of ethics has been suggested for the development of a model of care and treatment. Athar (1998) states that the major roles of the ethicist in the area of patient care are:

- Understanding the needs and concerns of the patient, family and significant others and transmitting them to healthcare professionals involved in the decision-making process.
- Interpreting the Qur'aan as it applies to specific concerns of the patient.
- Consoling and comforting the patient and his or her family or significant others so that they can accept the present situation as a will of Allah and pray for a better life in the hereafter. (Author's comment – There is also the duty of Muslims to pray for a cure or improvement in health.)
- Taking care of the needs of the family (spiritual, psychological and financial) after the death of the loved one.

Athar (1993, 1998) also stated that the principles followed by Islamic ethics are the preservation of faith, sanctity of life, alleviation of suffering, enjoining what is good and permitted, and forbidding what is wrong and prohibited. There is a need to respect patients' autonomy and heterosexual marriage, while achieving social justice without harm. The patient, family and significant others need to be consulted in the implementation of care and intervention strategies. When asked what actions are most excellent, Prophet Muhammad replied: 'To gladden the hearts of human beings, to feed the hungry, to help the afflicted, to lighten the sorrow of the sorrowful, and to remove the sufferings of the injured' (Bukhari [b]).

Diversity in caring

It is worth remembering that the Muslim population around the globe is not a homogeneous entity. Rather, there is a wide diversity of culture and local customs. As most countries in the world become more ethnically and racially diverse, there is a need for healthcare systems and providers to reflect and respond to an increasingly heterogeneous patient base. Diversity has been described as having four layers: (1) personality; (2) internal dimensions (such as gender, country of origin, race, physical ability); (3) external dimensions (such as religion, parental status, recreational habits, geographical location); and (4) organisational dimensions (such as management occupation, department, specialty) (Gardenswartz and Rowe, 1994). It is stated that this framework brings our attention to the less visible aspects of diversity, as each layer of diversity is salient for how we approach our healthcare practices. For example, a patient who, as a result of his or her ethnicity, culture and/or religion, believes that death is just another spiritual journey, may find the conversation about informed consent less stressful than one who fears death and believes modern medicine should alleviate all risks (Salisbury and Byrd, 2006).

According to Salleh (1994a), diversities are a blessing and a benefit to humanity if they are integrated into a given system. Those responsible towards a caring system must respect diversities and handle the system in a holistic way. Islam recognises differences, diversities and tolerance. There is absolutely no contradiction in respecting and caring for non-Muslim patients whether in Saudi Arabia or in Europe. One function of the Islamic law is to protect the privileged status of non-Muslims and minorities. According to Pickthall (1927), the tolerance within the body of Islam was, and is, something without parallel in history; class, race and colour ceasing altogether to be barriers. Anti-discriminatory practices and equality are laid down in Islam and they are regarded as fundamental expectations and requirements of Muslims be they patients or nurses. Racism is incomprehensible in Islamic thought and practice, for the Noble Qur'aan speaks of human equality in the following terms:

☐ *O mankind! We have created you from a male and a female, and made you into nations and tribes, that you may know one another. Verily, the most honourable of you with Allah is that (believer) who has At-Taqwa* [i.e. one of the *Muttaqun* (pious)]. (Al-Ḥujurāt [The Rooms] 49:13)

Understanding and appreciating Islam's concern for caring enhances one's interest to promote caring in all aspects of intentions, thoughts and actions. Islam insists on its adherents acquiring knowledge and expertise in any field of endeavour that is beneficial for all living things. Islamic caring through practice and management in nursing means that consideration is given to elements of sex, dress code, personal values, code of conduct and ethics, dietary requirements, family planning and life, healthy and safe living (Salleh, 1994b), and spiritual development. During the time of the Prophet, Rufaidah Al-Asalmiya practised as a nurse, established the first school of nursing, and developed the first code of nursing ethics. Lovering points out in Chapter 3 that Rufaidah's narrative symbolises many aspects of caring in Islamic nursing today: the attributes of empathy, kindness, patience and human touch; helping the needy and disadvantaged. Within the Islamic perspective, the concept of care, based on the '*Tawheed* Paradigm', is regarded as a spiritual dome where the basic needs of the patients are met according to the Holy Qur'aan and the statements (Hadiths) of the Prophet (Rassool, 2000).

The process of developing cultural competence is a means of responding effectively to the racial and ethnic demographic shifts and changes that are confronting the healthcare system of many countries. Cultural competence is a defined set of policies, behaviours, attitudes and practices that enable individuals and organisations to work effectively in cross-cultural situations (Salisbury and Byrd, 2006). To become culturally competent both personally and organisationally requires a well-planned and sustained integrated multicultural approach. A culturally competent healthcare setting should include an appropriate mix of the following (Anderson et al., 2003):

- A culturally diverse staff that reflects the community/communities served.
- Providers or translators who speak the clients' language(s).
- Training for providers about the culture and language of the people they serve.
- Signage and instructional literature in the clients' language(s) and consistent with their cultural norm.
- Culturally specific healthcare settings.

Conclusion

Islam is a natural religion applicable to Muslim and non-Muslim communities. It is fully capable of fulfilling the needs of the time and of satisfying the demands of new circumstances without any changes in the religion. What is called for, in caring for Muslim patients, is not mutual rivalry in the understanding of the needs of Muslim patients but mutual engagement and collaboration with providers of health care and nursing. In addition, we need to leave our cultural baggage behind and tailor the delivery of care to meet patients' social, cultural, linguistic and religious needs when caring for Muslim patients. Finally, it is valuable to note that developing culturally competent care is not a strategy to accommodate Muslim patients into the healthcare system and service provision that exist in our community but it is about transforming those systems to meet the needs of the service users.

Reflective Activity 2.2

- Spiritual needs and concerns are expressed by many patients, especially Muslim patients. What is meant by spiritual needs?
- Identify the spiritual resources and practices, beliefs, objects and/or relationships that people often turn to for help in times of crisis or concern.
- What do spiritual needs and resources have to do with caring for Muslim patients?
- How would you, as a nurse, assess the spiritual dimension of nursing care?
- How would you incorporate the spiritual dimension of care in the nursing environment?
- How might the patient's religious or spiritual views affect medical decision-making?
- Identify the barriers in providing spiritual care to hospitalised patients.
- How can your own spirituality (or religiosity) affect the delivery of nursing care?

References

American Holistic Nurses' Association (AHNA) ([1992] revised 1998) *Description of Holistic Nursing* (Flagstaff, AZ: Author).

Anderson, L.M, Scrimshaw, S.C., Fullilove, M.T., Fielding, J.E. and Normand, J. (2003) 'Culturally Competent Healthcare Systems: A Systematic Review', *American Journal of Preventive Medicine* 24 (3S), 68–79.

Athar, S. (1993) *Islamic Perspectives in Medicine. A Survey of Islamic Medicine: Achievements and Contemporary Issues* (Indianapolis: American Trust Publications).

Athar, S. (1998) *Ethical Decision-Making in Patient Care: An Islamic Perspective* (Lombard, IL: Islamic Medical Association of North America).

Bukhari [a], volume 46, no. 730, http://searchtruth.com/book_display.php?book=46&translator=1&start=0&number=730, date accessed 29 July 2013.

Bukhari [b] volume 1, 2, no. 10, http://searchtruth.com/book_display.php?book=46&translator=1&start=0&number=730, date accessed 29 July 2013.

Dyson, J., Cobb, M. and Forman, D. (1997) 'The Meaning of Spirituality: a Literature Review', *Journal of Advanced Nursing* 26, 6, 1183–8.

Erickson, H.L. (2007) 'Philosophy and Theory of Holism', *Nursing Clinics of North America* 42, 139–63.

Gardenswartz, L. and Rowe, A. (1994) *Diverse Teams at Work* (Chicago, IL: Irwin).

Hutchison, M.G. (1997) *Healing the Whole Person: The Spiritual Dimension,* http://members.tripod.com/marg_hutchison/nurse-4.html, date accessed 30 July 2013.

Philips, A.A.B. (1994) *The Fundamentals of Tawheed (Islamic Monotheism)* (Riyadh: International Islamic Publishing House).

Pickthall, M. (1927) Lecture on 'Islamic Tolerance in Islam', in *The Cultural Side of Islam* (Lahore: Sh.M. Ashraf Publishers).

Rassool, G. Hussein. (2000) 'The Crescent and Islam: Healing, Nursing and the Spiritual Dimension. Some Considerations towards an Understanding of the Islamic Perspectives on Caring', *Journal of Advanced Nursing* 32, 6, 1476–84.

Salisbury, J. and Byrd, S. (2006) Why Diversity Matters in Health Care.

CSA Bulletin, http://dc3.middlewaygroup.org/Members/patelashok/diversity healthcare.pdf, date accessed 29 July 2013.

Salleh, K.M. (1994a) *The Islamic Perspectives of Caring.* Proceedings of the First International Nursing Conference: Education for Caring. Pengiran Anak Puteri Rashidah Sa'adatul Bolkiah, College of Nursing Brunei, Darussalam, 1994, pp. 12–20.

Salleh, K.M. (1994b) *The Islamic Perspectives of Caring. Resolutions and Recommendations. Islamic Caring Practices and Management in Nursing.* Proceedings of the First International Nursing Conference: Education for Caring. Pengiran Anak Puteri Rashidah Sa'adatul Bolkiah, College of Nursing Brunei, Darussalam, 1994.

Simsen, B.J. (1985) *Spiritual Needs and Resources in Illness and Hospitalization.* (Manchester, UK: University of Manchester Press), p.10.

Tirmidhî, 1924, andAbu-Dawud, 494; classed as saheeh by al-Albani; cited in http://islamqa.info/en/105343, date accessed 14 October 2013.

www.mentalhealth.org.uk,Spirituality, cited in www.mentalhealth.org.uk/help-information/mental-health-a-z/S/spirituality/, date accessed 30 July 2013.

Caring as an Act of Spirituality: a Nursing Approach

3

S. Lovering

Learning Outcomes:

- Examine the meaning of caring from the perspective of Muslim nurses.
- Have an awareness of the legitimacy of Muslim nursing identity.
- Identify the relation between God and caring from an Islamic perspective.
- Discuss how the nursing identity in religious values is shared between nurses and patients.
- State how the sharing of the Muslim faith with their patients underpins the nurses' caring actions.

Reflective Activity 3.1

State whether the following statements are true or false. Give reasons for your answers.

	True	False
1 Caring and religion are inseparable for Muslim nurses.		
2 The foundation of the relationship between the nurse and patient is not founded on a shared Muslim worldview.		
3 Rufaidah Al-Asalmiya developed the first code of nursing ethics and was an advocate for health education and preventative care.		

	True	False
4 For Muslim nurses, the relationship between the nurse and God is not a central theme within the nurse–patient therapeutic relationship.		
5 Rufaidah Al-Asalmiya set up the first school of nursing before Florence Nightingale.		
6 Islam does not support nursing as a career choice.		
7 In Islam, the status of women in the nursing role was raised before the transformation of Western nursing.		
8 A fundamental belief in Islam is that you must live your life in preparation for reward in the afterlife.		
9 Nurses' caring actions include use of religious words, reading the Qur'aan, praying with patients, and support for end-of-life rituals.		
10 The use of religious words such as *Bismillah* is limited to Muslim nurses caring for Muslim patients.		
11 The focus of caring is to assist the patient's belief in and relationship with God.		
12 Sharing the Muslim faith with their patients underpins the nurses' caring actions.		
13 The nurse's professional and personal identity is separable from Islam.		
14 Islamic caring is based on building the patient's trust in God.		

Introduction

In nursing, care and caring are defined from a variety of perspectives reflective of the Western Judeo-Christian tradition (Holden and Littlewood, 1991; Narayanasamy and Owens, 2001; Rassool, 2000), with an assumption that nursing has a universal belief system. However, there is growing literature from non-Western cultural contexts that presents nursing frameworks grounded within distinct cultural systems, such as examples from Chinese (Chen, 2001; Pang et al., 2004; Wong et al., 2003), Korean (Shin, 2001), and Native America nurses (Hunter et al., 2006; Struthers and Littlejohn, 1999). Generally, nurses provide care to Muslim patients based on the nursing framework from the Judeo-Christian tradition. Mebrouk (2004) described the impact of Islam on nurses' practice, where 'Islam provides their framework upon which they base their scientific based nursing care and moral considerations involved in their decision making.' Caring and religion are inseparable for Muslim nurses where a shared Muslim worldview is the foundation of the relationship between the nurse and patient. The meaning of caring begins with the nurses' relationship with God. This chapter explores the meaning of caring for Muslim nurses, through presentation of findings from an ethnographic study (Lovering, 1996). The findings of the study indicated that Muslim nurses' caring actions support the spiritual and physical health of the patient, where caring is a spiritual action.

Nursing comes from the Prophet

In the Middle East, the history of nursing in Islam contributes to the nursing identity and shapes the caring role of Muslim nurses. As explained by one nurse, 'nursing comes from our Prophet Mohammad so we have to be careful when we touch the patient and how we will deal with the patient'. However, during the time of Prophet Muhammad, Rufaidah Al-Asalmiya was requested to place her tent in his mosque, which became the first Islamic health clinic. Thus, nurses caring for patients in the mosque symbolises acceptance of nursing within Islam. An important part of Rufaidah's narrative is the recognition given to the early nurses who participated in the Holy wars. Al-Osimy (1994) states: 'The status of the women participating as nurses in the wars was so highly honoured by the Holy Prophet that he considered their effort as a form of Jihad in the cause of Allah. He used to give them their share of the war loots just [as] he gave men theirs.' The symbolism of sharing equally in the war booty gives the message that nursing is worthy in Islam and raises the status of women in the nursing role.

The story of Rufaidah Al-Asalmiya: nursing as a means to practise Islam

Rufaidah Al-Asalmiya (also referred to as Rufaidah bint Saad) practised as a nurse during the wars when the Prophet Muhammad established Islam in the seventh century AD. Rufaidah was the daughter of Saad Al-Asalmi, a healer in Yathrib (modern-day Madinah in Saudi Arabia). She assisted her father and developed her nursing skills before she became Muslim (Jan, 1996). At the time of her reversion, there were many wars to protect and defend the Islamic state and religion in the area of Madinah. When there was a call for support in the Holy wars, Rufaidah saw nursing as a means to express her faith and commitment to the Prophet Muhammad and organised a group of women to assist in the wars in a nursing role. She began to teach her friends about nursing. During the Badr invasion, the first war in Islam in January 624, Rufaidah and her friends provided the Muslim soldiers with water, dressed the wounds of the injured and transported the dead back to Madinah. The first Islamic health clinic was in a tent in the Prophet's mosque where health education to the community was delivered.

Rufaidah set up the first school of nursing, developed the first code of nursing ethics and was an advocate for health education and preventative care (Jan, 1996). In this period of Islam, the female nurse was called Al-Assiyah from the verb *assaa*, which means to cure wounds. The Islamic verb *qaama*, which means to take care of patients, was applied to both male and female nurses (Al-Osimy, 1994). The narrative of Rufaidah (Al-Osimy, 1994; Bryant, 2003; Karaha, 2004; Mebrouk, 2008) shows aspects about caring that continue as a thread in Islamic nursing today. Rufaidah's narrative can be interpreted according to the following themes: nursing as a means to practise Islam, acceptance of nursing in Islam, legitimisation of nursing and foundation of the nurses' professional identity.

Legitimisation of nursing and nursing identity

There are parallels in the legitimisation of nursing in the Middle East through Islam and the transformation of Western nursing at the time of Florence Nightingale. At the time of Florence Nightingale, nursing gained legitimacy through linking nursing with a religious calling, a high moral ground, a mission to serve humanity and an emphasis on nurses' special womanliness (Brodie, 1994; Nelson, 2001). Nursing became an acceptable career for women rather than a domestic role carried out by women of questionable morality. Jaleesah (2004) notes the similarities in Western and Islamic nursing history: 'Nursing holds at its core a tradition of caring and responsibility at great personal sacrifice. We have in our collective history stories of nuns caring for the poor, infirm and outcast. Our rich history in Islam gives a reason for pride and a radical tradition to which we must set our sights.' The importance of Rufaidah as the first nurse in Islam is the foundation of the nursing identity for Muslim nurses. As Jan (1996, p. 268) explains, 'Because of Rufaidah we realise that nursing is a noble career for Muslim women in accordance to Islamic tradition. Indeed, Rufaidah is a great role model for us today. We, who are Muslims, should not forget our historical tradition and the example of Rufaidah – our first nurse, nurse educator, nurse leader, and founder of our first nursing school and clinics.' Hussain (2004) noted that 'Rufaidah was the mother of human medication [medicine] and nursing in the world 1400 years ago. Centuries later Florence Nightingale followed the steps of Rufaidah.'

The relationship between the nurse and God

Similar to the example of Rufaidah, Muslim nurses practise through their faith in God. This faith is the basis of their commitment to nursing and shapes the nature of their relationship with their patients with whom they share the same values. Mebrouk (2008) noted that nurses entered a relationship with their patients based on shared humanity including religion. The relationship between the nurse and God is the starting point for the caring experience. The nursing pledge spoken by graduates of the Dar Al Hekma College School of Nursing, Jeddah, Saudi Arabia, illustrates the centrality of faith in the nurses' commitment to the profession. The beginning point of this nursing pledge is the relationship of the nurse with God.

> In the name of Allah, the Almighty, Who granted me wisdom as a means in life; Whose name is high and holy, who endowed on Himself the name and description of mercy; I pledge to be faithful to my religion, king, and nation; To offer myself to this profession through my faith in God. (Dar Al Hekma College School of Nursing graduation ceremony, 2006)

The relationship between the nurse and God is a central theme within the nurse–patient therapeutic relationship. Al-Osimy (2005) described the duties of the Muslim nurse as: duty to God, duty of the Muslim to himself, duty of Muslim nurses to increase knowledge of science and nursing and the need to connect to the past and present. She encouraged Muslim nurses to be faithful, "pray as it leads to self-instruction and inner peace, work hard, and seek God's forgiveness and satisfaction as 'God looks into your heart." Nurses should be afraid of God and be faithful to God. Al-Osimy (2005) linked worship of God to the nursing role and the society's benefit.

Caring is an act of spirituality

In the study of Muslim nurses' experiences of 'the meaning of caring' (Lovering, 2008, p. 12), spirituality became a significant concept and this translates into the nurses' caring experiences. Caring is a spiritual action, and in turn, the nurse receives reward from God. The picture of caring as spiritual action emerges through exploring the relationship between the nurses and God, and the nurses' responsibility to assist the patient's belief in God as caring action. Nurses' caring actions include use of religious words, reading the Qur'aan, praying with the patients, and support for end-of-life rituals. In essence, nurses are guardians of the patient's spiritual, physical and psychosocial health through caring as an act of spirituality.

Sharing the Muslim faith with their patients underpins the nurses' caring actions. The focus of caring is to assist the patient's belief in and relationship with God. One nurse summarised the focus of her caring as 'building a relationship between the human [patient] and God" ' which is about the nurse being an agent or facilitator of the faith. The role of the nurse as a facilitator of the faith in caring for Muslim patients has been endorsed. Al-Osimy (2005) encouraged nurses to mention God and remind others to mention God at all times. She linked the giving of advice for health to the act of prayer, 'religion is advice, giving advice is like a prayer, and advice is the core of the religion'. She advised Muslim nurses to remember and give thanks to God and to remind patients of the greatness of God. According to Al-Osimy (2005), the role of the nurse is to console the patient and 'to remind the patient that the Prophet said everything is good for Muslims, including fever'. If having trouble with a patient, 'it is the duty of the nurse to forgive and forget the bad words from the patient. Take God's word and find a suitable solution.' Similar beliefs guide the education of nurses. Al-Osimy (2005) noted that nursing 'education is a part of prayer. It is important that faculty are believers [of Islam] and experienced in education. Teachers are like prophets on earth.' There is a narration from by Abu al-Darda' (Allah be pleased with him) recounting that the Messenger of Allah said, 'Scholars are the inheritors of the prophets' (Tirmidhî). The training of nurses must be within an Islamic environment, depending on Islamic principles and ethics. An example of the caring action as the facilitation of the faith is threaded through the narratives in Lovering's study (2008). One nurse explained the way she responds to a patient who asks her to do something that is against the religion and her role as a nurse.

> Sometimes the patient will ask you something that is not acceptable. You can't do it as a nurse, but if you say no to him directly, there will be trouble for you and the patient. ... Give him the view from the religion and he will accept it very easily.

Building the patient's trust in God is another aspect of caring action. A paediatrician explained the importance of building the patient's trust through a story of breaking the news to parents following the birth of a disabled child (Soby, 2004). He talked about a mother going through pregnancy with dreams of a child and their future. When a baby is born with a disability, that dream is shattered, and there is a need to break the news about the baby in a certain way. He started his advice on breaking the news by talking about the importance of belief in God, which is 'the most important thing'. You must present the baby as a gift from God. Secondly, the mother's belief in God may be harmed. The mother often thinks that she did something bad, not just in pregnancy, but in her life, and that this disabled baby is a punishment from God. 'Why did God do this, God is punishing me?' and this in turn affects her belief in God. Therefore, you must focus on the belief in God, and on fixing the notion that the parents are being punished. 'It is very important, as belief in God is the most important thing to the human being' (Lovering, 2008, p. 109).

Many nurses shared examples of the integration of their shared faith into the care of patients using religious teaching and religious words. The nurses used the word *Insha'Allah* (it is God's will) and prayer to calm patients' anxieties about having surgery or treatment. The nurses explained that as the outcome for the patient is already predestined, religious words support and reinforce the patient's belief in God, giving comfort and strength to the patient. Nurses also assist patients in reading the Qur'aan to relax the patient. An intensive care nurse used tape recordings of the Qur'aan to calm her patients. She 'went around with earphones to ICU patients and put on tapes with the Qur'aan'. Nurses also linked religious teachings from the Qur'aan to patient teaching. The use of prayers and reading of the Qur'aan were common caring actions in Mebrouk's study on Muslim nurses' caring (Mebrouk, 2008). One nurse encouraged palliative care patients to receive comfort from listening to recitations of the Noble Qur'aan or watching Islamic lessons on television. Another explained that when she 'gives him the anti-emetic and I am here beside him and I am reading the Noble Qur'aan for him, so it will make it much different, because we all believe in the Qur'aan and the role of it, the spiritual feeling' (Mebrouk, 2008, p. 154). Nurses also linked the emphasis given by the Prophet on cleanliness as a reason to clean the patient's skin prior to an injection, and use of Zam Zam water (Holy water from Makkah) instead of regular water to give oral medications (Mebrouk, 2008). A nurse discussed the use of Zam Zam water as part of her spiritual care. She explained,

> In the neonatal intensive care unit (NICU), the father will give you Zam Zam water to feed to the NICU baby. You may only give the baby a drop, or wash their face with it, or bathe the baby. This is spiritual care. The non-Muslim nurse does not understand how important this is to do. (Lovering, 2008, p. 111)

Nurses spoke of the importance of prayer and saying the *Ash-Shahadah* when a patient is dying. The *Ash-Shahadah* is the basic creed of Islam or testimony of faith, meaning 'There is no true God but Allah, and Muhammad is His Messenger' (Huseini, 2006, p. 58). One nurse said: 'If dying, say the *Ash-Shahadah* for the patient ... give them a smile, tell the patient if the nurse sees good signs. If there are bad signs, don't tell the family. Nurses must mention

God in the last breath, and say the Islamic *Ash-Shahadah.*' Another nurse spoke about taking care of a Muslim patient in an intensive care unit in Ireland. She would say *Ash-Shahadah* in the ear of the patient when the team was trying to save the patient's life. Patients also seek religious advice and support from the nurses. Patients ask for advice on performing ablutions (ritual washing) before prayer, ways to perform prayer when unable to bend or kneel, and the direction to face for prayer.

The nurses' narratives highlighted the use of religious words as a caring action and connecting to the patient relationship. The words *As-salamu Alaykum* (peace be upon you), *Bismillah* (by the name of God), and *Insha'Allah* (God's willing) were used to make a spiritual connection with the patient and to connect nurses' caring actions with the name of God as the basis of the trust between nurse and patient. The use of religious words such as *Bismillah* is not limited to Muslim nurses caring for Muslim patients, but can be used by all nurses prior to any procedure for a Muslim patient. A Muslim nurse explained that non-Muslim nurses should know that to say *Bismillah* is an action to calm the patient to establish trust between the patient and nurse. Muslim nurses consider the use of *Bismillah* as a form of prayer for their patients, regardless of a shared belief system. 'We will say *Bismillah* and will pray for our patients, even if they are not Muslim.' So, their spiritual caring is not specific only to the Muslim, but 'that is how we treat all of our patients'.

Reward for nursing actions

A fundamental belief in Islam is that you must live your life in preparation for reward in the afterlife. It follows that the belief in reward in the afterlife underpins the nurse's caring role. The nurses linked the importance of their caring actions to a verse in the Qur'aan that gives significance to saving another's life (interpretation of the meaning):

☐ *If anyone has saved a life, it would be as if he has saved the life of the whole of mankind.* (Al-Mā'idah [The Table Spread] 5:32)

Muneera Al-Osimy (2005), in a keynote address on 'Morals and Practices of the Muslim Nurse', began with the following excerpt from the Qur'aan (interpretation of the meaning):

☐ *Whoever works righteousness, whether male or female, while he (or she) is a true believer (of Islamic Monotheism) verily, to him We will give a good life (in this world with respect, contentment and lawful provision), and We shall pay them certainly a reward in proportion to the best of what they used to do (i.e. Paradise in the Hereafter).* (An-Nahl [The Bee] 16:97)

The use of this verse clearly links nursing care with righteousness, Islam and reward for good work. Further, Al-Osimy (2005) emphasised the importance of reward from God for nursing and advised nurses not to complain or be dissatisfied. She noted that good behaviour and conduct, relieving problems for others, visiting the patient, and showing the patient where to face for prayer, were all actions making the nurse deserving of entering heaven. Receiving recognition and reward from God and appreciation from the patient were frequent themes in the narratives of the nurses. According to the nurses, helping a patient to have a longer life brings greater reward over time to the nurses for their good work. The reward and recognition from God accumulates as you care for more patients. A nurse explained this concept:

> I did something good for this patient, for example I saved his life or I did a good dressing. It will increase his life maybe 15 or 20 years. All the good things that he is doing [over his lifetime] mean I will get benefit from it. God will reward me for it. God will not reward me for what I did just once. For example, if the patient is having a cardiac arrest, I help him to get back to life. He comes back to life, he does good things, and then I will get benefit as he is doing good at the same time. God is giving, and God will see how many patients you are dealing with. There are many good things you will receive from God. (Lovering, 2008, p. 117)

Another nurse talked about the patients appreciating and giving thanks to God for the nurses' caring. This makes nursing special as it comes from their shared religious values.

> One of the things that really make me like nursing: if the patient is in pain and says to you: 'Thank you, God Bless you.' That's a perfect thing for me. There are a lot of people that when you're doing something for them, they are really praying to God, saying your name all the time. 'God bless you, God help you.' This is something, I could receive all the money, but it's the religion that is important for me. (Lovering, 2008, p. 118)

Conclusion

The history of nursing in Islam grounds the nursing identity in the religious values shared between nurses and patients. While acknowledgement of this nursing history is recent in the region, the validation of the nursing role in Islam provides the foundation for caring as an act of spirituality. Rufaidah's narrative symbolises many aspects of caring in Islamic nursing today: the attributes of empathy, kindness, patience and human touch; helping the needy and disadvantaged. The belief that nursing is a means to express and practise the Muslim faith underpins caring as a spiritual action. Islam is the foundation of the shared values of the nurse and patient, and expressed through caring action. Thus, the nurse's professional and personal identity is inseparable from Islam (Mebrouk, 2008). Faith in God is the basis of the nurses' commitment to their profession and their patients. As with all Muslims, the first duty of the individual is to God, then to their own faith and worship of God. The nurse's relationship with God forms the beginning point of caring for the patient and actions to assist the patient's belief in and relationship with God. Caring actions include reading from the Qur'aan and use of religious teaching. The verse in the Qur'aan [An-Nahl 5:23]: *'if anyone has saved a life, it would be as if he has saved the life of the whole of mankind'* is significant to the belief that nursing is a spiritual action that will bring rewards in the afterlife. Receiving recognition and reward from God are central goals for all Muslims, and caring is a means of achieving this outcome. Muslim nurses are guardians of a patient's spiritual and physical health. The following Hadith captures the link between a Muslim nurse's own spirituality and the caring role. One companion of the Prophet asked him: 'What actions are excellent?' He replied: 'To feed the hungry, to help the afflicted, to lighten the sorrow of the sorrowful, and to remove the sufferings of the injured' (Bukhari).

Reflective Activity 3.2

- After reading this chapter, what is the most important thing you take out of this?
- How are your values expressed through your nursing care practice?
- What sorts of things make you feel uncomfortable in relation to meeting the spiritual needs of the Muslim patients? Why?
- How does your understanding of cultural competence impact on the nursing approach to care?
- Why might it be important to establish what beliefs, values and theories you are aligned with?
- How do you reconcile differences in beliefs, values and attitudes?
- Reflect on the role of Muslim nurses and on your own role in caring as an act of spirituality.

References

Abu Dawood, At-Tirmidhi and Ibn Hibbaan [this is the wording found in his collection, in abridged form]. Al-Bukhari mentioned in his Saheeh Collection in his Book of Knowledge, Chapter: 'Knowledge precedes Speech and Action', the part from it: 'The scholars are the inheritors of the Prophets'.

Al-Osimy, M. (1994) *Nursing in Saudi Arabia* (Jeddah, Saudi Arabia: King Fahd National Library), p. 18.

Al-Osimy, M. (2005) *Morals and Practices of the Muslim Nurse*. 3rd International Nursing Conference, Muscat, Oman.

Brodie, B. (1994) 'Nursing's Quest for Professionalism', in J.M. Closkey and H. Grace (eds), *Current Issues in Nursing* (4th edition) (Philadelphia, PA: Mosby-Year Book), pp. 559–65.

Bryant, N. (2003) *Women in Nursing in Islamic Societies* (Oxford: Oxford University Press).

Bukhari, cited in *The Best Hadith Collection, Holy Prophet Muhammad*, www.ummah.com/forum/showthread.php?290923-The-best-hadith-collection-holy-prophet-muhammad-%28p-b-u-h-%29, date accessed 29 July 2013.

Chen, Y. (2001) 'Chinese Values, Health and Nursing', *Journal of Advanced Nursing* 36, 2, 270–3.

Holden, P. and Littlewood, J. (1991) 'Introduction', in P. Holden and J. Littlewood (eds), *Anthropology and Nursing* (London: Routledge), pp. 1–6.

Hunter, L., Logan, J., Goulet, J.G. and Barton, S. (2006) 'Aboriginal Healing: Regaining Balance and Culture', *Journal of Transcultural Nursing* 17, 1, 3–22.

Huseini, S.F. (2006) *Islam and the Glorious Ka'abah* (Jeddah, Saudi Arabia: King Fahd National Library).

Hussain, S. (2004) 'The First Nurse in Islam', in M. Al-Osimy (ed.), *The First Nurse* (Jeddah, Saudi Arabia: King Fahd National Library), pp. 16–19.

Jaleesah, R. (2004) *The Nursing Profession in Islam. Windows into the World of Nursing*, 1st International Nursing Conference. Jeddah, Saudi Arabia, 2004.

Jan, R. (1996) 'Rufaidah Al-Asalmiya, the First Muslim Nurse. Image', *Journal of Nursing Scholarship* 28, 3, 267–8.

Karaha, S. (2004) 'First Nurse in Islam: Koaiba Al-Aslamia – Rofaida Alaslamia', in M. Al-Osimy (ed.), *The First Nurse* (Jeddah, Saudi Arabia: King Fahd National Library), pp. 5–35.

Lovering, S. (1996) *Saudi Nurse Leaders: Career Choices and Experiences* (Master's thesis) (Palmerston North, New Zealand: Massey University).

Lovering, S. (2008) *Arab Muslim Nurses' Experiences of the Meaning of Caring* (PhD dissertation) (Sydney, Australia: University of Sydney).

Mebrouk, J. (2004) *Perceptions of Nursing Care: Views of Saudi Arabian Female Nurses* (Master's thesis) (Adelaide, Australia: Deakin University).

Mebrouk, J. (2008) 'Perception of Nursing Care: Views of Saudi Arabian Female Nurses', *Contemporary Nurse* 28, 1–2, 149–61.

Narayanasamy, A. and Owens, J. (2001) 'A Critical Incident Study of Nurses' Responses to the Spiritual Needs of their Patients', *Journal of Advanced Nursing* 33, 4, 446–55.

Nelson, S. (2001) *Say Little, Do Much. Nursing, Nuns, and Hospitals in the Nineteenth Century* (Philadelphia, PA: University of Pennsylvania Press).

Pang, S., Wong, T., Wang, C., Zhang, Z., Chan, H., Lam, C. and Chan, K. (2004) 'Towards a Chinese Definition of Nursing', *Journal of Advanced Nursing* 46, 6, 657–70.

Rassool, G. Hussein. (2000) 'The Crescent and Islam: Healing, Nursing and the Spiritual Dimension. Some Considerations towards an Understanding of the Islamic Perspectives on Caring', *Journal of Advanced Nursing 32*, 6, 1476–84.

Shin, K.R. (2001) 'Developing Perspectives on Korean Nursing Theory: the Influence of Taoism', *Nursing Science Quarterly* 14, 4, 346–53.

Soby, A. (2004) 'International Nurses Day', *Breaking the News* (Riyadh, Saudi Arabia).

Struthers, R. and Littlejohn, S. (1999) 'The Essence of Native American Nursing', *Journal of Transcultural Nursing* 10, 2, 131–5.

Tirmidhî, 2606; classed as saheeh by al-Albani; cited in www.huda.tv/fatawa-bank?sobi2Task=sobi2Details&catid=45&sobi2Id=450, date accessed 15 October 2013.

Wong, T., Pang, S. and Wang, C. (2003) 'A Chinese Definition of Nursing', *Nursing Inquiry* 10, 2, 79.

Ethical Dimensions in Caring **4**

S. Lovering and G. Hussein Rassool

Learning Outcomes:

- Discuss how the spiritual and cultural values are embedded within Islamic caring practices.
- Have an awareness of the ethical dimensions in caring within the Muslim healthcare context.
- Identify the principles of Islamic bio-ethics.
- Identify the core elements of the 'Ethical decision-making in an Islamic healthcare context'.

Reflective Activity 4.1

State whether the following statements are true or false. Give reasons for your answers.

	True	False
1 A universal set of ethical principles are applicable to all cultures.		
2 Ethical principles are culturally derived.		
3 The mother's role in the family is as the key decision maker.		
4 The Western bio-ethical perspective gives priority to the values of autonomy and patients' rights.		
5 Muslim nurses are guided by the primary principles of preserving their faith and protecting the sanctity of life.		

	True	False
6 Muslim and non-Muslim nurses approach ethical dilemmas from the same ethical perspectives.		
7 Visiting the sick is an important cultural, social and religious obligation.		
8 Spiritual and cultural values are separable within Islamic caring practices.		
9 In Islam, the avoidance of harm does not take priority over the accrual of benefit as the primary principle when determining ethical action.		
10 The psychosocial and spiritual needs of the patient and family are at the centre of nursing care.		
11 Culture determines moral belief systems, and personal and professional values.		
12 For Muslim nurses, spiritual and cultural values are separable within their caring practices.		
13 Muslim nurses must maintain their faith in all caring actions, and use Islamic teachings to guide their moral decision-making and ethical action.		

Introduction

Globally, nurses from diverse cultural and religious backgrounds care for Muslim populations from a distinctive perspective based on their worldview. The blending of cultural views leads to a healthcare environment rich in cultural diversity and complexity. However, there are similarities as well as differences in the ethical principles applied by nurses in caring for Muslim patients (Lovering, 2008). The literature guiding the care of Muslim patients, from an ethical perspective, tends to focus on the ethical issues including organ transplantation, genetic manipulation, termination of pregnancy and end-of-life care (Al-Qattan, 1992; Daar and Khitamy, 2001; Gatrad and Sheikh, 2001; Hedayat and Pirzadeh, 2001; Rispler-Chaim, 1989; Sachedina, 2005; Sahin, 1990). Within the nursing literature, there is limited discussion on Islamic bio-ethics as applied to nursing practice, with the exception of Rassool (2000, 2004) and Moawad (2006). Understanding the different perspectives of ethical decision-making by Muslim nurses helps to reduce misunderstanding and conflict between non-Muslim nurses and their Muslim nursing colleagues and patients.

This chapter will explore the ethical dimensions in caring for Muslim patients and examine the debate on ethical principles applied in an international context. It will present an introduction to the principles of Islamic bio-ethics and an overview of Islamic medical codes of ethics to guide practice. The ethical considerations examined in this will enable nurses to have a greater awareness and understanding of ethical decision-making while caring for Muslim patients.

Ethics: an international perspective

An understanding of what constitutes ethical decision-making is based on principles including beneficence, non-malfeasance, respect for autonomy, fidelity, and justice (Taft, 2000). The foundation values that dominate ethical perspectives in the bio-medical and nursing fields include: respect for persons, the right of the person to act autonomously, respect for dignity, and the moral demand that the rightness of an ethical act depends on the action, rather than the consequences (Ray, 2010). However, these principles are derived from Judeo-Christian traditions and form the basis of international ethical guidelines such as the Declaration of Helsinki and various nursing codes of ethics of national nursing associations (Harper, 2006; Pacquiao, 2003; Taft, 2000). There is recent recognition that Western ethical principles may or may not reflect the values of developing countries or non-Western cultures (Harper, 2006; Ray, 2010; Tschudin, 2005). In the international milieu, there is debate on whether there is a universal set of ethical principles applicable to all cultures; whether culture defines ethical principles; or whether a basic set of principles exists that can be modified to fit the cultural context (Harper, 2006; Ray, 2010). Within the nursing context, it is suggested that respect for persons, beneficence and justice should be applied universally (Harper, 2006; Ketefian, 2008; Mill and Ogilvie, 2002; Olsen et al., 2003). However, this perspective is not universally agreed upon. Christakis (1992) argues that culture shapes both the content and forms of moral and ethical systems, and ethical behaviour needs to fit within the framework of the local context. That is, ethics are culturally bound.

Muslim and non-Muslim nurses approach ethical dilemmas, such as assisting with organ donation, end-of-life practices with a critically ill patient, and assisting with procedures such as abortion and sterilisation, from different ethical perspectives (Lovering, 2008). In relation to organ transplantation, this is supported by the non-Muslim (Western) bio-ethical perspective. In contrast, many Muslims believe that organ transplantation is prohibited by Islamic law.

However, a great number of Muslim religious scholars permit organ donation and this holds true for donating organs to non-Muslims as well (Ghaly,
2012). Organ donations and transplantations are examined in Chapter 16.
Muslim and non-Muslim nurses face different ethical dilemmas in the decision
to discontinue medical treatment for patients who are clinically dead. Non-
Muslims perceive continuation of life support as causing unnecessary suffering
(Halligan, 2006; Gebara and Tashjian, 2006). In contrast, Muslims believe that
life is sacred and Allah decides the time of death, so life saving measures
should not be withdrawn, but neither should treatment be offered that is futile
and causes suffering (Aramesh and Shadi, 2007; Rassool, 2004). Muslim and
non-Muslim (Western) ethical perspectives on sterilisation and abortion procedures highlight different views on the value of patient autonomy and the
sanctity of life. Sterilisation is not supported in an Islamic bio-ethical view, as
it is interpreted as interfering with reproduction and God's will. Abortion is
prohibited, as God gives human life, and life cannot be taken away by human
action. The only exception is when the mother's life is at risk, as the mother's
life takes precedence over that of the unborn child (Moawad, 2006; Rassool,
2000). A reflection on the different ethical perspectives of Muslim and non-
Muslim nurses highlights that the moral systems underpinning nurses' ethical
behaviour are culturally determined, suggesting that there is not a universal
set of ethical principles in nursing.

Islamic codes of nursing ethics

Codes of ethics for nurses have been established to guide the practice of
Muslim nurses in the Middle East (Moawad, 2006). In the Middle East, the
Gulf Co-operation Council (GCC) Code of Professional Conduct for Nursing
focuses on the core values of accountability, dignity, privacy and confidentiality but does not articulate the principles of Islam inherent in the code of
ethics. In another Islamic context, Sanjari et al. (2008) identified the need for a
national code of ethics for nurses in Iran, based on Islamic principles. In Saudi
Arabia, work began on a code of ethics for nursing based on Islamic teachings.
Overall, while there is some discussion on the need for a code of ethics based
on Islamic principles to guide Muslim nurses in caring for Muslim patients,
there is yet to be such a code developed on an international or national level.

Islamic bio-ethical perspective

Islamic bio-ethics emphasises the duties and obligations of the Muslim to
adhere to Islamic principles. The most important obligations for a Muslim are
to preserve the faith and to protect the sanctity of life (Al-Swailem, 2007; Daar
and Khitamy, 2001; Hanson, 2008). Ethical decision-making is guided by the

values of Islam, teachings of the Qur'aan and interpretation of Islamic law. Islamic principles that apply to bio-ethical decision-making include: preservation of life, protection of the species, preservation of mental facilities, preservation of wealth, and the need to maximise the good and minimise harm or evil. In addition, the principle of justice requires that benefits and burdens are fairly distributed so that individuals receive that which they deserve and which they are entitled to (Al-Swailem, 2006, 2007). According to Rassool (2000), the principles of Islamic ethics applied in nursing are the preservation of the Islamic faith, preservation of life, alleviation of suffering, promoting what is good (beneficence), and forbidding what is wrong (non-malfeasance). Islamic bio-ethics speaks about the call to virtue, referring to *Ihsaan* (striving to perfection). For Muslims, *Ihsaan* is a continuous attempt to do all things well, drawing nearer to perfection.

Developing an ethical decision-making approach

There is a dearth of literature on the nursing ethics decision-making model using Islamic principles. The majority of models use a Western bio-medical rights-based approach, supporting the principle of preserving an individual's autonomy and client choice (Hook and White, 2003; Mylott, 2005; Pacquiao, 2003). Pacquiao's (2003) culturally competent model of ethical decision-making, based on Leininger's (1991) theory of culture care, supported the ethical values common to both Western and Islamic bio-ethics. Pacquiao's (2003) model aims to preserve human rights and incorporate the ethical principles of beneficence, non-malfeasance and justice as part of the values of the patient, and so has consistency with the Islamic perspective. However, the model assumes that the care giver is of a different culture from the recipient, and does not appear to guide the priority of Islamic principles (preservation of the faith, protecting the sanctity of life) in ethical decision-making.

In the absence of a suitable model from the nursing literature, an illustration was produced to guide 'Ethical decision-making in an Islamic healthcare environment' (Figure 4.1). The ethical decision-making diagram evolved through discussions on the interaction of Islamic values, culture and ethical decisions, and testing the evolving diagram with Muslim nurses and an expert on Islamic bio-ethics. The diagram was used as the framework for discussion of ethical dilemmas faced by Muslim and non-Muslim nurses caring for patients in a Muslim healthcare context (Al-Swailem and Lovering, 2007).

The core elements of the 'Ethical decision-making in an Islamic healthcare environment' diagram (Figure 4.1) are Islam, culture and the patient–family unit. Islamic values are the foundation of decision-making. Islamic values impact on culture of the patient and family, and guide the practice of the nurse, the physician, and the organisation. The patient and family are located

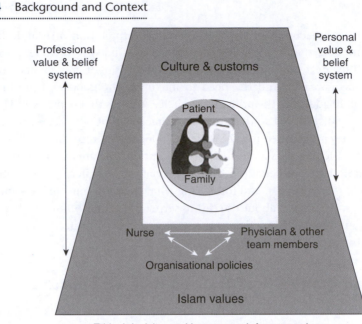

Ethical decision-making approach for nurses in an
islamic predominant healthcare environment

Figure 4.1   Ethical decision-making in an Islamic healthcare environment

in the centre as the focus of care, and are cradled by the crescent. The patient and family are also influenced by culture and customs within the ethical situation, and there may be conflicts between cultural and religious requirements. The nurses' professional values and personal belief systems are placed outside the core as the religious and cultural perspectives are more central to the worldview of Muslim nurses (Lovering, 2008).

Reflective Activity 4.2

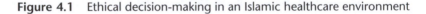

The following case study highlights the ethical dilemmas faced by nurses in a paediatric intensive care setting when caring for a Muslim child and family, in the decision to donate the child's organs. The interaction of spiritual, cultural, professional and personal values in ethical decision-making is highlighted, as are the different ethical perspectives of Muslim and non-Muslim nurses.

Case Study

A six-year-old female child was admitted to the paediatric intensive care unit in critical condition following a house fire. The child had experienced severe smoke inhalation and burns; and a few days later the child was confirmed to be brain dead. A request for organ donation was made to the family, and after long deliberations, permission was given. The child was later taken to the operating room for removal of several organs.

When nurses are faced with an ethical situation the following questions are asked to clarify aspects of the situation:

- What are the values in Islam that guide this situation?
- What are the cultural values impacting on the situation?
- What are the perspectives of the nurse, the physician, and organisational policies?
- What are the professional values that guide this situation (such as a code of ethics)?
- What are the nurse's personal beliefs?

Comments on Reflective Activity 4.2

The Muslim nurses raised this case as it was the first time they had dealt with the ethics of organ transplantation. As noted earlier, many Muslims believe that Islam does not permit organ transplantation (Daar, 1989; Sahin, 1990). The nurse caring for this child and family explained that he did not know if organ transplantation was acceptable in Islam. Consistent with the ethical principle that the Islamic faith must be maintained in ethical decisions, the nurse first went to the hospital's religious advisors to find out if organ transplantation was permitted. He was advised that there was a religious ruling (*fatwa*) giving permission for organ transplantation.

The nurse could now feel comfortable participating in the care of the patient and supporting the family. The most important obligations for a Muslim are to preserve the faith and to protect the sanctity of life (Al-Swailem, 2006, 2007; Daar and Khitamy, 2001). The nurse could discuss transplantation with the family as it was acceptable in the religion and, in turn, he could support the family in their religious beliefs. He has also met his own obligation to preserve his faith by following the *fatwa* on organ donation. After he had met his religious obligations to himself and the family, he considered the cultural needs of the family. These cultural needs included working with the family through the key decision maker of the family (in this case the father of the child), giving time for family discussion and consultation with religious experts as well as elders in the family. After meeting the cultural needs, the organisational requirements (as guided by policy for informed consent) and professional aspects were considered in planning for the eventual organ removal.

While assured there was a *fatwa* permitting organ transplantation, another Muslim nurse felt ethical discomfort with the decision for the child to be an organ donor. He explained that Muslims believe the body must be whole when meeting God on the Day of Judgement, and removing organs from the body meant violation of the sanctity of the body. He believed it was his religious and ethical obligation to protect the child's body from mutilation. In his view, there were conflicting ethical principles and obligations within his faith in caring for the child and family. However, an Islamic bio-ethics expert explained that the Islamic principles (as expressed through the *fatwa*) take precedence, and that organ transplantation did not constitute mutilation of the body as it was giving life to another, thereby meeting the obligation to preserve life and accrue benefit.

A non-Muslim nurse who professed a strong Christian belief also cared for the child and family during the decision to support organ donation. From her perspective, there were no ethical dilemmas, as organ donation was consistent within her professional and personal belief system. Her priorities for care included meeting the cultural and psychological needs of the family and the physical needs of the child. Placing the organ donation decision within the Islamic belief system for the family was not part of her caring action; however, she expressed a spiritual aspect to her caring from her Christian belief system (to provide care, as God would want her to be caring).

(1) What are the values in Islam that guide this situation?

In analysing this case study, many of the elements of Islamic bio-ethics are present. The two primary principles of maintaining the faith (ensuring that transplantation was permissible), the sanctity of life and the accrual of benefit (transplantation was to save the lives of others) guided the Muslim nurses' actions. The principle of beneficence (promoting the good) and the call to virtue (doing right in the sight of Allah) apply as well. In contrast, the non-Muslim nurse did not experience ethical conflict in her caring as the Islamic spiritual aspect (is organ donation permissible?) was not a factor. While she cared from her own sense of spirituality, the understanding of the importance of meeting the family's spiritual dimension in relation to organ donation did not inform her caring action or ethical decision-making.

(2) What are the cultural values that have an impact on the situation?

The primary cultural needs of this family related to support for the family decision-making process consistent with Muslim values. For most Muslims, there are specific roles for family members, and the family functions as part of an extended family unit. The father's role in the family is to be the key decision-maker. The mother's role is to provide caring support to the child and the rest of the family members. Within the extended family, the elder family members are consulted on all major decisions impacting on the family (Zahr and Hattar-Pollara, 1998). For Muslims, visiting the sick is an important cultural, social and religious obligation (Halligan, 2006; Lawrence and Rozmus, 2001; Rashidi and Rajaram, 2001; Wehbe-Alamah, 2008). The nurses' actions needed to include permitting extended family members to visit the child in the intensive care unit, as well as providing an area where family members could receive visitors and provide support during the difficult decision-making time.

(3) What are the perspectives of the nurse, the physician and organisational policies?

In this case, there were conflicting values for the Muslim nurses taking care of the child, while the non-Muslim nurse did not experience ethical conflict. The physicians caring for the child were also Muslim, so also needed to confirm that organ donation was acceptable from the religious point of view. The organisational policies primarily concerned ensuring informed consent for the organ donation.

(4) What are the professional values that guide this situation (such as a code of ethics)?

The national or international code of ethics would guide the professional values. From an Islamic perspective, it is stated in the Noble Qur'aan that:

☐   *If anyone has saved a life, it would be as if he has saved the life of the whole of mankind.* (Al-Mā'idah [The Table Spread] 5:32)

In the context of the Middle Eastern countries, the GCC code would be applicable. The GCC code specifies the following primary values to guide ethical caring by nurses: accountability, dignity, privacy and confidentiality. The GCC code defines dignity as 'a fundamental value of nursing practice. The nurse strives to promote, protect and advocate the dignity and self-respect of those patients/clients who are vulnerable and incapable of protecting their own interests' (GCC Health Minister's Council, 2001, p. 7). Within the behavioural directive of dignity, the nurse must 'Help and support patients/clients to enable them to live with as much physical, emotional and spiritual comfort as possible and maximize the values they treasure in life' (2001, p. 7). While not guiding the nurses on the specific cultural and spiritual requirements (such as the application of the Islamic principles requiring them to maintain the faith and preserve the sanctity of life), nevertheless the nurse is directed to place the psychosocial and spiritual needs of the patient and family at the centre of nursing care.

(5) What are the nurse's personal beliefs?

For Muslim nurses, spiritual and cultural values are inseparable within their caring practices (Lovering, 2008). As illustrated by the Muslim nurse who experienced ethical conflict over his obligation to preserve the body of the child upon death (during removal of the organs), there is inseparability of personal view, religious interpretation (which principle has greater priority) and professional obligations. Through reflection on this case study, the integration of Islamic ethical beliefs into Muslim nurses' caring is apparent. Muslim nurses must maintain their faith in all caring actions, and use Islamic teachings to guide their moral decision-making and ethical action. The beginning point for ethical decisions is determination of the Islamic principles that apply, followed by the cultural perspective. On many occasions, it is difficult to separate religious from cultural needs as Islam and most Muslim cultural practices are often inseparable (Lovering, 2008) and religious expert advice may be needed.

Conclusion

Religion determines moral belief systems, personal and professional values that guide all nurses' ethical reasoning. Nursing ethics based on the Western belief system focus on the value of autonomy (Elliott, 2001). In contrast, Muslim nurses are guided by the primary principles of preserving their faith and protecting the sanctity of life (Al-Swailem, 2006; Daar and Khitamy, 2001; Rassool, 2000). Islamic and Western bio-ethical systems consider the actions and outcomes of ethical decision-making and share the principles of doing good (beneficence); avoiding harm (non-malfeasance); and fairness and equity (justice). Spiritual, cultural and professional values intertwine to guide Muslim nurses' ethical caring in their daily work. The ethical framework used by Muslim nurses has not been adapted from a universal set of principles or principles modified for the cultural context. These insights support the ethical relativist view that ethical principles are culturally bound and context dependent.

References

Al-Qattan, S.M. (1992) 'Islamic jurisprudential judgment on human organ transplantation', *Saudi Medical Journal* 13, 6, 483–7.

Al-Swailem, A. (2006) *Bio-ethics from the Islamic Point of View*. Bio-ethics and Regulatory Aspects of Bio-medical Workshop (Jeddah, Saudi Arabia).

Al-Swailem, A. (2007) *Nursing and Nurses' Ethical Issues from Islamic Perspectives*. Building Bridges to the Future, 2nd International Nursing Conference (Jeddah, Saudi Arabia).

Al-Swailem, A. and Lovering, S. (2007) *Ethical Perspectives at the Bedside*. Building Bridges to the Future, 2nd International Nursing Conference (Jeddah, Saudi Arabia).

Aramesh, K. and Shadi, H. (2007) 'Euthanasia: an Islamic Medical Perspective', *Iran J Allergy Asthma Immunol* 6 (Suppl. 5), 35–8.

Christakis, N. (1992) 'Ethics are Local: Engaging Cross-cultural Variations in the Ethics for Clinical Research', *Social Science & Medicine* 35, 9, 1070–91.

Daar, A.S. (1989) 'Ethical Issues: a Middle East Perspective', *Transplantation Proceedings* 21, 1, 1402–4.

Daar, A.S. and Khitamy, A. (2001) 'Bio-ethics for Clinicians: 21. Islamic Bio-ethics', *Canadian Medical Association Journal* 164, 1, 60–3.

Elliott, A.C. (2001) 'Health Care Ethics: Cultural Relativity of Autonomy', *Journal of Transcultural Nursing* 12, 4, 326–30.

Gardiner, P.A. (2003) 'Virtue Ethics Approach to Moral Dilemmas in Medicine', *Journal of Medical Ethics* 29, 297–302.

Gatrad, A.R. and Sheikh, A. (2001) 'Medical Ethics and Islam: Principles and Practice', *Archives of Disease in Childhood* 84, 1, 72–5.

Gebara, J. and Tashjian, H. (2006) 'End-of-Life Practices at a Lebanese Hospital: Courage or Knowledge?' *Journal of Transcultural Nursing* 17, 4, 3818.

Ghaly, M. (2012) 'Religio-ethical Discussions on Organ Donation among Muslims in Europe: an Example of Transnational Islamic Bioethics', *Medical Health Care Philosophy* (May) 15, 2, 207–20.

Gulf Cooperation Council (GCC) Health Minister's Council (2001) *Executive Board Code of Professional Conduct for Nursing. 2001.* www.qatar.ucalgary.ca/files/GCC%20code%20of%20professional%20conduct%20for%20nursing%20-%202001.pdf, date accessed 22 July 2013.

Halligan, P. (2006) 'Caring for Patients of Islamic Denomination: Critical Care Nurses' Experiences in Saudi Arabia', *Journal of Clinical Nursing* 15, 12, 1565–73.

Hanson, H. (2008) 'Principles of Islamic Bioethics', in A. Sheikh and A.R. Gastrad (eds), *Caring for Muslim Patients*, 2nd edn (Oxford: Radcliffe Medical Publishing), pp. 45–53.

Harper, M. (2006) 'Ethical Multiculturalism: an Evolutionary Concept Analysis', *Advances in Nursing Science* 29, 2, 110–24.

Hedayat, K. and Pirzadeh, R. (2001) 'Issues in Islamic Biomedical Ethics: a Primer for the Pediatrician', *Pediatrics* 180, 4, 965–71.

Hook, K. and White, G. (2003) *Code of Ethics for Nurses with Interpretive Statements: An Independent Study Module*, www.nursingworld.org/mods/mod580/code.pdf?q=code-of-ethics-code-of-ethics, date accessed 25 July 2013.

Ketefian, S. (2001) 'Ethical Concerns in International Nursing Research', *International Journal of Nursing Practice* 6, 8, 354.

Ketefian, S. (2008) 'Ethical Concerns in International Nursing Research', *International Journal of Nursing Practice* 6, 6, 354.

Lawrence, P. and Rozmus, C. (2001) 'Culturally Sensitive Care of the Muslim Patient', *Journal of Transcultural Nursing* 12, 3, 228–33.

Leininger, M. (1991) *Culture Care Diversity and Universality: A Theory of Nursing* (New York: National League for Nursing Press).

Lovering, S. (2008) *Arab Muslim Nurses' Experiences of the Meaning of Caring* (Professional Doctorate) (Sydney, Australia: University of Sydney), http://hdl.handle.net/2123/3764, date accessed 15 July 2013.

Mill, J.E and Ogilvie, L.D. (2002) 'Ethical Decision Making in International Nursing Research', *Qualitative Health Research* 2, 6, 807–15.

Moawad, D. (2006) *Nursing Code of Ethics: An Islamic Perspective*, www.cis.psu.ac.th/fathoni/cis/nursing.html, date accessed 4 April 2013.

Mylott, L. (2005) 'The Ethical Dimension of the Nurses' Role in Practice', *Journal of Hospice & Palliative Nursing* 7, 2, 113–18.

Olsen, D., Arend, Drought, T., Eby, M., Fasting, U., Gastmans, C. et al. (2003) 'Ethical Considerations in International Nursing Research: a Report from the International Centre for Nursing Ethics', *Nursing Ethics* 10, 2, 122–37.

Pacquiao, D. (2003) 'Cultural Competence in Ethical Decision-making', in M. Andrews and J. Boyle (eds), *Transcultural Concepts in Nursing Care*, 4th edn (Philadelphia, PA: Lippincott Williams & Williams), pp. 503–32.

Rashidi, A. and Rajaram, S. (2001) 'Culture Care Conflicts among Asian-Islamic Immigrant Women in US Hospitals', *Holistic Nursing Practice* 16, 1, 55–64.

Rassool, G. Hussein (2000) 'The Crescent and Islam: Healing, Nursing and the Spiritual Dimension. Some Considerations towards an Understanding of the Islamic Perspectives on Caring', *Journal of Advanced Nursing* 32, 6, 1476–84.

Rassool, G. Hussein (2004) 'Commentary: An Islamic Perspective', *Journal of Advanced Nursing* 46, 3, 281.

Ray, M. (2010) 'Transcultural Caring Ethics', in M. Ray (ed.), *Transcultural Caring Dynamics in Nursing and Health Care* (Philadelphia, PA: F.A. Davis), pp. 62–92.

Rispler-Chaim, V. (1989) 'Islamic Medical Ethics in the 20th Century', *Journal of Medical Ethics* 15, 203–8.

Sachedina, A. (2005) 'End-of-life: the Islamic View', *Lancet* 366, 774–9.

Sahin, A.F. (1990) 'Islamic Transplantation Ethics', *Transplantation Proceedings* 22, 3, 939.

Sanjari, M., Zahedi, F. and Larijani, B. (2008) 'Ethical Codes of Nursing and the Practical Necessity in Iran', *Iranian Journal of Public Health* 37, 1 (Suppl.), 22–7.

Taft, S. (2000) 'An Inclusive Look at the Domain of Ethics and its Application to Administrative Behavior', *Online Journal of Issues in Nursing* 6, 1, http://cms.nursingworld.org/MainMenuCategories/ANAMarketplace/ ANAPeriodicals/OJIN/TableofContents/Volume62001/No1Jan01/Article PreviousTopic/DomainofEthics.aspx, date accessed 25 July 2013.

Tschudin, V. (2005) 'Cultural and Historical Perspectives on Nursing and Ethics: Listening to Each Other – Report of the Conference in Taipei, Taiwan, 19 May 2005, organised by ICNE and Nursing Ethics', *Nursing Ethics*, 13, 3, 304–22.

Wehbe-Alamah, H. (2008) 'Bridging Generic and Professional Care Practices for Muslim Patients through Use of Leininger's Culture Care Models', *Contemporary Nurse* 28, 1–2, 83–97.

Zahr, L. and Hattar-Pollara, M. (1998) 'Nursing Care of Arab Children: Consideration of Cultural Factors', *Journal of Pediatric Nursing* 13, 6, 349–55.

5 Understanding the Muslim Family System

G. Hussein Rassool and C. Sange

Learning Outcomes:

- Discuss the role of the family in the care of the Muslim patient.
- Examine the practices and values that a Muslim family shares.
- Discuss the objectives of modesty and privacy in relation to Muslim patients.
- Discuss the issues of contraception and abortion for Muslim women.
- Discuss the bases of care for the Muslim elders.

Reflective Activity 5.1

State whether the following statements are true or false. Give reasons for your answers.

	True	False
1 The family is the fundamental component within Muslim culture that determines acts and behaviours.		
2 Islam gives a specific age for marriage, either for the husband or for the wife.		
3 Marriages are financial contracts which bring rights and obligations to both parties.		
4 Whether the family live together with their children or with the extended family or separately, parents are usually consulted in all decision-making processes.		

	True	False
5 Muslim men are encouraged to grow their beards long and trim the moustache.		
6 Plural marriage is not permissible in Islam.		
7 The value of modesty is regarded as a must in Islam by both sexes.		
8 The right of females to seek knowledge is different from that of males.		
9 According to the Qur'aan, men and women are equal and should be treated as such.		
10 Islam allows men and women to meet each other for 'free mixing'.		
11 Most Muslim authorities permit contraception for the purpose of preserving the mother's health and the well-being of the family through spacing of births.		
12 After the third stage, and after four months have passed, it is not permissible to abort a pregnancy.		
13 It is not permissible for a mother with HIV/AIDS to take care of and breastfeed her healthy child.		
14 It is permissible for elderly women or women past childbearing to uncover their faces.		
15 Muslim children who have reached puberty are not obligated to fast during Ramadan.		
16 A child's guardian is responsible for decision-making regarding medical or psychological treatment.		

Introduction

Nurses who have a basic understanding of the Muslim family system can motivate other nurses to adopt culturally acceptable behaviours, strengthen nurse–patient relationships and optimise therapeutic outcomes. In this chapter, we will examine the concept of the Muslim family, the practices and values that each Muslim family shares. In addition, the roles of Muslim men, women and children will also be examined in relation to the Islamic texts and the orientalist view.

The Muslim family

There have been remarkable changes in family structures and dynamics in Western Europe and North America in the twentieth century. The extended family, the backbone of society, has now been replaced by the nuclear family. Generally, Islam's family system is still based on the extended family structure. A harmonious social order is created by the existence of extended families, which determines acts and behaviours and brings the rights of the husband, wife, children, and relatives into a fine equilibrium. The stability of the extended Muslim family is greatly valued, and it is seen as essential for the spiritual growth of its members. It is stated that 'The piety of a family is dependent on the piety of individual members of the family, and the piety of a community is likewise dependent on the piety of the families who make up the community' (Ath-Thubaytie).

In the UK, British Muslims are characterised by more traditional family patterns than other faith groups (Hussain, 2008). For Muslims, the traditional patterns include higher proportions living in extended or three-generation households, early marriage for girls, giving birth at a younger age than other groups and conceiving and giving birth within marriage. In Muslim families of Asian origin (Indo-Pakistan subcontinent), couples usually continue to live with their parents after they have started a family of their own (Anwar, 1994). An extended structure offers many advantages, including stability, coherence, and physical and psychological support, particularly in times of need (Dhami and Sheikh, 2000). However, the pattern of the family is changing in Muslim communities. Many second-generation Muslim migrants have grown up in nuclear families, not having first-hand familiarity with the richness and complexity of living within extended family networks (Dhami and Sheikh, 2000). It has been suggested that the individual freedom offered by a nuclear family structure far outweighs any benefits of living in an extended family for some younger Muslims (Anwar, 1994).

Islam's family system brings the rights of the husband, wife, children, and relatives into a fine equilibrium as the decrees of family living are clearly stated in the Qur'aan. Whether the family live together with their children or with the extended family or separately, parents are usually consulted in all decision-making processes. It has been stated that all actions, decisions and judgements ought to be family orientated and culturally derived (Halligan, 2006). Despite the many pressures it faces, the Muslim family institution remains strong. The structure and organisation of family relationships are based on the husband–wife relationship and parent–children relationship. The husband–wife relationship is based on sacrifice, love, loyalty, and obedience. This is well documented in the Qur'aan, and the following verse depicts the right Islamic tone (interpretation of the meaning):

☐ *And among his signs is this: He created for you spouses from yourselves that you might find rest in them, and He ordained between you love and mercy.* (Ar-Rūm [The Romans] 30:21)

The Prophet Muhammad also stressed these meanings when he said: 'The best of you is he who is best to his family, and I am the best among you to my family' (Tirmidhî [a]). Islamic traditions also prescribe a much stronger participation of the family in the contracting and preservation of marriages.

Marriage is considered a solemn and sacred contract with God. Islam does not give a specific age for marriage, either for the husband or for the wife. The Qur'aan clearly indicates that marriage is a sharing between the two halves of society, and that its objectives, besides perpetuating human life, are emotional well-being and spiritual harmony. Sheikh Ibn Baaz said in Majmoo' al-Fataawa (20/421): 'What is required is to hasten to get married, and no young man or young woman should delay marriage for the sake of studies, because marriage does not prevent any such thing. It is possible for a young man to get married in order to protect his religious commitment and morals, and enable him to lower his gaze. Marriage serves many purposes, especially in this day and age.' Allah says in the Qur'aan (interpretation of the meaning):

☐ *They (your wives) are your garment and you are a garment for them.* (Al-Baqara [The Cow] 2:187)

This verse of the Qur'aan reveals the basic purpose and concept of marriage in Islam. The verse has been explained as follows: 'Just as a garment hides our nakedness, so do husband and wife, secure each other's chastity. The garment gives comfort to the body; so does the husband find comfort in his wife's company. The garment is the grace, the beauty, the embellishment of the body, so too are wives to their husbands as their husbands are to them' (Rahman). Indeed, spouses are like garments to each other because they provide one another with protection, comfort, support, and the adornment that garments provide to humans (Sheikh Adhami).

The importance attached to marriage and family life in Islam is reflected in the many Islamic decrees and laws aimed at protecting the institution of the family. In the United Kingdom (UK), a Muslim couple should have an Islamic (religious) wedding and a civil ceremony needed for the marriage to be recognised under British law. A growing number of young Muslims in the UK are entering marriages that are not legally recognised (BBC Asian Network, 2010). However, Muslims who marry without legal registration are putting their womenfolk at some risk, and their children are not legitimate in the eyes of the law of the particular country. In the United States, it is possible to obtain a civil marriage before a local civil authority, such as a mayor, judge, deputy marriage commissioner or other public official, conducted in the town hall or local courthouse. As part of such ceremonies, a religious official such as an *Imam* may be given the authority to conduct the marriage by the state, thus unifying the religious with the civil ceremony. In most European countries there is a civil ceremony requirement. Following the civil marriage ceremony, couples are free to marry in a religious ceremony. In many countries in the Middle East, Africa, the Indian Sub-continent and the Far East, marriages are conducted by religious authorities, and are registered by civil authorities.

The male Muslim

During hospitalisation, for a male Muslim patient, there is an overriding objective of modesty and privacy. They may prefer having a male to assist in more 'personal care'. Some Muslim men will often wear a head covering in the form of a brimless cap. Muslim men are encouraged to grow their beards long and trim their moustache. The definition of the beard (*al-lahyah*) as stated by the scholars of the (Arabic) language is the hair of the face, jawbone and cheeks, in the sense that everything that grows on the cheeks, jawbone and chin is part of the beard (Sheikh Ibn 'Uthaymin, p. 36). Muslim men may be reluctant to shave their beards before an operation. Like any other patient, their permission must be obtained to shave any part of the beard. For a male Muslim, the dress code is to cover the region between the waist and knees, which must be covered at all times. A Muslim man may be reluctant to expose this area even to a male member of staff. A hospital gown that securely covers this area will help male Muslim patients feel more at ease.

Muslim men are permitted to have up to four wives and this permission is given by God. Allah says in the Qur'aan (interpretation of the meaning):

☐ *And if you fear that you shall not be able to deal justly with the orphan-girls then marry (other) women of your choice, two or three, or four; but if you fear that you shall not be able to deal justly (with them), then only one or (the slaves) that your right hands possess. That is nearer to prevent you from doing injustice.* (Al-Nisa' [The Women] 4:3)

This Qur'aanic text above shows that plural marriage is allowed. According to Islamic jurisprudence (*shari'ah*), a man is permitted to marry one, two, three or four wives, in the sense that he may have this number of wives at one time. It is not permissible for him to have more than four. There is consensus among Muslims on this point, with no differing opinions (Sheikh Muhammed Salih Al-Munajjid, Fatwa 14022). It should be noted that there are conditions attached to plural marriage. (For a discussion on the wisdom behind permitting plural marriage, see http://islamqa.info/en/ref/14022/.) All wives must be treated equally. Prophet Muhammad said: 'Among the Muslims the most perfect, as regards his faith, is the one whose character is excellent, and the best among you are those who treat their wives well' (Tirmidhî [b]).

The female Muslim

The status of women in Islam has been the subject of much controversy as Islam is often misunderstood by people who believe that it degrades and oppresses women. This misperception is based on prejudice and ignorance. Cultural practices within the Muslim communities have articulated this belief, although the Qur'aan clearly states otherwise. Chapter 4 of the Qur'aan is dedicated specifically to women in Islam and provides clear evidence that women are equal to men in the sight of Allah in terms of their rights and responsibilities. Allah says in the Qur'aan (interpretation of the meaning):

☐   *Never will I allow to be lost the work of any of you, be he male or female.* (Āli'Imrān [The Family of Imran] 3:195)

The Prophet rejected all stigma attached to a woman by virtue of her gender, and willed, in his last sermon, that women be treated with respect and kindness. Islam gives women equal rights: the automatic right to inheritance, the right to own businesses, the right to choose a husband, the right to divorce, the right to take paid employment, the right to education (Barlas, 2002) and many other rights that might surprise non-Muslims. Allah says in the Qur'aan (interpretation of the meaning):

☐   *And they (women) have rights (over their husbands as regards living expenses, etc.) similar (to those of their husbands) over them (as regards obedience and respect, etc.) to what is reasonable, but men have a degree (of responsibility) over them.* (Al-Baqara [The Cow] 2:228)

The statement 'men have a degree (of responsibility) over them', has caused many orientalists and others to consider women to have no, or limited, human rights or say in any activities. This notion refers to the natural ability and differences in the two sexes but it does not imply any form of superiority or inferiority. According to Abdul-Ati, 'the rights and responsibilities of a woman are equal to those of a man but they are not necessarily identical with them. Equality and sameness are two quite different things. This difference is understandable because man and woman are not identical but they are created equals.' She added that 'Islam has given woman rights and privileges, which she has never enjoyed under other religious or constitutional systems.' Thus, Islam elevated the position of woman in society and in some cases, as a mother for instance, clearly gave her precedence over man. Women as mothers are regarded graciously in Islam. When the Prophet Muhammad was asked: 'Who is most entitled to be treated with the best companionship by me?' the Prophet replied, 'Your mother.' The man asked, 'Who is next?' The Prophet said, 'Your mother.' Again the man asked, 'Who is next?' The Prophet repeated, 'Your mother.' The man asked for a fourth time, 'Who is next?' The Prophet then replied, 'Your father' (Bukhari [a]). That is why Islam made paradise under the feet of mothers. In terms of religious obligations, such as the daily prayers, fasting, poor-due, and pilgrimage, woman is no different from man. In some cases indeed, woman has certain advantages over man. For example, the woman is exempted from the daily prayers and from fasting during her menstrual periods and up to forty days after childbirth. She is also exempted from fasting during her pregnancy and when she is nursing her baby if there is any threat to her health or her baby's. If the missed fasting is obligatory (during the month of Ramadan), she can make up for the missed days whenever she can. She does not have to make up for the prayers missed for any of the above reasons. Although women could and did go into the mosque during the days of the Prophet, thereafter attendance at the Friday congregational prayers has been optional for them while it is mandatory for men (Badawi, 1998).

Women in Islam are equal to men in the pursuit of education and knowledge. Prophet Muhammad said: 'Seeking knowledge is mandatory for every Muslim' (Al-Bayhaqi and Ibn-Majah). In this context, Muslims include both males and females. A woman has the right to seek employment in Islam as long as the sanctity of the family remains intact and a women's honour is not compromised (Al-Musnad, 1996, p. 313). It is permissible for a woman to go out of her house for work, but that is subject to certain conditions. Some of the conditions include: there should be no mixing with non-*mahram* men (anyone who a Muslim is not allowed to marry is *mahram*); whilst at work she should observe complete *jilbāb* (which refers to any long and loose-fitting coat or garment); her work should not lead to her travelling without a *mahram*; and her going out to work should not involve committing any *haram* action, or wearing perfume where non-*mahrams* can smell it (Sheikh Muhammed Salih Al-Munajjid, Fatwas 106815; 6742). However, her role in society as a mother and a wife is regarded as the most sacred and essential. According to Islamic law, woman's right to her money, real estate, or other properties is fully acknowledged (Badawi, 1998).

The media have also placed great emphasis on Muslim women and the 'hijab'. The hijab is another important aspect of the life of Muslim women.

There are two types of hijab: external, which refers to clothes, and internal, which refers to attitudes and behaviour (Khattab, 2001). Two such obligations for women's dress codes are: Islamic dress consists of the covering of the whole head and body, including the face and hands. The clothes should be thick enough to conceal the colour of the woman's skin and the shape of the body (Khattab, 2001, pp. 15–19). In relation to dress code, Allah says in the Qur'aan (interpretation of the meaning):

☐ *And tell the believing women to lower their gaze (from looking at forbidden things), and protect their private parts (from illegal sexual acts) and not to show off their adornment except only that which is apparent (like both eyes for necessity to see the way, or outer palms of hands or one eye or dress like veil, gloves, head-cover, apron, etc.), and to draw their veils all over Juyubihinna (i.e. their bodies, faces, necks and bosoms) and not to reveal their adornment except to their husbands, or their fathers, or their husband's father, or their sons, or their husband's sons, or their brothers or their brother's sons, or their sister's sons, or their (Muslim) women (i.e. their sisters in Islam), or the (female) slaves whom their right hands possess, or old male servants who lack vigour, or small children who have no sense of feminine sex. And let them not stamp their feet so as to reveal what they hide of their adornment. And all of you beg Allah to forgive you all, O believers, that you may be successful. (An-Nūr [The Light] 24:31)*

Another piece of evidence from the Qur'aan is Verse 59 of Al-'Aĥzāb (The Combined Forces) (33:59) (interpretation of the meaning).

☐ *Prophet, tell your wives and your daughters and the women of the believers to bring down over themselves [part] of their outer garments. That is more suitable that they will be known and not be abused.*

There is a unanimous agreement (*ijma*, consensus) among all Islamic scholars on the obligation that the dress code for women in Islamic societies is the covering of the whole body including the face and hands. The tradition of the Islamic mode of clothing has been continued in today's Western society, and is considered to impart a sense of belonging and identity. However, it should be pointed out that not all Muslim women follow this dress code and wear the hijab.

Modesty in Islam is regarded as freedom from vanity and showiness, which includes language, dress and attitude (Ramji, 2007). The importance of modesty is stated by the Messenger of Allah in an authentic tradition: 'Verily for every religion there is a characteristic, and the characteristic of Islam is

Haya`a (modesty, shyness, bashfulness)' (Ibn Majah 4171/2). That is, modesty, shyness and bashfulness all constitute woman's attire (Khattab, 2001, p. 18). Whether a Muslim woman wears a hijab or not she should still strive to adopt Islamic behaviours and etiquette. In relation to men and women mixing freely, it is also absolutely clear from the texts that Islam does not allow men and women to meet each other, or 'free mixing'. There is evidence in the Qur'aan about the prohibition of mixing, and intermingling, of men and women in one place (Al-'Aḥzāb [The Combined Forces] 33:53). Islam has, according to Sheikh Sami al-Majid (2010), placed clear regulations and restrictions upon such behaviour and has defined the limits of interaction between men and women. These acts are prohibited because they are among the causes for *fitnah* (temptation or trial, which implies evil consequences), the arousing of desires, and the committing of indecency and wrongdoing (Sheikh Muhammed Salih Al-Munajjid, Fatwa 1200).

Touch is another act which is strictly prohibited with members of the opposite sex, even shaking hands (Al-Musnad, 1996, p. 373). It is not permissible for a man who believes in Allah and His Messenger to put his hand in the hand of a woman who is not permissible for him or who is not one of his *mahrams*. Whoever does that has wronged himself (for example, sinned) (islamqa, Fatwa 21183). In Anglophone countries, the 'hand-shake' is a sign of politeness and is used to greet somebody, which cannot be avoided unless contact with the outside world is avoided all together. In casual non-business situations, men are more likely to shake hands than women. These ideas are especially challenging for Muslims born outside the Islamic countries.

Women: Contraception and abortion

Contraception

One of the major purposes of marriage in Muslim and other religions is procreation. The question that arises is, then, should procreation be unlimited or should it be controlled according to the couple's needs and economic abilities? The institution of marriage and the desire to have children was the custom of the best of creation, the Prophets and Messengers chosen by Allah. Allah says about them (interpretation of the meaning):

☐ *And We have already sent messengers before you and assigned to them wives and descendants.* (Ar-Ra`d [The Thunder] 13:38)

These Prophets and Messengers are the people whom Muslims should look to emulate. Allah says (interpretation of the meaning):

☐ *Those are the ones whom Allah has guided, so from their guidance take an example.* (Al-'An`ām [The Cattle] 6:90)

The best example for the believers is the example of the Prophet Muhammad, who married and had children. The Prophet made this clear when he told those companions who were considering ascetic forms of life: 'I fast and break my fast, I do sleep and I also marry women. So he who does not follow my tradition in religion, is not from me (not one of my followers)' (Bukhari [b]). The Prophet not only encouraged marriage but he encouraged marrying those women who are capable of child-bearing. He stated: 'marry the loving, child-bearing women for I shall have the largest numbers among the prophets on the day of Resurrection' (Ahmad and ibn Hibban). Islam, being strongly pro-family, regards children as a gift from God. Allah says in the Qur'aan (interpretation of the meaning):

☐ *And one of [God's] signs is that He has created for you mates from yourselves, that you may dwell in tranquillity with them, and has ordained between you Love and Mercy.* (Al-Rum [The Romans] 30:21)

Allah says (interpretation of the meaning):

☐ *And God has made for you mates from yourselves and made for you out of them, children and grandchildren.* (Al-Nahl [The Bee] 16:72)

Teachings regarding contraception are to be understood within the context of marriage since sexual intercourse outside of marriage is forbidden (*haram*). The Qur'aan does not refer directly to contraception but some scholars refer to verses in the Qur'aan related to infanticide as the basis for banning contraception. Allah says in the Qur'aan (interpretation of the meaning):

☐ *And do not kill your children for fear of poverty. We provide for them and for you. Indeed, their killing is ever a great sin.* (Al-Isrā' [The Night Journey] 17:31; Al-'An`ām [The Cattle] 6:151)

Thus, there have been multiple opinions from Muslim scholars regarding the levels of preventing a pregnancy from occurring. Some believe that it is equal to infanticide (an extreme view), while others approve some of the natural methods of birth control such as breastfeeding, since the Qur'aan encourages women to nurse their children (interpretation of the meaning):

☐ *Mothers may breastfeed their children two complete years for whoever wishes to complete the nursing [period].* (Al-Baqara [The Cow] 2:233)

Still others approve any contraceptive method as long as it is not of a permanent nature. In practice, most Muslim authorities permit contraception for the purpose of preserving the mother's health and the well-being of the family through spacing of births. Contraceptive methods that disrupt the natural hormonal or menstrual cycle of a woman in order to prevent pregnancy and that are temporary and are agreed to by the husband are generally acceptable by the majority of Muslim scholars (Roudi-Fahimi, 2004). Such methods include the calendar method, Combined Oral Contraceptives (the Pill), injections to produce temporary sterility, patches, cervical caps, condoms and intrauterine devices.

Contraceptive methods are also acceptable if they do not have a permanent effect such as sterilisation including vasectomy (when the *Vas deferens* of a man are cut and tied to prevent the passage of sperm from the testicles to the semen) and hysterectomy (surgical removal of the uterus). Thus, it is forbidden to 'permanently' end a man's or a woman's ability to produce children, such as by having a hysterectomy or vasectomy, unless it is called for by circumstances of necessity according to the Islamic framework. However, it is permissible to control the timing of births with the intent of distancing the occurrences of pregnancy or to delay it for a specific amount of time, if there is some need (*shari'ah*) for that, in the opinion of the spouses, based on mutual consultation and agreement between them (Zarabozo). There are conditions attached to the control of timing of births as it has to be done by means that are approved in the *Shari'ah* and it must not do anything to oppose a current and existing pregnancy.

One of the methods of birth control used during the time of the Messenger of Allah was called *al-Azel*, that is, *coitus interruptus*, 'when a man withdraws his penis from the vagina prior to ejaculation to prevent insemination of the ovum'. Some scholars point out that it should not be practised without the approval of the woman since it deprives her of sexual fulfilment and the right to have children if she desires (Maguire, 2003). These requirements indicate the need for mutual sexual fulfilment as well as consultative decision-making between the married couple regarding family planning (Shaikh, 2003).

Abortion

Islam's approach to the issue of birth control and abortion is very balanced. In principle, although the Qur'aan does not explicitly mention abortion, Allah condemns the killing of humans except in the case of defence or as capital punishment. However, Islam allows women to prevent pregnancy but forbids them to terminate it. 'Aborting pregnancy is not permissible, whether the soul has been breathed into the foetus or not, but after the soul has been breathed into it, the prohibition is more emphatic. If the soul has been breathed into this foetus and it has begun to move, then the mother aborted it after that and it died, then the mother is regarded as having killed a soul, so the mother must offer expiation. That applies if it was four months old, because in that case the soul had been breathed into it but if the mother has an abortion after that, then she must offer expiation' (Sheikh Salaah al-Fawzaan Al-Muntaqa, 5:301–2). There is a ruling on aborting a pregnancy in the early stages. The Council of Senior Scholars (Al-Fataawa al-Jaami'ah, 3:1056) issued the following statement:

> It is not permissible to abort a pregnancy at any stage unless there is a legitimate reason, and within very precise limits. If the pregnancy is in the first stage, which is a period of forty days, and aborting it serves a legitimate purpose or will ward off harm, then it is permissible to abort it. But aborting it at this stage for fear of the difficulty of raising children or of being unable to bear the costs of maintaining and educating them, or for fear for their future or because the couple feel that they have enough children – this is not permissible. It is not permissible to abort a pregnancy when it is an 'alaqah (clot) or mudghah (chewed lump of flesh) (which are the second and third periods of forty days each) until a trustworthy medical committee has decided that continuing the pregnancy poses a threat to the mother's wellbeing, in that there is the fear that she will die if the pregnancy continues. It is permissible to abort it once all means of warding off that danger have been exhausted. After the third stage, and after four months have passed, it is not permissible to abort the pregnancy unless a group of trustworthy medical specialists decide that keeping the foetus in his mother's womb will cause her death, and that should only be done after all means of keeping the foetus alive have been exhausted. A concession is made allowing abortion in this case so as to ward off the greater of two evils and to serve the greater of two interests.

The *Shar'iah* allows abortion only when doctors declare with reasonable certainty that the continuation of pregnancy will endanger the woman's life. This permission is based on the principle of the lesser of the two evils, known in Islamic legal terminology as the principle of *al-ahamm wa 'l-muhimm* (the more important and the less important). In this case, abortion is permitted to save a life (Syed).

However, the situation is quite different when it comes to a woman who has had sexual intercourse outside of marriage (*Zina*) and has become pregnant. If abortion of a pregnancy resulting from a proper marriage is forbidden (*haram*) under normal circumstances, then it is even more so in cases where the pregnancy results from immorality, because permitting abortion of pregnancy which results from immorality would encourage evil actions and the spread of immorality. But

> it is permissible to resort to aborting the foetus of a woman who has committed this evil action but now wants to repent sincerely, and is very afraid. This is a major principle of shari'ah, and is subject to the condition that this be done as early in the pregnancy as possible, and that this fatwa be given only in individual cases and not be treated as a general fatwa, lest this concession becomes a means of encouraging evil in the Muslim society. And Allah knows best. (Umar ibn Muhammad ibn Ibraaheem Ghaanim, Fatwa 13331)

With regard to the ruling on aborting a child whose mother has HIV/AIDS, this is not permissible (Islamqa, Fatwa 4038). This is because HIV is not usually transmitted by a mother to the foetus until the later stages of pregnancy – after the soul has been breathed into the child – or during delivery, thus it is not permissible according to *shari'ah* for her to abort the foetus. It is, however, permissible for a mother with HIV/AIDS to take care of her healthy child and breastfeed him. Current medical knowledge indicates that there is no definite risk to the child from a mother who has HIV/AIDS. So, from the point of view of *shari'ah*, there is no reason why the mother should not take care of her child and breastfeed him, so long as there is no medical report to state that she should not do so.

The Muslim elders

There can be no doubt that Islam has given the elderly a special status, as there are texts which urge Muslims to respect and honour them. Family elders are looked upon as heads of the family, and are respected for their accounts of their life experiences. Caring for one's parents is considered an honour and a blessing. When Muslim parents reach old age, they are treated mercifully, with kindness and selflessness. In Islam, serving one's parents is a duty second only to prayer, and it is their right to expect it. This belief is also emphasised in the Qur'aan (interpretation of the meaning):

> □ *And your Lord has decreed that you worship none but Him. And that you be dutiful to your parents. If one of them or both of them attain old age in your life, say not to them a word of disrespect, nor shout at them but address them in terms of honour. And lower unto them the wing of submission and humility through mercy, and say: 'My Lord! Bestow on them Your Mercy as they did bring me up when I was small.'* (Al-Isrā' [The Night Journey] 17:23–4)

The Prophet said, 'He is not of us who does not have mercy on young children, nor honour the elderly' (Tirmidhî [c]). Ahmed (2010) suggested that we need to recognise the status of the elderly and give them due respect. He added that 'when walking with them, walk slightly behind, to their right. Let them enter and exit first. If you meet them, greet them properly and respectfully. If you discuss something with them, let them speak first, and listen to them attentively and graciously. If the conversation involves debate, you should remain polite, calm, and kind-hearted and you should lower your voice. Never forget to remain respectful.'

In an authentic saying, the Prophet said: 'If a young man honours an elderly on account of his age, Allah appoints someone to honour him in his old age' (Tirmidhî [d]). Being dutiful to one's parents is one of the greatest obligations and duties. Sheikh 'Abd-Allah ibn Baaz stated that 'Allah has commanded us to treat our parents well, and He has linked this to the command to worship Him and the prohibition of associating anything in worship with Him.' Allah says (interpretation of the meaning):

☐ *Do not worship except Allah; and to parents do good.* (Al-Baqarah [The Cow] 2:83)

And one of the deeds loved by Allah, according to the Prophet, is: 'To be good and dutiful to one's parents' (Bukhari and Muslim). Respecting the elderly and honouring them are characteristics of Muslim society. The Prophet said: 'Part of glorifying Allah is honouring the grey-haired Muslim' (Abu Dawud). In Islam, the care of the elderly is based on a number of focal points, including the following (islamqa, Fatwa 33680): 'Man is an honoured creature and has an honourable status in Islam [al-Isra' 17:70]; Muslim society is the society of mutual compassion and coherence [al-Fath 48:29]; the Muslim society is a society of cooperation and mutual support; the elderly person has a high status before Allah if he adheres to the laws of Allah. The Prophet said: The one who lives a long life and does good deeds' (Tirmidhî [e]). The ways in which Muslim society takes care of the elderly are: enjoining good treatment of parents and enjoining honouring one's parents' friends even after the parents have passed away, and regarding that as part of honouring one's parents (islamqa, Fatwa 33680). It is permissible for an elderly woman or for women past childbearing to uncover their faces before non-*mahram* men, but it is better and safer for them to observe hijab (Islam Q&A, islamqa, Fatwah 111940). Caring for the elderly is part of the family's function and many Muslims, despite all the difficulties and constraints, are reluctant even to consider placing an aging family member in a residential home for the elderly. The following case study illustrates the traditional model of a full-time stay-at-home caregiver for the Muslim elderly.

Case Study

A 61-year-old elderly Somali man was taken to the Accident and Emergency Department after collapsing in the local supermarket. He was diagnosed as suffering from a stroke. He regained consciousness after a couple of days but had paralysis of the right face and arm, loss of sensitivity to touch on the skin of the right face and arm, and inability to answer questions but ability to respond to what was said to him. After suffering multiple strokes he was bed-bound and all his basic needs had to be met by the nurse. The family did not want him to be transferred to the local rehabilitation centre for the elderly and said they would prefer to look after him at home with support from the community and social services. He was able to be cared for at home and looked after by his extended family.

Muslim children

There is a dearth of literature on Muslim children as patients. One of the most indisputable rights of the child in Islam is a right to life and equal chances in life. No discrimination of any kind is permitted as children have the right to be treated equally vis-à-vis their siblings. Parents are essentially responsible for the moral, ethical, and basic and essential religious teaching of their children. This means that children should be given sound and adequate religious, ethical and moral guidance to last them for their entire life. They should be imbued with true values, the meaning of right and wrong, true and false, correct and incorrect, appropriate and inappropriate, and so forth and so on (Sheikh Al-Uthaymin, *The Rights of Children in Islam*). It is a religious injunction that children have the right to be fed, clothed, and protected until they reach adulthood; they must have respect, and be able to enjoy love and affection from their parents. Parents have an obligation to seek medical examination and treatment for their children. A child's guardian is responsible for decision-making regarding medical or psychological treatment.

Muslim children who have reached puberty are obligated to fast during Ramadan. Prior to puberty, children are encouraged by their parents to practise fasting. Around the age of seven, children may fast a half-day or at weekends, increasing the length of the fast each year.

Circumcision is performed on all male children. The timing of this varies but it must be done before puberty.

In relation to praying, Muslim children should start performing daily prayers when they reach the age of seven years. By the age of ten, they should perform the five daily compulsory prayers. The Messenger of Allah said: 'Tell your children to pray when they are seven years old and smack them (lightly) if they do not pray when they are ten, and separate them in their beds' (Abu Dawud and Ahmad).

Adoption of children is of two types, forbidden and not forbidden. The forbidden type means adopting a child in the sense that the child is considered to be the child of the adopting parent and subject to the rulings on children (Sheikh Muhammad ibn Ibraaheem, Fatwa 10010). Allah stated in the Qur'aan that (interpretation of the meaning):

☐ *...nor has He made your adopted sons your real sons...* (Al-'Aḥzāb [The Combined Forces] 33:4)

The kind which is prescribed, according to Sheikh Muhammad ibn Ibraaheem (Fatwa 10010), means 'being kind towards the child and giving him a righteous religious upbringing and sound direction, teaching him that which will benefit him in this world and the next. But it is not permitted to hand a child over except to one who is known to be trustworthy, religiously-committed and of good character, who will take care of the child's interests.' He added that the person(s) 'should also be a local resident, so that he will not take the child away to a country where his presence may be a cause for his religious commitment being lost in the future'.

Conclusion

Islamic values give immense importance to the family, and extended family systems are encouraged, to provide extra care for the young and the elderly. In addition, the family structure is one where every individual plays a vital role, in the growth, the values, the practices and the beliefs of Islam. A stable family brings peace and security and is an essential part of the spiritual growth of the family members. Islam notes the vital role of a Muslim woman as a mother and a wife as the most sacred and essential one. Islam provides clear evidence that women are equal to men in the sight of Allah in terms of their rights and responsibilities. The implications for nurses are that they need to be fully cognisant of and sensitive to Muslims' customs and religious beliefs. Understanding the Muslim as an individual with special needs and implementing sensitive and culturally appropriate nursing care will enhance positive health outcomes.

Reflective Activity 5.2

Case Study

Maryam is 21 years old and has just had her second baby girl (Ayesha). While caring for her, you notice that her mood is low and that she is preoccupied with her thoughts. You sit and talk to her and you find out that she is concerned and worried that she may get pregnant once her periods start. Maryam is afraid to use contraceptives because her husband would like to have a large family. She tells you that her friends and relatives keeps pressuring her and tell her she should keep getting pregnant till she has a boy since men are inclined to remarry if their wife does not give them a boy.

Source: Dr Sawsam Majali, Head of Nursing Program, Dar Al Hekma College Jeddah, Saudi Arabia (personal communication). (Reproduced with permission.)

- What is the role of the nurse in this situation?
- Do you believe that Maryam has the right to use a contraceptive, but you don't want to cause her problems with her husband?
- From your readings related to Islam's position on family planning, how can you help Maryam and her husband while respecting their values and beliefs?
- What other resources can you use in helping Maryam with her concerns?
- Addressing the cultural and religious beliefs around the issue of family planning has been a big challenge for nurses and other healthcare workers. Discuss this statement in relation to the provision of health education in family planning.

References

Abdul-Ati, H. 'The Status of Woman in Islam', *Islam in focus* www.mission islam.com/discover/status_of_women.htm, date accessed 31 July 2013.

Abu Dawud, 4843, Hasan by al-Albani, in *Saheeh Abi Dawood*, 4053.

Abu Dawud (459) and Ahmad (6650), Sahih by al-Albani in *al-Irwa'* (247).

Ahmad and ibn Hibban, Sahih by al-Albani. *Irwa al Ghaleel fi Takhreej Ahadeeth Manaar al-Sabeel* (Beirut: al-Maktab al Islami, 1979), vol. 6, p. 195.

Ahmed (2010) Social Manners with the Elderly, www.haqislam.org/social-manners-with-the-elderly/, date accessed 31 July 2013.

Al-Bayhaqi and Ibn-Majah, quoted in M.S. Afifi, *Al-Mar'ah Wa Huququha Fil-Islam* (in Arabic) (Cairo: Maktabat Al-Nahdhah, Cairo, Egypt, 1988), p. 71.

Al-Musnad, M. (1996) *Selected Invocations* (Riyadh, Saudi Arabia: Dar-us-Salaam Publications).

Anwar, M. (1994) *Young Muslim's in Britain: Attitudes, Educational Needs and Policy Implication* (Leicester: Islamic Foundation).

Ath-Thubaytie, A.B. The Family in Islam, http://alminbar.com/khutbaheng/2062.htm, date accessed 1 August 2013.

Badawi, J.A. (1998) *The Status of Women in Islam* (Birmingham: Islamic Vision IPCI).

Barlas, A. (2002) *Believing Women in Islam, Unreading Patriarchal Interpretations of the Quran* (Austin, TX: University of Texas Press), pp.139–49.

BBC Asian Network (2010) *Wedding Trouble as UK Muslim Marriages not Recognised*, 3 February 2010, http://news.bbc.co.uk/2/hi/8493660.stm, date accessed 24 July 2013.

Bukhari [a] Book 8, Volume 73, Hadith 2.

Bukhari [b] Book 62, Volume 7, Hadith 1.

Bukhari and Muslim, cited in 'The Virtues of Dutifulness to Parents', http://wathakker.info/english/flyers/print/1163, date accessed 31 July 2013.

Council of Senior Scholars. *Ruling on Aborting a Pregnancy in the Early Stages.* Al-Fataawa al-Jaami'ah, 3/1056, http://islamqa.info/en/ref/42321, date accessed 31 July 2013.

Dhami, S. and Sheikh, A (2000) 'The Muslim Family: Predicament and Promise', *Western Journal of Medicine* 173, 5, 352–6.

Halligan, P. (2006) 'Caring for Patients of Islamic Denomination: Critical Care Nurses' Experiences in Saudi Arabia', *Journal of Clinical Nursing* 15, 1565–73.

Hussain, S. (2008) *Muslims on the Map: A National Survey of Social Trends in Britain* (London: I.B. Tauris Academic Studies).

Ibn Majah 4172, authenticated by Al Albānī and al Hilālī.

islamqa, Fatwa 111940. Fataawa al-Mar'ah al-Muslimah (1/424). *Is it permissible for an elderly woman to uncover her face before men who are not her mahrams?* http://islamqa.info/en/ref/111940, date accessed 31 July 2013.

islamqa, Fatwa 21183. *Shaking hands with a non-mahram woman*, http://islamqa.info/en/ref/21183, date accessed 31 July 2013.

islamqa, Fatwa 4038. *Ruling on aborting or caring for a child whose mother has AIDS*, Majma' al-Fiqh al-Islami, pp. 204–6, http://islamqa.info/en/ref/4038, date accessed 31 July 2013.

islamqa, Fatwa 33680, http://islamqa.info/en/ref/33680, date accessed 1 August 2013.

Khattab, H. (2001) *The Muslim Women's Handbook* (London: Ta-Ha Publishers).

Maguire, D.C. (2003) 'Contraception and Abortion'. Excerpt from Chapter 9, in D. Maguire (ed.), *Sacred Choices: The Case for Contraception and Abortion in World Religions* (Oxford: Oxford University Press).

Rahman A.I. Doi. *Women in the Quran and the Sunna*, http://islamtomorrow.com/women/Muslimah.htm, date accessed 26 July 2013.

Ramji, H. (2007) 'Dynamics of Religion and Gender amongst Young British Muslims', *Sociology* 41, 6, 1171–89.

Roudi-Fahimi, F. (2004) *Islam and Family Planning* (Washington DC: Population Reference Bureau).

Shaikh, S. (2003) 'Family Planning, Contraception and Abortion in Islam: Undertaking Khilafah: Moral Agency, Justice and Compassion', in D. Maguire (ed.), *Sacred Choices: The Case for Contraception and Abortion in World Religions* (Oxford: Oxford University Press).

Sheikh Abdullah Adhami. *To the Prospective Muslim Husband: What is a Wife?* Madrasa In'aamiyyah, www.qiran.com/marriage/a_wife.asp, date accessed 26 July 2013.

Sheikh Al-Uthaymin. *The Rights of Children in Islam*, www.missionislam.com/family/childrensrights.htm, date accessed 31 July 2013.

Sheikh Ibn Baaz, Majmoo' al-Fataawa (20/421), cited in http://islamqa.com/en/ref/82968, date accessed 1 August 2013.

Sheikh Muhammad ibn Ibraaheem. From Fatawa Samaahat, Fatwa 10010, http://islamqa.info/en/ref/10010/adoption, date accessed 31 July 2013.

Sheikh Muhammed Salih Al-Munajjid, Fatwa 14022, *The ruling on plural marriage and the wisdom behind it*, http://islamqa.info/en/ref/14022/muslim%20men%20and%204%20wives, date accessed 31 July 2013.

Sheikh Muhammed Salih Al-Munajjid, Fatwa 1200, *Evidence Prohibiting of Mixing of Men and Women*, http://islamqa.info/en/ref/1200, date accessed 31 July 2013.

Sheikh Muhammed Salih Al-Munajjid, Fatwas 106815; 6742, www.islamqa.com/en/ref/106815, date accessed on 31 July 2013.

Sheikh Saalih al-Fawzaan Al-Muntaqa (5/301, 302), http://islamqa.info/en/ref/82334, date accessed 31 July 2013.

Sheikh Sami al-Majid (2010) *Prohibition of Free-Mixing Between Men and Women; 2001*, www.islamcan.com/youth/prohibition-of-free-mixing-between-men-and-women.shtml, date accessed 31 July 2013.

Sheikh Ibn 'Uthaymin, Fataawa Hammah, p. 36. *What is the definition of the beard according to sharee'ah?* http://islamqa.info/en/ref/12740/moustache, date accessed 31 July 2013.

Syed, I.B. *Abortion*. Islamic Research Foundation International, www.irfi.org/articles/articles_101_150/abortion.htm, date accessed 31 July 2013.

Tirmidhî [a], Hadith 3252. Narrated by Aisha; Abdullah ibn Abbas.

Tirmidhî [b], Hadith 628. Narrated by Abu Hurayrah.

Tirmidhî [c], http://1000gooddeeds.com/2009/09/01/good-deed-12-have-mercy-on-children/, date accessed 31 July 2013.

Tirmidhî [d], Hasan by Al-Albani. Cited in www.onislam.net/english/shariah/muhammad/manners/442090-the-prophets-mercy-towards-the-elderly.html.

Tirmidhî [e], 2329, Sahih by al-Albani in *Saheeh al-Tirmidhî*, 1899.

Umar ibn Muhammad ibn Ibraaheem Ghaanim, Ahkaam al-Janeen fi'l-Fiqh al-Islami. Fatwa 13331, http://islamqa.info/en/ref/13331, date accessed 31 July 2013.

Zarabozo, J. *Family Planning Allowed in Islam?* http://islamic-world.net/sister/h8.htm, date accessed 31 July 2013.

6 Health Behaviours in Islam

G. Hussein Rassool and C. Sange

Learning Outcomes:

- Discuss the role of personal hygiene in the life of a Muslim patient.
- Discuss the practical aspects of looking after Muslim patients in relation to issues of hygiene, purification, and medications.
- Discuss briefly the etiquette of eating a nutritional and balanced food.
- Identify some of food that is permissible and non-permissible for the Muslim patient.
- Discuss the nursing implications in caring for Muslim patients with special dietary needs.

Reflective Activity 6.1

State whether the following statement are true or false. Give reasons for your answers.

	True	False
1 In Islam, cleanliness is 'half of faith'.		
2 Islamic law does not regulate lifestyle and behaviours that are hazardous to health, and does not prescribe behaviours.		
3 Islam places great emphasis on hygiene, in both physical and spiritual terms.		
4 Purification is not obligatory in Islam prior to worship.		

	True	False
5 Muslims must wash with water after urination or defecation.		
6 Toilets should be equipped with a small water container to assist with washing.		
7 A beaker of water should be made available to a bed-bound Muslim patient whenever they use a bedpan.		
8 Islam has no rules about the types of food that are prohibited (*haram*) for Muslims.		
9 Muslims follow dietary requirements that may affect compliance with prescriptions.		
10 In case of dire necessity, *haram* (forbidden) food and beverages are not allowed.		
11 During the initial assessment before admission, the nurse should determine the extent to which the patient follows *halal* requirements.		
12 Gelatine from an animal source that is not *halal* is acceptable.		
13 The main prohibited foods are pork and its by-products, alcohol, animal fats, and meat that has not been slaughtered according to Islamic rites.		
14 There are some foods which are usually *halal* that may contain ingredients and additives that can make them *haram*.		
15 For the majority of Muslims, eating *halal* beef is forbidden.		
16 Islam also forbids cooking, eating or drinking from any pans, dishes, cups or table utensils that have been used to prepare food containing pork or alcohol. They cannot be used to prepare or serve food for Muslims until they have been thoroughly washed.		

Introduction

Health behaviour is the most fundamental component of Islamic principles and practice. It is the actions undertaken by an individual for the purpose of attaining, maintaining and preventing ill health. Some common health behaviours include exercising regularly, eating a balanced diet, and personal hygiene. In the Western world, a lot of emphasis is now focused on a healthy lifestyle with the potential to obtain better physical and psychological health. Islam places great emphasis on both physical and spiritual health, and Muslims are encouraged to maintain a balanced diet, and remain active and healthy. In this chapter, the focus will be on aspects of nutrition, personal hygiene and exercise in relation to religious principles derived from the Qur'aan and the teachings of the Prophet Muhammad and their implications for nursing care and interventions.

Personal hygiene

A simple definition of personal hygiene is regular bathing, regular washing of hands, a clean and tidy appearance and clothes, care of the feet, nails and teeth, covering the mouth when coughing or sneezing – basically, to maintain a high standard of personal care. Personal hygiene considered through the Islamic viewpoint is a fundamental part of faith (*Imaan*). It has been stated that 'the soul can reside only in a clean body, by maintaining the outer cleanliness, one can obtain inner purity' (*Shams*). Though cleanliness is regarded as a pleasing attribute, Islam insists on it 'as cleanliness is half of faith' (Muslim). Cleanliness is so important in Islam that it is written in the Qur'aan itself (interpretation of the meaning):

> ☐ *Truly, Allah loves those who turn unto Him in repentance and loves those who purify themselves (by taking a bath and cleaning and washing thoroughly their private parts, bodies, for their prayers, etc.).* (Al Baqarah [The Cow] 2:222)

The traditions of Prophet Muhammad include advice about actions that are part of a natural way to maintain personal hygiene. Five practices are characteristics of the *Fitra* (natural disposition of a human): circumcision (for men); shaving the pubic hair; cutting the moustache short; clipping the nails; and depilating the hair of the armpits (Bukhari). Hence, it becomes imperative for any Muslim to maintain a high level of cleanliness, as neither prayer nor the worship of Allah is acceptable without purification.

Purification is obligatory in Islam prior to worship. Muslims are required to wash the exposed body parts five times a day. Although this is an act of purification, it also suggests the importance of safeguarding oneself from infectious diseases and bacteria. While this act of purification is a set routine that Muslims will follow, the Western emphasis is now also placed on maintaining a high standard of personal hygiene, to provide safe and effective health care, for example, the reduction of infections in hospital settings, through the correct technique of hand washing. The act of purification for a Muslim consists of many stages, which we will consider in more depth. Purification can be any cleansing act, whereas ablution (*wudu*) is the act of cleansing oneself prior to performing prayers or worship, which consists of washing the exposed body parts. 'Exposed parts' in this instance refers, for example, to the hands, face, mouth, nose, ears, head, arms and feet. Now let us consider the importance of washing these body parts both within an Islamic framework and from a medical perspective.

The Hands: not washing your hands is the commonest means to transfer bacteria from person to person. The hands are the part of the body with which we touch, feel, reach out etc. There is considerable emphasis in healthcare institutions upon the correct hand hygiene for patients, medical staff and visitors, as this is one of the best ways to avoid spreading infections. The correct method of hand washing for the purpose of ablution requires the performer to wash both hands, including the back of the hand and in between the fingers, up to each wrist.

The Mouth and Nose: this is the ideal location for micro-organisms to multiply as the environment of the mouth is dark, wet and warm. The mouth, if not cared for properly, can become home to many bacteria, viruses, fungi and protozoa. Most bacteria are harmless; however, mouth bacteria are responsible for some of the most common mouth diseases. The use of a tooth-stick (*siwak*) is recommended. In particular, a *siwak* is to be used while rinsing the mouth with water during ablution, in order to ensure the cleanliness of the mouth and to be ready for worship and prayers (Sheikh Al-Fawzan, 2009). Gargling water in the mouth is also part of ablution and can only be beneficial as it can help reduce the likelihood of harmful bacteria multiplying.

The Face is the first feature another person will see. Washing the face appears to be the simplest of tasks; however, failing to cleanse thoroughly can promote skin infections and acne. Cleansing the face allows old surface skin cells, dirt and dust, grime, make-up and bacteria to be removed, and can keep the skin pores free from clogging. Cleansing the face also aids circulation. In preparation for prayers the Muslim will wash the face from the top of the forehead to the bottom of the chin, from one ear to the other, and make sure the whole face surface is washed with fresh running water.

The Arms: Muslims will wash both arms from the tips of the fingers to above the elbows. This ensures sweat and sebaceous gland secretion near the hair glands are removed. Deposits of sweat can clog the pores and cause infections, or even acne, on the arms. Although this appears especially in warmer months, it is not common.

The Head: likewise, the head is an ideal place for the body to produce sweat and where dust particles can reside, causing skin allergies and infections.

The Ears: caring for the ears is a very important part of personal hygiene. Maintaining hygiene of the ears on a regular basis or while a Muslim is performing ablution involves cleansing the outer ear. It is not advisable to place any foreign body, for example, cotton buds, further into the ear as this can cause damage.

The Feet contain many sweat glands that produce fluid, which either lies on the skin or is absorbed into the materials around it, such as socks or shoes. Throughout the day the feet are contained within shoes; the bacteria in the fluid are left to multiply and create odours, conditions which promote fungal and bacterial growth. Such conditions can cause dryness, redness, and blisters, itching and peeling. To prevent such symptoms developing or progressing further, the feet must be kept clean and dry. When ablution is performed relating to cleansing the feet, the performer will wash both feet up to the ankles, including the soles of the feet and between the toes. This procedure is beneficial for maintaining the hygiene of the feet.

This is the last stage of ablution. Ablution is performed five times a day at a minimum, prior to performing prayers (*Salaat*). Taking the act of ablution into consideration, we can appreciate that these practices are tried and tested for the prevention of illness. These procedures are now becoming universal and many health organisations have made this a priority. While people generally consider cleanliness a desirable attribute, Islam insists on it, making it an indispensable and fundamental part of faith – and taking it much beyond the superficial concept of personal hygiene.

Purification

In Islam, cleanliness and purification are not only requirements for the performance of worship, or when embracing Islam, but are part of a Muslim's faith. The act of purification prior to performing prayers is mandatory; there are three broad categories of purification:

1 Purification from impurity.
2 Cleansing one's body, dress or place from an impurity of filth.
3 Removing the dirt or grime from body parts.

The importance of purification has been discussed above; the second most important act of purification is a ritual bath (*ghusal*). The ritual bath is required of every Muslim after sexual intercourse, after wet dreams, after post-partum bleeding, and each month after the menstruation. Before a ritual bath is performed one must make known the intention (*niyyat*) to cleanse oneself from impurities. However, there are compulsory acts involved in the ritual bath that must be completed by all Muslims:

- Make known the intention to cleanse oneself
- Rinse the mouth
- Rinse the nostrils, and
- Completely wet the entire body.

Physical cleanliness, as stated previously, relates also to environmental cleanliness, which includes, water, house, clothes, and public places. Muslims are required to keep their homes clean and free from clutter and impurities. Environmental cleanliness is as vital as personal physical cleanliness. The third type of cleanliness is spiritual cleanliness. Spiritual cleanliness means being free from polytheism, hypocrisy, ill manners, love of wealth, love of fame and other carnal desires. Spiritual cleanliness is cleansing of the heart, the mind and the soul, which is the ultimate goal of Islam. To achieve spiritual cleanliness a Muslim undertakes fasting during the month of Ramadan, by giving charity (*zakat*) and ultimately through regular remembrance of God (Allah).

The rules governing balanced nutrition

In Islam, there are health promoting regulations which include: moderate eating, abstinence from alcohol and tobacco consumption and other psychoactive substances, regular exercise (idleness is prohibited for Muslims), prayers, fasting, ablution and bathing, breastfeeding and many other injunctions (El-Kadi, 1993). A healthy balanced diet is a matter of faith in Islam as it allows Muslims to contemplate the relationship of the mind, the soul and the body. For this reason, Islam has prohibited some foods (*haram*) and beverages, due to their ill effects. Allah says in the Qur'aan (interpretation of meaning):

☐ *He has only forbidden to you dead animals, blood, the flesh of swine, and that which has been dedicated to other than Allah. But whoever is forced [by necessity], neither desiring [it] nor transgressing [its limit] – then indeed, Allah is Forgiving and Merciful. (An-Nahl [The Bee] 16:115)*

The above verse states the foods that Muslims are strictly forbidden to consume. According to the Islamic (*shari'ah*) law, 'in cases of necessity, *haram* foods are permitted' to a limit. This means that a Muslim cannot consume any noted *haram* food or beverages under any circumstances, except in cases of necessity. By necessity, one is referring to cases of starvation, when there are no other forms of food. This is only in cases where the follower has had no food or drink for a number of days. This all depends upon the individual ability and capacity to remain hungry or thirsty for a period of time. Intoxicants such as illegal drugs and consuming alcohol are also strongly forbidden in Islam (see Chapters 13, 14), as they are listed as harmful to health. A list of the permissible and non-permissible food is presented in Table 6.1.

Table 6.1   Guide to permissible (*halal*) and non-permissible (*haram*) food

APPROVED (HALAL)	FORBIDDEN (HARAM)
Meat, fish and substitutes	
Chicken, beef, lamb killed according to Islamic ritual.	Pork and all pork products (bacon, ham salami).
	Animals that died through an accident or disease, or that were not slaughtered in the name of Allah.
	Carnivorous animals and birds of prey.
	Blood and blood by-products (blood puddings).
Fish and other seafood	
Eggs (cooked in water, butter, vegetable margarine or vegetable oil).	Canned beans, peas and lentils containing pork.
Dried beans, peas and lentils.	Meat and meat alternative dishes prepared with alcohol, pork products or animal shortening.
Pizza prepared without *haram* foods and ingredients.	
Soups made without pork, ham or animal fats.	Any soup made with pork, ham or animal fats.
Fats and oils	
Butter, vegetable margarine, vegetable oils, olive oil, peanut oil, mayonnaise, and some salad dressings.	Lard, dripping, suet, other animal fats (except butter), and any other foods made with or cooked in them.

(*Continued*)

Table 6.1 Continued

APPROVED (HALAL)	FORBIDDEN (HARAM)

Grain and grain products

Rice, Pasta, wheat, oats, cornmeal, barley or any other cereal grain.
Any grain product, such as bread, breakfast cereal, cakes, and biscuits or baked goods, prepared without *haram* ingredients.

Any grain products prepared with *haram* ingredients such as alcohol, animal shortening, lard, or pure and artificial vanilla extract (prepared with alcohol).

Fruit and vegetables

All fruit or vegetables that are raw, dried, frozen or canned.
Vegetables and fruit cooked or served with water, butter, or vegetable oils.
All juices.

Any vegetables and fruit prepared with alcohol, animal shortening, bacon, gelatine, lard, or some margarines which contain monoglycerides or diglycerides from an animal source.

Milk or milk products

Milk, yoghurt, cheese, sherbet, and ice cream made without animal fat, gelatine or microbial enzymes such as microbial rennet.

Cheese, yoghurt, ice cream, frozen tofu desserts made with animal rennet, gelatine, lipase, pepsin, pure or artificial vanilla extract or whey (whey is *haram* if prepared with non-microbial enzymes).

Beverages

Tea, coffee, water, fruit juices, soft drinks, carbonated drinks, mineral and soda water, cordials (fruit-flavoured drinks).

Alcoholic beverages: beer, wine, cider, liqueur. Cordials with alcohol or liqueur.
Alcohol and foods cooked with alcohol, e.g. trifles, puddings, sauces.

Desserts

Any without alcohol, lard, dripping or suet, or gelatine, e.g. fruit-based desserts, sherbets, custards or puddings made with butter or vegetable margarine; egg dishes; rice dishes.

Any with alcohol, lard, suet and dripping, or gelatine; ice cream with animal fat.

(Continued)

Table 6.1 Continued

APPROVED (HALAL)	FORBIDDEN (HARAM)
Miscellaneous	
Coconut milk, spices, chilli, curry powder.	Gelatine (pork product), vanilla essence (alcohol base).
Pickles, chutneys. Sweeteners: honey, sugar, syrup, chocolate liquor (roasted ground cocoa bean syrup)	Chocolates, sweets or candies made with alcohol or pure or artificial vanilla extract. Sweeteners: chocolate liqueur (made with alcohol.
Additives	
	E120 Cochineal: A red colour obtained from female insects. This additive is always *haram* because the consumption of blood and insects is forbidden.
	E422 Glycerol / Glycerin / Glycerine: *Haram* if obtained from pork or non-*halal* meat sources.
	E441 Gelatin / Gelatine: Derived from the bones and/or hides of cattle and/or pigs or non-*halal* meat sources. Gelatine-containing food products, multivitamins and fish oils are not *halal* unless they contain fish gelatine. A vegetarian alternative is available.
	E470 to E483 Emulsifiers: *Haram* if obtained from pork or non-*halal* sources.
	E542 Edible Bone Phosphate: An extract from animal bones. *Haram* if obtained from pork or non-*halal* meat sources.
	E904 Shellac (Glazing agents): *Halal* if it is not treated with alcohol.

Allah in the Qur'aan, in addition to the verse quoted above, said (interpretation of meaning):

■ *O mankind, eat from whatever is on earth [that is] lawful and good.* (Al-Baqarah [The Cow] 2:168)

- *It is Allah who made for you the grazing animals upon which you ride, and some of them you eat.* (Ghāfir [The Forgiver] 40:79)
- *Lawful to you is game from the sea and its food as provision for you.* (Al-Mā'idah [The Table Spread] 5:96)
- *So eat of that [meat] upon which the name of Allah has been mentioned, if you are believers in His verses.* (Al-'An`ām [The Cattle] 6:118)
- *We give pure milk, palatable to drinkers.* (An-Nahl [The Bee] 16:66)
- *And He it is who causes gardens to grow, [both] trellised and untrellised, and palm trees and crops of different [kinds of] food and olives and pomegranates, similar and dissimilar.* (Al-'An`ām [The Cattle] 6:141)
- *And the earth He laid [out] for the creatures. Therein is fruit and palm trees having sheaths [of dates]. And grain having husks and scented plants.* (Ar-Raḥmān [The Beneficent] 55:10–13)

The Qur'aan and Hadiths not only both provide recommendation on forbidden foods and beverages but also advise on how to maintain a healthy, well balanced diet. Religious ethics encourage the believer to eat in moderation, not to overeat or to starve the body of nourishment. We may deduce from the above verses from the Noble Qur'aan that these recommended foods will certainly fulfil the daily protein, carbohydrate, fat and vitamin requirements. Foods that are high in protein, as well as fruit and vegetables are encouraged by both the Hadiths and the Qur'aan. The prohibitions not only include harmful categories of food but also recommend limiting one's intake of food, in a moderate manner, to maintain health. It has been recommended in the Qur'aan by Allah (interpretation of the meaning):

- *And be not excessive. Indeed, He does not like those who commit excess.* (Al-'An`ām [The Cattle] 6:141)
- *Eat of the good things ... We have provided for your sustenance, but commit no excess therein.* (Ta-ha [Ta-ha] 20:81)

Besides, there are numerous spiritual benefits of a restricted diet, such as achieving humility of the heart, strengthening of understanding, weakening of base desires, lessening of personal opinions and anger, while overeating induces the opposites of all of those (Islamicweb).

Washing of hands prior to preparing food and eating is also a recommendation. There are general rules that many Muslims across the world follow when consuming food. It is obligatory to mention the name of Allah, The Almighty, before eating by saying *'Bismillah'* (in the name of Allah) when starting to eat. It is obligatory for the Muslim to eat with his right hand; he should not eat with his left hand. The Prophet stated that: 'No one among you should eat with his left hand, or drink with it, for the devil (*Shaytaan*) eats with his left hand and drinks with it' (Muslim). This implies that eating with the left hand is not permissible (*haram*). However, this is applicable so long as there is no valid excuse; if a patient cannot eat or drink with his right hand, due to sickness or injury, then there is nothing wrong with his eating with his left hand. Eating slowly is recommended for health. Slow eating reduces the consumption of food, as it postpones much of the meal to a time when the absorption of nutrients begins to produce physiological signals of satiety. Slow eating helps in chewing the food well. Thus, there are fewer incidences of heartburn and similar ailments and discomfort (Islamicweb). Hence, when caring for a Muslim patient it is important to understand why certain acts are carried out, and why compliance or non-compliance with treatment may occur.

Exercising and physical activity

Physical health is as important as spiritual health in Islam. Undertaking the five daily prayers is in itself a form of exercise, with its gentle prescribed movements, which target the muscles and joints. Obesity, a poor diet and lack of exercise are all discouraged in Islam. Although exercise and physical activity are encouraged, it should not transgress Islamic rulings. Attending gyms or classes that incorporate both sexes is forbidden, and wearing clothing that exposes parts of the body or that is tight fitting should also be avoided. Exercise, like diet, should be within moderation; it should not delay or hinder family time or religious observances. Muslims are encouraged through the teachings of the Prophet Muhammad to put aside some time daily or weekly to maintain their physical health, and to encourage competition in sports involving physical exercise and discipline.

Nursing implications

Nurses or healthcare professionals providing care for the Muslim patient should have an awareness of the patient's needs and customs, whether that is related to a religious aspect of care or whether it is a cultural belief. People of all ages, race, religion, creed, nationality, or gender all have personal beliefs that are vital to who they are, and if not fulfilled can hinder their health outcomes. For example, *haram* or 'forbidden', for the Muslim patient, does not only refer to food products but also to other products that may contain ingredients that are also forbidden. It is stated by the the scholars of the Standing Committee that 'if a Muslim is certain or thinks it most likely that meat, fat or ground bones of a pig have got into any food, medicine or toothpaste etc., then it is not permissible for him to eat it, drink it or use it. In the case of doubt, then he should not use it, because the Prophet said: "Leave that which makes you doubt for that which does not make you doubt"' (Sheikh 'Abd al-'Azeez ibn Baaz et al., Fataawa al-Lajnah al-Daa'imah 22/281).

Many prescribed medications and over-the-counter drugs contain pork products or alcohol in their ingredients. Medications for use in the treatment of the sick are permissible, but it is unlawful (*haram*) to use prohibited products based on alcohol or pork. Islamic rulings also need to be considered in the context of prescribing decisions involving Muslims (Sattar et al., 2004). In emergencies, this rule does not apply if an alternate drug is not available, but this should be explained to the patient. If the medication is absolutely necessary, then Islam permits its use. For a comprehensive account of medications derived from pigs and their clinical alternatives, see 'An Introductory Guide for Patients and Carers' from /www.mcb.org.uk/uploads/PBEnglish.pdf.

A practical way of ensuring that health professionals have sufficient information about treatment options available would be for the British National Formulary (BNF) or other alternative to clearly indicate which preparations contain blood, animal, and alcohol derivatives, and, where possible, suggest suitable alternatives (Gatrad et al., 2005).

Conclusion

The teaching and principles of Islam are designed to benefit all of humankind. Rules and recommendations for personal hygiene, nutrition, and exercise promote the well-being of individuals and communities. Infection control is inherent in Islamic hygiene behaviour, similar to eating in moderation, and maintaining an active life through exercise. Caring for Muslim patients means that considerations are given to elements of gender, dress code, personal care, dietary requirements, family planning, 'rites de passage' from birth to death, prayers, fasting and spiritual development. A holistic assessment of a patient includes both cultural and religious beliefs. When prescribing medications, a level of awareness of the parent's religious sensitiveness need to be considered. Understanding the Muslim patient is an essential aspect in the provision of holistic care (physical, psychological, social, and spiritual).

Caring for Muslim patients involves meeting the needs of the patients in the context of their own culture and beliefs. Religious practices that may seem insignificant to some healthcare providers can make a major difference in how patients perceive health care or whether they choose to avoid care (Steefel, 2005). Therefore, a Muslim patient will have hope that Allah will provide a cure for him. It has been stated that 'Certainty and despair both remove one from the religion, but the path of truth for the people is that a person must fear and be conscious of Allah's reckoning as well as be hopeful of Allah's mercy' (Imam Abu Ja'far al-Tahawi). Muslim individuals, families, professionals, *Imams*, local communities and organisations need, through engagement of the health service providers and other stakeholders, to highlight the health issues of Muslim communities. Above all, in a multicultural society, we need to recognise diversity and provide optimal care to our patients regardless of race, ethnicity, religion, sex, or national origin.

Reflective Activity 6.2

Case Study 1

Mrs Ayesha Jamaal Khan, a 60-year-old Muslim, was admitted to the local general hospital for a swallowing disorder (dysphagia) following a stroke. After assessment, the dietician prescribed a clear liquid diet and the nurse offers the patient a choice of several jellies. However, the patient refuses the jelly, even though she stated earlier that she was hungry.

- What are the immediate health care needs of Mrs Khan?
- If Mrs Khan speaks little English, how would you communicate with her?
- Mrs Khan refused to eat the jelly. Why?
- What would be an alternative substitution for Mrs Khan?
- If Mrs Khan insists that she would like to eat home food, what would be your response?

Case Study 2

Abdul Gaffur, a 56-year-old man with a history of type 2 diabetes, was admitted through the Accident and Emergency (A&E) department with pneumonia. He was transferred to a medical unit. During nursing assessment, Mr Abdul Gaffur's son, who was concerned about his father's diet, informed the nurse that Muslims don't eat pork. During mealtime, Mr Abdul Gaffur was served chicken, potatoes and vegetables. He refused to accept the food on the ground that it was not *halal* food.

- What are the immediate healthcare needs of Mr Gaffur?
- Why did Mr Gaffur refuse to accept the meal served?
- What would be an alternative substitution for Mr Gaffur?
- Even when a suitable food substitute (*halal* food) was served, he refused to take it on the ground that it was mixed with pork or horse products. How would you respond to this situation?

Case Study 3

Safiyya, a 21-year-old devout Muslim, was admitted to an orthopaedic ward following an accident. During mealtime, she always reminded the nurse that she would only eat *halal* food or a Muslim meal. However, on one occasion, she was provided with non-*halal* food. She refused the food and asked the nurse to remove the offending items of food from her plate. She completely refused the offer. Subsequently, she refused to eat hospital food.

- What are the immediate healthcare needs of Safiyya?
- How you would meet her spiritual needs?
- Safiyya refused to eat hospital food. Why?
- How would you respond in this situation?

Comments on Case Study 1

Swallowing disorders, in which patients experience difficulty with swallowing, can lead to a variety of problems from malnutrition to difficulty speaking. Muslims will reject this type of food as it is not considered *halal*. Therefore, the dietician should understand this cultural reason for avoiding such food items and offer alternatives. Gelatine is made from pig bones. Gelatine is used in the preparation of baked goods, ice cream, yogurt, jellies, and gelatine Jell-O. The use of gelatine is only acceptable in Islam if derived from a vegetarian or *halal* source.

Comments on Case Study 2

It is very common for nurses and other healthcare professionals to perceive "not eating pork" as being the only food restriction for a Muslim diet. Chicken, lamb and other meat products are often believed to be OK (*halal*) because they are not pork. This is a misconception. All foods are considered *halal* except the following (which are *haram*):

- Swine/Pork and its by-products
- Animals improperly slaughtered or that died through an accident or disease
- Alcoholic drinks and intoxicants
- Carnivorous animals, birds of prey and certain other animals
- Foods contaminated with any of the above products

A vegetarian option is the least that ought to be on offer to patients and staff who are Muslim or belong to other ethnic groups if a specific meal is not available for them.

Comments on Case study 3

It is common in hospitals (or airlines) for the nurse to remove the non-*halal* item from the plate. Muslims would refuse to eat food that is *halal* served on the same plate as non-*halal* food. An example of poor practice in this context would be placing meat and vegetarian foods on the same serving platter, or using alcohol in the cooking or preparation of food without clear labelling of such. The transfer of serving utensils from one bowl or dish to another is also not acceptable. Those used for serving 'forbidden' food must not be used to dish out other foods, otherwise 'cultural cross-contamination' will occur. Some Muslim patients may find hospital food bland compared with their usual home diet. There is also a need to consider allowing a patient's family or friends to bring in food for them as this is often more acceptable, but before doing so, check hospital policy or the treatment regime if there are dietary restrictions.

References

Bukhari, http://islamic-dictionary.tumblr.com/page/9, date accessed 3 August 2013.

El-Kadi, A. (1993) 'Health and Healing in the Qur'an', in S. Athar (ed.), *Islamic Perspectives in Medicine. A Survey of Islamic Medicine: Achievements and Contemporary Issues* (Indianapolis: American Trust Publications), pp.117–18.

Gatrad, A.R., Mynors, G., Hunt, P. and Sheikh, A. (2005) 'Patient Choice in Medicine Taking: Religious Sensitivities must be Respected', *Archives of Disease in Childhood* 90, 9, 983–4.

Imam Abu Ja'far al-Tahawi. Aqeedah al-Tahawiyah. *The Creed of Imam Tahawi*, www.masud.co.uk/ISLAM/misc/tahawi.htm, date accessed 3 August 2013.

Islamicweb. Food for Thought: Prophet Muhammad Recommendations regarding Food, www.islamweb.net/ver2/engblue/ebooks/en/Prophet%20Muhammads%20Recommendations%20Regarding%20Food.pdf, date accessed 3 August 2013.

Muslim: Book 2, 'Al-Taharah', Number 0432.

Muslim 2020, http://islamqa.com/en/ref/6503, date accessed 3 August 2013.

Sattar, S.P., Shakeel, A.M., Majeed, F., et al. (2004) 'Inert Medication Ingredients Causing Non Adherence due to Religious Beliefs', *Annals of Pharmacotherapy* 38, 621–4.

Shams, A.M. Concept of Health and Hygiene in Islam, www.biharanjuman.org/health_islam.htm, date accessed 3 August 2013.

Sheikh 'Abd al-'Azeez ibn Baaz, Sheikh 'Abd al-Razzaaq 'Afeefi, Sheikh 'Abd-Allaah ibn Ghadyaan, and Sheikh 'Abd-Allaah ibn Qa'ood.

Fataawa al-Lajnah al-Daa'imah (22/281)., http://islamqa.info/en/ref/97541/products%20with%20alcohol, date accessed 3 August 2013.

Sheikh Al-Fawzan, S. (2009) *A Summary of Islamic Jurisprudence*, volume 1 (Riyadh, Saudi Arabia: Al-Maiman Publishing House), p. 39.

Steefel, L. (2005) 'Cultural Care Makes a Difference', *Nursing Spectrum*, 24 October, www.nursingspectrum.com, date accessed 3 August 2013.

7 Islamic Belief and Practices Affecting Health Care

G. Hussein Rassool and C. Sange

Learning Outcomes:

- Discuss the Muslim patient's view of illness and health.
- Examine the Islamic framework and prescription for good health.
- Have an awareness of the religious beliefs that affect the attitudes and behaviours of Muslim patients in hospital.
- Describe the problems and issues concerning the following: (a) medical consultation and examination; (b) privacy and mixed ward; (c) food; and (d) prayer.

Reflective Activity 7.1

State whether the following statements are true or false. Give reasons for your answers.

	True	*False*
1 There are no restrictions of any kind for the purposes of medication, treatment, preventative or health care measures for the Muslim in life threatening situations.		
2 Language, family values and norms, and religion have no significant influence on an individual's understanding of concepts such as 'health' and 'illness'.		
3 Muslims believe that cure comes solely from Allah.		
4 A Muslim believes and understands that suffering and dying are not a part of life and a test from Allah.		

	True	False
5 When ill, Muslims are encouraged to seek medical treatment.		
6 Spiritual health is considered by Muslims to be the most important aspect as compared with physical, psychological, or social well-being.		
7 The value placed on modesty and premarital virginity contributes to the reluctance of Muslim women to seek health care.		
8 Muslims believe an illness is something that is viewed in a negative sense rather than as a positive event that purifies the body.		
9 There is a conflict between seeking medical treatment and seeking help from Allah.		
10 Islamic beliefs do not affect healthcare delivery and interventions.		
11 Islam requires that Muslims seek treatment from a same gender person whenever it is possible.		
12 Muslim women may avoid direct eye contact during a conversation or assessment.		
13 The right or the left hand may be used for feeding, administering medications, or handing something to a Muslim patient.		
14 Muslim men and women are obliged to recite prayers five times each day.		
15 Touching may be acceptable between Muslim members of the opposite gender.		
16 A Muslim woman may wear the head covering (hijab or nikab) during a medical examination or while in the hospital, removing it only when necessary.		
17 Islam bans treatment or testing by a doctor, nurse, or technician of the opposite sex if it cannot be avoided.		
18 Naming conventions in some Muslim communities may differ greatly from those in Western nations.		
19 A Muslim may eat meat from the regular menu as long as it is not pork.		
20 For Muslims, regular performance of ritual obligations, prayer, and Qur'aan reading are therapeutic resources.		

Introduction

Nurses will encounter Muslim patients in a variety of healthcare settings. There are certain issues and problems which are specific to being a Muslim patient in a non-Muslim country or institution. The preservation of life overrides all the guidelines presented in this chapter. Islam allows exceptions to its rules in emergency situations but these must truly be life threatening. Under emergency and life threatening situations, there are no restrictions of any kind for the purposes of medication, treatment, preventative or healthcare measures, etc., for Muslim patients (Qur'aan, 5:3, 6:145). In this chapter, we will help the reader to understand the Muslim patient's view of illness and disease and their beliefs that may affect healthcare delivery and interventions.

Islamic framework of health

The Qur'aan considers 'Imaan', faith in Allah, as the foremost necessity for physical, spiritual and mental health development. From an Islamic perspective, health is viewed as one of the greatest blessings that God has bestowed on humankind. Indeed, the greatest blessing after belief is health. The Prophet Muhammad states: 'Ask Allah for forgiveness and health, for after being granted certainty, one is given nothing better than health' (Tirmidhî). As with the development of nursing in the Islamic tradition, Muslim physicians have also shared with other physicians in the development of the field of medicine. Abu-Bakr Mohammed Ibn-Zakaria Al-Razi, was one of the greatest Muslim physicians, who focused on three aspects of medicine, namely: public health, preventive medicine, and treatment of specific diseases. He wrote a treatise on measles and smallpox, used alcohol as an antiseptic and made medical use of mercury as a purgative. His book *Kithab al-Hawi'*, a masterpiece in clinical medicine, was one of the main textbooks in the medical school in Paris, France, especially its 9th volume on pharmacology. 'It was translated into Latin under the auspices of Charles I of Anjou by the Sicilian Jewish physician, Faraj ibn Salim (Farragut) in 1279 and was repeatedly printed from 1488 onwards. *Al-Hawi'*, was known as 'Continens' in its Latin translation. "By 1542 there had appeared five editions of this vast and costly work, besides many more of various parts of it. Its influence on European medicine was thus very considerable" ([Arnold, 1931] *The Legacy of Islam*, pp. 323–5)' (Zahoor).

Another famous physician and philosopher is Avicenna (Ibn-Sina – his full name is Abu-Ali Husayn Ibn-Abdullah Ibn-Sina). He wrote 100 treatises and a book named *Al-Qanon fi Al-Tibb* (*Canon of Medicine*, 5 volumes). The *Canon of Medicine* remained a medical authority up until early nineteenth century (Haque, 2004). It set the standards for medicine in Europe and the Islamic world. Ibn Sina created a holistic system of medicine which involved physical and psychological factors, drugs and diet.

An individual's understanding of concepts such as 'health', 'illness' or 'disease' arises from a complex interaction between personal experiences and a range of cultural factors that may include, among other things, language, family values and norms, and religion (Helman, 2001). These factors are of great significance in determining one's perception on health. In Muslim communities, where people retain a sense of the sacred, the influence of religion on shaping individual and communal views is often quite considerable (Rahman, 1998). Muslims believe that cure comes solely from Allah. Even if this is practically in the form of a health professional, it is still, ultimately, achieved through prayers and the powers of Allah. Illness and well-being are closely interconnected with Islam and every Muslim believes and understands that suffering and dying are a part of life and a test from Allah (interpretation of the meaning):

☐ *And certainly, We shall test you with something of fear, hunger, loss of wealth, lives and fruits, but give glad tidings to As-Sabirin (the patient ones, etc.).* (Al-Baqarah [The Cow] 2:155)

Illness has three possible meanings in Islam, 'a natural occurrence', 'punishment of sin', or 'a test of the believer's patience and gratitude' (Ibn Musa, 1982). Regardless of the cause, it is obligatory for the sufferer to seek treatment. There are many prophetic sayings which encourage Muslims to seek medical treatment, including: 'There is no disease that Allah has created, except that He also has created its treatment' (Bukhari [a]). The Prophet also stated that: 'Verily, Allah has not let any malady occur without providing its remedy. Therefore, seek medical treatment for your illnesses' (Nasa'i and al-Hakim). In another saying, the Prophet said: 'There is a cure for every disease. Whenever an illness is treated with its right remedy, it will, by Allah's permission, be cured' (Muslim). The health of the Muslim is very important, as the healthier the Muslim, the more they worship Allah. Health in Islam is built on a hygienic regime, which aims to create a community that is healthy and immune against disease (Al-Fangary, 2008).

Prescription for good health

Islam not only provides guidance in spiritual matters but also places considerable emphasis on health and the prevention of ill health. Ali ibn Al-Abbas, ten centuries ago, defined health as 'A state of the body in which functions are run in the normal course'. The World Health Organisation (WHO) defines health as 'A state of complete physical, mental, and social well-being and not merely the absence of disease and infirmity'. Thus, the holistic nature of health was emphasised. However, it is argued that the definition of health is utopian, inflexible, and unrealistic (Saracci, 1997), and ignores the social, political, and economic factors. Proponents of holistic health believe that the time has come to give serious consideration to the spiritual dimension and to the role it plays in health and disease. According to Al Khayat (1999), health within the Islamic framework is described as a 'state of complete physical, psychological, social and spiritual well-being'. The additional element in Al Khayat's definition is the spiritual dimension of health, which he considered to be the most important aspect. Thus, Islam as an ethical and holistic way of life, deals with the spiritual and physical aspects of an individual's life. One of the principles of Islamic health care is to prevent suffering and disease prior to any clinical symptoms. Muslims are accountable to Allah for their health (Al Khayat, 1999). This suggests that they should maintain a healthy lifestyle. The World Health Organisation (WHO, 1996), in conjunction with Islamic organisations, established health promotion strategies that are culturally sensitive to the Muslim community, with the Amman Declaration on Health Promotion (see Table 7.1). The WHO has recognised the role that spiritual well-being plays in promoting good health, in the Ottawa Charter (De Leeuw and Hussein, 1999).

From the Islamic perspective, there are three approaches in promoting health (Al Khayat, 1997; El-Kadi, 1996). The first one is the legal approach; that is, legal injunctions concerning what is permissible and what is forbidden. The second approach is identified as a guiding approach for individuals in their daily lives. The healing effect of the Qur'aan is identified as the third approach. Many Muslims may employ 'Prophetic medicine' as part of their lay system of health care based on the recommendations of the Prophet Muhammad. According to Nagamia, in the realm of health, hygiene, prevention and treatment of maladies, the Prophet employed both popular and spiritual remedies. The latter comprised recitation of verses of the Holy Qur'aan, *duahs* or prayers (*nafl* prayers) on various occasions, with successes recorded from his actions by various companions. Thus, his was a true 'holistic' approach to problems of health. He was able to set broad guidelines for the use of household remedies (like honey), the usefulness of dietary discretion, the use of herbal remedies (like the black seed or *nigella sativa*), and give valuable advice on keeping away from areas afflicted by epidemics or contagion (like the plague) (Nagamia). Some Muslims, particularly from South Asia, may practise forms of traditional Arabic or Unani (lit., 'Greek') medicine. Unani medicine, unlike modern Western medicine, is based on a humoural theory of wet/dry, hot/cold humours in the body, whose balance defines health.

Table 7.1   The Amman Declaration on Health Promotion

- First: Health is a blessing from God, which many people do not appreciate, as is mentioned in the Hadith.
- Second: Health is but one element of life, and cannot be complete unless the other major elements are provided, including: freedom, security, justice, education, work, self-sufficiency, food, water, clothing, housing, marriage and environmental health.
- Third: People can preserve their health, as enjoined in the Qur'aan, by maintaining a moderate health balance in a state of dynamic equilibrium, neither exceeding the bounds, nor falling short in that balance.
- Fourth: Every human being is in possession of a certain health potential, which they must develop in order to enjoy complete well-being and ward off disease, as is mentioned in the Hadith.
- Fifth: The lifestyles followed by human beings have a major impact on their health and well-being.
- Sixth: Islamic lifestyles embrace numerous positive patterns promoting health and rejecting any behaviour which is contradictory to health.
- Seventh: Islam, as defined in the Qur'aan, is the natural course of life which God has bestowed on humanity. Hence, adhering to Islamic lifestyles is, in itself, a realisation of the true nature of the human being, and ensures harmony with the laws of God in body and soul, in the individual, the family and community, and between human beings and their environment.
- Eighth: A list of the Islamic lifestyles derived from the Qur'aan and the Sunnah of the Prophet (PBUH), and affecting health development and human development in general. (Ablution, basic needs, behaviour, circumcision, cleanliness, disability, drug abuse, ethics, family planning, food contamination, healthy lifestyles, legislation and human rights, marriage, mental health, mother–child care, nutrition, oral hygiene, physical fitness, pollution, water work.)

Source: WHO (1996) *Health Promotion through Islamic Lifestyles: The Amman Declaration* (The Right Path to Health: Health Education Through Religion, No. 5) (Alexandria, Egypt: WHO Regional Office for the Eastern Mediterranean). (With kind permission.)

In healing, foods and herbs are also classified according to the four humours and are to re-establish proper equilibrium, forming the basis of this practice. Traditional doctors are known as *hakims*, and their practice usually includes aspects of complementary or alternative medicine such as herbal medicine, homeopathy, naturopathy, and chiropractic.

Understanding health and illness for the Muslim patient

People from different cultures often make very different attributions about health, viewed from that individual's perspective. From a religious perspective, Muslims understand recovery from any condition or deterioration as being only in the hands of God, because God meant it to be that way. It is reported that the Prophet Muhammad said that: 'A Muslim does not encounter fatigue, tiredness, concern, sorrow, injury or grief, or even a thorn which pricks him without Allah expiating his errors for him by that' (Bukhari [b]). However, seeking treatment for ill health does not conflict with seeking help from Allah.

Many Muslims do not seek help, as they believe illness can and will purify the body. For this reason many Muslims discard 'depression' as an illness, as it is seen to be related to a lack of faith (Fonte and Horton-Deutsch, 2005). Research has identified that some Muslims do not comply with medical treatments (Bashir et al., 2001; Khokhar et al., 2008). A survey of Muslim patients with glaucoma on their use of prescribed eye drops during the month of fasting (Ramadan) found that treatment compliance was significantly reduced in patients who kept the fast (American Academy of Ophthalmology, 2008). This lack of adherence to a treatment or medication regime may influence the treatment outcomes. However, religious injunctions do not allow the use of particular medications, and specify certain procedures to be undertaken. For example, Muslims will not take some medications because many modern medications contain pork extracts or alcohol, which are strictly forbidden in the Islamic religion. This issue will be examined in detail in another section of this chapter. Religious and cultural beliefs, such as the value placed on modesty and premarital virginity, contribute to a reluctance to seek health care (Matin and LeBaron, 2004). A recent study on help-seeking behaviour and urinary incontinence in Muslim women found that many women felt it was religiously forbidden to seek help; however, many were unaware of the above statement that seeking treatment for ill health does not conflict with seeking help from Allah (Sange, 2009).

Islamic beliefs affecting health care

There are a number of Islamic religious beliefs that will affect the attitudes and behaviours of Muslim patients in hospital and community settings. It is important that nurses have some understanding of these attitudes and beliefs so that more culturally appropriate care may be provided. The following are some of the religious beliefs affecting nursing or medical interventions.

Medical consultation and examination

Muslim men and women, due to modesty, may be reluctant to expose their bodies to a nurse or other healthcare professional for a medical examination. Islam requires that Muslims seek treatment from a person of the same gender whenever it is possible. A summary of the regulations is as follows: 'Priority should be given to the treatment of men by men and women by women. When a sick woman needs to be uncovered (for medical treatment), preference should be given to a qualified female Muslim doctor; if such is not available, the order of preference is then a female non-Muslim doctor, a male Muslim doctor, and lastly, a male non-Muslim doctor. If it is sufficient to be treated by a female doctor, she should not go to a male doctor even if he is a specialist. If a specialist is needed, she should go to a female specialist, but if one is not available, then the female patient may uncover in front of a male specialist. If the female specialist is not qualified to treat the problem and the situation calls for the involvement of a highly skilled, qualified male specialist, then this is permissible. If there is a male specialist who is more highly skilled and more experienced than the female doctor, the female patient should still not go to him unless the situation requires this extra level of experience and skill. Similarly, a man should not be treated by a woman if there is a man who is able to carry out the treatment (Sheikh Muhammed Salih Al-Munajjid).

In cases of necessity, things that are ordinarily forbidden are permitted. The scholars have agreed that it is permissible for a male doctor to look at the site of illness in a woman when necessary, within the limits set by Islamic laws (*shari'ah*). Similarly, a male doctor may look at the *awrah* (what is between the navel and the knees) of a sick man. However, he should look at the site of the complaint only as much as is necessary (and no more). The rulings apply to female doctors as to male doctors. This ruling is based on the idea of giving priority to the principle of saving life over the principle of covering the *awrah*, in cases where there is a conflict between the two (Sheikh Muhammed Salih Al-Munajjid). This tenet of Islam is further elaborated by the fact that if the doctor is of the opposite sex, a female patient's husband, or a male relative must be present. This is obligatory also for males, who must be accompanied by a female family member, especially when health care is sought from female professionals. The medical treatment can be sought from a non-Muslim, however, but when a Muslim who is equally qualified is available, the Muslim patient is required to seek treatment from him/her.

Mixed wards and privacy

Privacy and modesty are two of the hallmarks of the Islamic religion, and the issue has already been discussed in the previous chapter. A key concern for many, especially female patients on mixed hospital wards, is their privacy and maintaining their decency. This is even more important when intimate procedures may need to be carried out or private medical discussions held. Islam requires both men and women to dress modestly when in public or in the presence of non-family members of the opposite sex. This standard may not be followed by all Muslims due to the interpretation of 'modesty' relative to the norms of the society, fashion, and the acculturation of Western culture. For a Muslim male patient, it is not permissible for him to take a bath naked in front of people, since exposing one's private parts (to other than one's spouse) is forbidden. However, if he covers himself with a knee-length shirt or sarong there is no problem, as there is no prohibition on bathing naked where people cannot see you. Women also are not permitted to bathe or use the bathroom while other women are present. These guidelines do not change when a woman is in hospital, in labour, or in delivery. When carrying out dressings or other nursing or medical procedures, it is important to keep the woman's body covered except those specific areas that need to be uncovered for specific procedures.

An important point to remember when dealing with unmarried women, regardless of their age, is that virginity is conceived of as the presence of an intact hymen in much of the Muslim world. This may necessitate a clear, tactful discussion of what certain procedures entail (see Muslim inpatient care, www.ethnicityonline). Wherever possible, Muslim patients must be admitted to a single-sex ward. A study (Maternity Alliance, 2004) examining Muslim parents' experiences of maternity services found that there were problems of acute discomfort and embarrassment amongst Muslim parents due to the lack of privacy in hospitals and there being too few female staff. Muslims would require extensive periods of privacy and seclusion to wash, pray and meditate on their condition. This needs to be fully acknowledged and respected by nursing personnel.

Food

Islam has rules about the types of food which are permissible (*halal*) and those which are prohibited (*haram*) for Muslims. The main prohibited foods are pork and its by-products, alcohol, animal fats, and meat that has not been slaughtered according to Islamic rites. In many European countries, for example in the UK, some hospitals serve *halal* foods to their Muslim patients. It has been suggested that 'providing picture menus and using symbols to indicate the meals that are suitable for particular diets (vegetarian/*halal*/kosher etc.) will help the patient to choose an appropriate dish. Meal times may clash with prayer times, so alternative arrangements may be required (Picker Institute

Europe, 2003). Some patients may prefer to have their meals brought from home, but this would be subject to its being allowed by patient protocol. It is important to discuss the issue of food with the patient, as *halal* food should be made available to Muslim patients. If this is not possible, Muslims should be given the choice of having seafood, eggs, fruits and vegetables. The left hand is considered unclean in many Muslim cultures. To avoid offence, use the right hand for feeding, administering medications, or handing something to a Muslim patient.

Prayer

Most hospitals offer a prayer room or multi-faith room for patients and visitors. Where there are large Muslim populations, prayer areas should be provided in hospitals for Muslim families. Some Muslim patients who are confined to bed may need assistance and help with their ritual washing (ablution) before performing their prayer. If their garments have become soiled, they will want to get changed before prayer and again may need assistance. Cleanliness is part of the Islamic faith. A Muslim cannot pray or hold a copy of the Qur'aan without having ablution. In general, Muslims prefer to wash in running water. If possible, allow your patients to use a shower for washing; however, if one is not available, or they are not able to use one, then providing a bowl and a jug of fresh water is a good alternative. There is a special format for prayer that can be carried out even while bedridden, removing the need to stand, kneel and bow. This is carried out using special hand gestures instead of the whole-body movements of normal prayers. The patient needs to be positioned in the direction of Makkah. The family of the patient may use a corner of the room to pray. The nursing staff should ensure privacy and respect for their religious practices.

Ramadan and fasting

Muslims fast during the holy month of Ramadan. Some Muslims may consider medication as food, from which they must abstain during Ramadan. The Qur'aan allows medical exemptions from fasting. A comprehension examination of Ramadan and health care is presented in Chapter 10.

Holy and festival days

Friday is a significant day to Muslims and a special prayer (*Salaat-ul-Juma'a*) is performed just after noon. Attendance is strictly incumbent upon all adult males who are legal residents of the locality. *Salaat-ul-Juma'a* in the presence of a congregation is not obligatory for female Muslims. According to Ibn al-Qayyim (Al-Jawaziya, *Zaad al-Ma'aad*, 1/376), Friday prayer is one of the most important obligations in Islam, and one of the greatest gatherings of Muslims. Gathering on Friday is more important and more obligatory than any other gathering apart from *Arafat* (during *Hajj* pilgrimage). Whoever neglects it, 'Allah will place a seal on his heart.'

There are two major festivals in the Islamic calendar: '*Eid al-Fitr*', falls on the first day of *Shawwal*, the tenth month of the Islamic year, and '*Id al-Adha*', falls on the tenth day of *Thul-Hijjah* and coincides with the *Yauman-Nahr*, 'Day of the Sacrifices' in the *Hajj* pilgrimage. The first festival, *Eid-al-Fitr* (the 'Festival of the Breaking of the Fast'), occurs as soon as the new moon is sighted at the end of the month of fasting, namely Ramadan. Like festivals in other religions, Muslim patients may wish to visit their homes during these times.

Visiting the sick

Strong emphasis is placed on the virtues of visiting the sick and this is a sign of much mutual love, mercy and empathy. More than that, visiting the sick is a major responsibility that every single Muslim is duty-bound to fulfil. The sick Muslim is usually happy to receive many visitors. It is a requirement of the family members of the sick Muslim to notify as many people as possible of the illness. This is usually done by the close relatives or significant others. However, there are rules and etiquette in visiting the sick. These include: to sit where you are told; keep the visit short; convey regards and wishes; ask the sick how they are doing; show compassion at every moment and opportunity; pray for their recovery; and leave immediately after bidding them farewell. There is no sin in a man visiting a non-*mahram* (an unmarriageable kin) woman, or a woman visiting a non-*mahram* man, so long as the following conditions are met: proper covering; no risk of improper behaviour; and not being alone together (islamqa, ref 71968). If the patient is dying, Muslims usually say, 'All of us belong to Allah and unto Him shall we return' (Ibn al-Qayyim, 1953).

Nurse–patient interaction

Muslim patients accord a great deal of authority to nurses and will be comforted by some degree of formality in speech and dress. Titles and formal address are usually preferable to first names and informality with the older generation but this may not be applicable to young Muslims. Some Muslims patients, especially women, will avoid direct eye contact during a conversation as a sign of respect for the speaker. The cultural norm of modesty discourages direct eye contact with unfamiliar males. It is inappropriate for women and men to shake hands. When nursing a Muslim patient, especially of the opposite gender, avoid unnecessary physical contact.

Reflective Activity 7.2

- List the Islamic beliefs that may affect healthcare or nursing interventions.
- A nursing intervention is unable to be carried out because the patient is praying. How would you respond to this situation?
- If a Muslim is an inpatient in a hospital ward, how do you facilitate his/her needs in regards to required prayer?
- When is it permissible for an opposite gender person to provide nursing or medical care to a Muslim patient?
- Why may a Muslim patient refuse some medications?
- A Muslim patient feels very uncomfortable exposing any part of the body which is not directly under examination. What would you do?

Comments on Reflective Activity 7.2

The Islamic beliefs that affect healthcare delivery or nursing interventions have been examined above. These beliefs dictate the practices used to preserve and maintain health. Other health beliefs and attitudes that have significant impact on health care are: mental health and/or cognitive dysfunction; embryo experimentation and stem cell research; sexual and reproductive health; death and dying; and transplants and organ donation. Beliefs and practices about these issues will be examined in other chapters. However, when the nurse is not familiar with even basic religious and cultural practices of the client, problems of professional practice become apparent. This may lead to misunderstandings between the nurse and the patient, which can develop and lead to ethical dilemmas, practice problems, and problems in communication (Catlin and Boffman, 1998). For a nursing intervention that cannot be carried out because the patient is praying, the simple response is to wait, as prayer takes only a few minutes. A case scenario illustrates this point.

Case Study

When the nurse entered the room of a Muslim patient, she found the patient huddled on the floor, mumbling. At first, she thought the patient had fallen out of bed, but when she tried to help her up the patient became visibly upset and distressed. She spoke no English and the nurse had no idea what the problem was. The patient had been praying. Since she was scheduled for surgery the next day, she thought it was especially important to pray. If the nursing staff had some understanding of Muslim customs, they could have arranged to provide the patient some privacy during certain times of the day so that she could pray.

Source: Adapted from Fernandez and Fernandez (1999). (With kind permission.)

Prayers are not lengthy, so, if you see the patient is in prayer, you should wait until they are finished. Muslim men and women are obliged to recite prayers five times each day, starting at dawn, until nightfall, and they pray in the direction of Makkah. Prayer can be made from the bed, or a chair, if the patient is not physically able to make it in the usual manner (ISOS, 2009). Praying or reading from the Qur'aan can bring comfort and hope, and the supplications get answered. In order to facilitate the needs of the patient in relation to prayer, a clean prayer mat, sheet, or towel and a quiet space in the patient's room or in the hospital should be provided. Nurses should be aware and not disturb the patient at prayer, unless it is an emergency.

It is permissible for ana person of the opposite gender to provide nursing or medical care to a Muslim patient, if it cannot be avoided. If a male nurse or doctor must examine a female patient, she may feel more comfortable in the presence of another female or a male family member. When a nurse or doctor of the same gender is available, that person must provide the treatment. However, women will especially appreciate treatment by another woman during gynaecological examinations and during childbirth.

A Muslim patient may refuse some medications because Muslim dietary regulations can affect patients' use of medications, especially drugs incorporating alcohol, gelatine or other animal products. A substance which causes intoxication in large amountsshould not be used, because Prophet Muhammad said, 'Whatever causes intoxication in large amounts, a little of it is forbidden (*haram*).' But if it does not cause intoxication, or large amounts of it would not cause intoxication, but it brings some relief and eases the pain, then there is nothing wrong with it (Sheikh Ibn Baaz, 6/18). Among the basic principles of Islamic law, on which the scholars are agreed, is that cases of necessity make forbidden things permissible. For example, if no other medication is available and if taking it is necessary to save the patient's life, then it is permissible to take the 'forbidden' (*haram*) medication. But certain conditions have to be met (islamqa, 130815). The dietary prohibition against alcohol has occasionally raised questions about Muslims' use alcohol-based hand rubs in the hospital. However, it is suggested that while the religious and cultural beliefs of Muslims, as for others, should be respected in healthcare policies, the appropriate use of alcohol-based hand rubs need not cause any concern to Muslim healthcare workers (Ahmed et al., 2006).This information may also be helpful to healthcare workers advising Muslim patients and their visitors. If a Muslim patient feels very uncomfortable exposing any part of the body which is not directly under examination, culturally sensitive interventions by the nurse will help the patient to relax. If a patient is feeling vulnerable, uncovered or exposed, close curtains or doors and alert staff to announce their presence before entering. A sign outside a patient's room asking others to knock and announce their presence before entering will allow the patient to cover the head or body (Boston University School of Medicine, Boston Healing Landscape Project).

Conclusion

Muslim patients have certain issues and problems which may affect nursing interventions. Islam not only provides guidance in spiritual matters but also places considerable emphasis on health and the prevention of illness. There are a number of Islamic religious beliefs that will affect the attitudes and behaviours of Muslim patients in hospital and community settings. It is important that nurses have some understanding of these attitudes and beliefs so that more culturally appropriate care may be provided. The preservation of life overrides all the guidelines because in emergency and life-threatening situations, there are no restrictions of any kind for the purposes of medication, treatment, and preventative or nursing interventions. Muslims believe that cure comes solely from Allah even if this is practically in the form of a health professional.

References

Ahmed, Q.A., Memish, Z.A., Allegranzi, B. and Pittet, D. (2006) Muslim Health-care Workers and Alcohol-based Handrubs, *The Lancet* 367, 9515, 1025–7.

Al-Fangary, A.S. (2008) The Impact of Islam on Health, www.islamset.com/hip/Al-Fangary.html#7, date accessed 2 August 2013.

Al Khayat, M.H. (1997) *Environmental Health: An Islamic Perspective* (Alexandria, Egypt: World Health Organisation).

Al Khayat, M.H. (1999) *Health: An Islamic Perspective – Setting the Balance*, www.emro.who.int/publications/healthedreligion/islamicperspective/chapter1.htm, date accessed 2 August 2013.

American Academy of Ophthalmology (2008) 'Could Religious Beliefs Affect Compliance with Ocular Treatment?' *ScienceDaily*, www.sciencedaily.com¬/releases/2008/11/081109074608.htm, date accessed 2 August 2013.

Arnold, T.W. (1931) *The Legacy of Islam* (Oxford: Clarendon Press).

Bashir, A., Asif, M., Lacey, F.M. et al. (2001) 'Concordance in Muslim Patients and Primary Care, *International Journal of Pharmacy Practice* 9 (Supplement), R78.

Boston University School of Medicine. Boston Healing Landscape Project, www.bu.edu/bhlp/Resources/Islam/health/guidelines.html, date accessed 2 August 2013.

Bukhari [a] Volume 7, Book 71, Number 582.

Bukhari [b] 28, 226, 492, Al-Adab al-Mufrad Al-Bukhari, www.sunnipath.com/library/Hadith/H0003P0028.aspx, date accessed 2 August 2013.

Catlin, A.J. and Boffman, J.H. (1998) 'When Cultures Clash: Review of Anne Fadiman "The spirits catch you and you fall down" ', *Pediatric Nursing* 24, 2, 170–3.

De Leeuw, E. and Hussein, A.A. (1999) 'Islamic Health Promotion and Interculturalization', *Health Promotion International* 14, 4, 347–53.

El-Kadi, A. (1996) *What Is Islamic medicine?* http://members.tripod.com/ppim/intro1.htm, date accessed 6 April 2013.

Fernandez, V.M. and Fernandez, K.M. (1999) *Transcultural Nursing: Basic Concepts and Case Studies* (online), www.culturediversity.org/, date accessed 2 August 2013. Used by permission.

Fonte, J. and Horton-Deutsch, S. (2005) 'Treating Postpartum Depression in Immigrant Muslim Women', *Journal of the American Psychiatric Nurses Association* 11, 1, 39–44.

Haque, A. (2004) 'Psychology from Islamic Perspective: Contributions of Early Muslim Scholars and Challenges to Contemporary Muslim Psychologists', *Journal of Religion and Health* 43, 4, 357–77.

Helman, C.G. (2001) *Culture, Health and Illness*, 4th edn (London: Arnold).

Ibn Al-Abbas, A. and Kamel as-Sina'ah (in Arabic), vol. 2, p. 3.

Ibn al-Qayyim, Al-Jawaziya. *Zaad al-Ma'aad* (1/376): http://islamqa.com/en/ref/13815, date accessed 2 August 2013.

Ibn Al-Qayyim, Al-Jawaziya (1953) *Zad al Ma'ad* (Cairo, Egypt: Al-Fiqi, M.H.).

Ibn Musa, A. (1982) Resakat al-dhahabiya (*The Golden Epistle of Health*) (Karachi, Pakistan: Peer Mohammed Ibrahim Trust).

Islamic Social Services of Oregon State (ISOS) (2009) *Health Care Training Handbook for Muslim Patients*. Islamic Social Services of Oregon State (ISOS) Aloha, Oregon, www.I-SOS.org.

Islamqa. *Visiting the sick – some etiquettes*, http://islam-qa.com/en/ref/71968, date accessed 2 August 2013.

Islamqa, Fatwa Number 130815. *Permissibility of haram things in the case of necessity and the conditions governing that*, www.islam-qa.com/en/ref/130815/medicine%20with%20alcohol, date accessed 2 August 2013.

Khokhar, W.A., Hameed, I., Sadiq, J. et al. (2008) 'To Trust or Not to Trust? Faith Issues in Psychopharmacological Prescribing', *Psychiatric Bulletin online*, 32, 4, 179–82.

Maternity Alliance (2004) *Experiences of Maternity Services. Muslim Women's Perspectives*, www.maternityaction.org.uk/sitebuildercontent/sitebuilder files/muslimwomensexperiencesofmaternityservices.pdf, date accessed 2 August 2013.

Matin, M. and LeBaron, S. (2004) 'Attitudes towards Cervical Cancer Screening among Muslim Women: a Pilot Study', *Women and Health* 39, 3, 63–77.

Muslim. Cited in As-Sayyid Sabiq (1991) *Fiqh Us-Sunnah*, S4.5 American Trust.

Muslim inpatient care. *Cultural Awareness in Healthcare*, www.ethnicityonline. net/islam_inpatient_care.htm, date accessed 2 August 2013.

Nagamia, H.F. Prophetic Medicine: 'A Holistic approach to Medicine', *International Institute of Islamic Medicine*, www.iiim.org/Files/Articles/ Prophetic%20Medicine%20Final.pdf, date accessed 2 August 2013.

Nasa'i, ibn Majah, and al-Hakim, cited in As-Sayyid Sabiq (1991) *Fiqh Us-Sunnah* S4.5 American Trust.

Picker Institute Europe (2003) 'Improving Patients' Experience', March 2003; issue 5, www.pickereurope.org/Filestore/Quality/Factsheets/cultural_ awareness_newsletter_mar03.pdf, date accessed 2 August 2013.

Rahman, T. (1998) 'Language, Religion and Identity in Pakistan: Language Teaching in Pakistani Madrassas', *Ethnic Report* XVI, 2, 197–213.

Sange, C. (2009) *I am not being awkward: A hermeneutic phenomenological study on the perceptions of South Asian Muslim women and urinary incontinence.* Unpublished doctoral thesis, University of Warwick.

Saracci, R. (1997) 'The World Health Organization Needs to Reconsider its Definition of Health', *British Medical Journal* 314, 7091, 1409–10.

Sheikh Ibn Baaz Majmoo' Fataawa li'l-Shaykh Ibn Baaz, 6/18, cited in www. islamqa.com/en/21718, date accessed 23 October 2013.

Sheikh Muhammed Salih Al-Munajjid,Fatwa, Fatwa 5693, cited in www.islam-qa.com/en/5693, date accessed 23 October 2013.

Tirmidhî, Hadith, 780. Compiled by Imam Abu Zakariya Yahya bin Sharaf an-Nawawi, transl. S.M. Madni Abbasi (Karachi, Pakistan: International Islamic Publishers, 1983).

WHO (1996) *Health Promotion through Islamic Lifestyles: The Amman Declaration* (Alexandria, Egypt: World Health Organisation).

Zahoor, A. 'Abu Bakr Muhammad bin Zakariya ar-Razi (Rhazes) (864–930 C.E.)', cited in www.unhas.ac.id/rhiza/arsip/saintis/razi.html, date accessed 23 October 2013.

8 The Crescent of Care – a Nursing Model to Guide the Care of Muslim Patients

S. Lovering

Learning Outcomes:

- Contrast the meaning of health in a Western and a Muslim worldview.
- Identify the spiritual and cultural values impacting on health, illness and healing for Muslim patients.
- Describe the 5 components of care within the Crescent of Care nursing model and way to meet the patient's care needs.
- Reflect on the use of the Crescent of Care nursing model to guide the care of Muslim and non-Muslim patients.

Reflective Activity 8.1

State whether the following statements are true or false. Give reasons for your answers.

	True	*False*
1 There is the view that the role of caring is not culturally constituted.		
2 In the Muslim worldview, Islam provides the basis for beliefs about health, disease, illness and healing.		

	True	False
3 Beliefs about health, illness and healing influence the way nurses care for patients but not the health behaviours of the patients.		
4 Nursing has a universal belief system, with care and caring defined from a Western Judeo-Christian perspective.		
5 Florence Nightingale placed health and the environment as central to her nursing theory.		
6 Modern concepts of nursing placed the person's health (or illness) as being a result of environmental influences.		
7 Muslims have a spiritual obligation to maintain health which is consistent with achieving health as a socio-cultural obligation.		
8 Historically, the Western worldview had a different health explanatory model from that of Islam.		
9 Within the humanistic paradigm, transcultural nursing theory places the concept of health within the socio-cultural context.		
10 For Muslims, response to medical treatment is not considered preordained by God.		
11 Beliefs about health, illness and healing influence the way health practitioners care for patients.		
12 Belief in the evil eye as a supernatural cause of disease or misfortune is common to many cultures.		
13 Belief in the *jinn* (good and bad) is another form of blending religion with cultural beliefs.		
14 For Muslims, spiritual and religious needs must take priority over cultural and social needs.		

Introduction

In the nursing literature, there is an assumption that nursing has a universal belief system, with caring defined from a Western Judeo-Christian perspective (Narayanasamy and Owens, 2001; Rassool, 2000). Alternatively, the view that the role of caring is culturally constituted is supported by research conducted within Eastern, Asian and Native American cultures (Chen, 2001; Holroyd et al., 1998; Lovering, 2008; Lundberg and Boonprasabhai, 2001; Shin, 2001; Spangler, 1991; Struthers and Littlejohn, 1999; Wong and Pang, 2000; Wong et al., 2003). Muslim nurses' cultural beliefs about health, disease and healing and how these explanatory models blended into the nurses' caring experiences have been examined in an ethnographic study by Lovering (2008). Explanatory models are culturally based explanations concerning the concepts of health, disease, illness and healing (Kleinman, 1980; Kleinman, Eisenberg and Good, 1978). These culturally derived models influence health-related behaviours and include beliefs about the causes of disease; responses to illness, injury or disability; use of various healing methods; and the role of others (especially family members) in the healing process (Fitzgerald et al., 1997). Beliefs about health, illness and healing influence the way nurses care for patients; these same belief systems influence the health behaviours of the patients.

In the Muslim worldview, Islam provides the basis for beliefs about health, disease, illness and healing. In Lovering's (2008) study, the nurses' definition of health reflected the Muslim worldview, with spiritual health at the centre of their caring model. The Muslim nurses translated their spiritually derived beliefs about health, illness and healing into a form of caring that is distinct from Western or Eastern nurses' caring models. The outcome of this study was the development of the Crescent of Care nursing model, which captures the centrality of Islam in Muslim nurses' practice (Lovering, 2012). As this model is grounded in the Muslim worldview and beliefs about health, illness and healing, the Crescent of Care model provides guidance in the care of Muslim patients by Muslim and non-Muslim nurses. This chapter explores health as defined in Western nursing theory, and the health meanings of Muslim populations. The Crescent of Care nursing model will be presented and a case study will be used to demonstrate the applicability of the model in practice.

Health as defined in Western nursing theory

Health is a central concept and is variously conceptualised as a state, a process, a continuum, an outcome and a style of life (Jones and Meleis, 1993; Meleis, 1990). Saylor (2003, 2004) argues that current health definitions reflect the dualistic Cartesian philosophy underlying the biomedical model and suggests that holistic care should incorporate Eastern traditions of mind–body integration, energy systems and balance. Meleis (1990) suggests that multiple definitions of health are required for the diversity of populations and clinical environments served by nursing, but argues that some aspects of health are universal. In the 1850s, Florence Nightingale (1992), the pioneer nursing theorist, placed health and the environment as central to her nursing theory. A century later, nursing theorists of the 1970s and 1980s moved from a biomedical perspective of health to a more phenomenologically informed humanist paradigm. The central concepts of nursing included: person, environment, health and nursing (Fawcett, 1984). Thorne (1993) coceptualises that health behaviours, illness experiences and nursing actions take place within the socio-cultural context that shapes their meaning. It has been stated that 'One of the most universal aspects of health in most of the world's cultures is its inseparability from the essence of the social fabric ... the individual cannot be fully understood in isolation from his or her community, natural environment and spirit world' (Fawcett, 1984, p. 1933). Within the humanistic paradigm, transcultural nursing theory places the concept of health within the socio-cultural context. Culture prescribes what a person recognises as health, illness or disease and definitions of health and disease are culturally determined (Andrews and Boyle, 2003). Leininger (1995) links the concept of culturally defined health with performance of social roles and defines health as a consequence.

Historically, the Western worldview had a similar health explanatory model to that of Islam. Spiritual health was an important part of healing, where spirituality, health and illness were complementary aspects (Dawson, 1997; Tinley and Kinney, 2007; VanDan, 2004). Healing occurred as an expression of divine action while purification came through suffering, and sickness and death resulted from sin. Dual roles were common in many cultures, where the roles of priest and healer were combined. Theologians and physicians had identical social and healing roles until recent times (Thorne, 1993). In the past few hundred years, the rise of positivism and the influence of Descartes led to medical healers separating the body and spirit in the healing process and a rationalistic approach to health in Western culture emerged (Dawson, 1997). This separation of mind and body affects the holistic approach to care in medicine as the integration of the human person has lost its value (Rashidi and Rajaram, 2001). However, while physicians no longer incorporate spiritual care as part of the medical role, the practice of faith healing by ministers or religious practitioners continues.

Health meanings in Islam: the Muslim worldview

Within the Muslim worldview, health beliefs are based on the concept of *Tawheed*. This complete integration of the Muslim worldview with health is summarised by Rassool: 'Central to Islamic teachings are the connections between knowledge, health, holism, the environment and the "Oneness of

Allah", the unity of God in all spheres of life, death and the hereafter' (Rassool, 2000, p. 1476). *Tawheed* requires that a Muslim lives in a way that reflects the unity of mind and body with Allah; and implies there is no separation of the physical and spiritual dimensions of health. Muslims have a spiritual obligation to maintain health (Mardiyono et al., 2011), and spiritual health is an essential component of the Muslim health explanatory model. Muslims also believe in predestination (*Qadar*, meaning life, unfolds according to Allah's will), and in life after death, when Allah judges a person on the Day of Judgement for their earthly deeds. *Tawheed*, and the belief in predestination and being judged be Allah in the afterlife, shape the health beliefs held by Muslims. Muslims have a spiritual obligation to practise healthy ways of living and find guidance for physical and spiritual health in the Qur'aan. In addition, Muslims are also required to maintain a balance (Daly, 1995; Emani, Benner and Ekman, 2001) and live a satisfactory life in preparation for the Day of Judgment.

In Islam, illness, suffering and dying are all part of life as predestined by Allah. Disease may be a sign from Allah for the person to take care of their body and achieve greater knowledge of God. Illness is a part of life, and considered a test of faith, or an opportunity for atonement of sins and greater reward in the afterlife if accepted with patience. While Allah predetermines disease and cure, a person should try to prevent disease and should pursue treatment. Response to medical treatment is also considered *Qadar*, or pre-ordained by God (Lovering, 2012). Death is the ultimate in suffering, and a natural and inevitable phenomenon of life's journey (Hedayat and Pirzadeh, 2001) to meet Allah on the Day of Judgement. The Qur'aan teaches that it is Allah who gives life and causes death (Qur'aan 3:156) and Allah who takes away the souls at death (Qur'aan 39:42). Illness and death should be received with patience, meditation and prayer (Al-Shahri, 2002; Hedayat and Pirzadeh, 2001; Lovering, 2012; Rassool, 2004; Webhe-Alamah, 2008).

Research on the health meanings of Muslim populations validates the integration of the Muslim worldview in the health experience. According to Brooke and Omeri (1999), Wehbe-Alamah (2008), and Lovering (2008), care is an act of worship derived from the Muslim worldview, and incorporates religious beliefs and actions to care for the person's own health. In her study of Syrian Muslims in the United States, Wehbe-Alamah (2008) highlighted the importance of spiritual health for promoting physical health and illness prevention. Brooke and Omeri (1999), Daly (1995), Wehbe-Alamah (2008) and Lovering (2008) found that health promotion is valued to maintain good health in order to be able to practise and meet the requirements of Islam. Illness is a caring practice from God to erase sins and avoid punishment in the afterlife (Wehbe-Alamah, 2008). Similarly, spirituality and health meanings were inseparable for Iranian Muslim immigrants in Sweden (Emani, Benner and Ekman, 2001).

The findings from Lovering's research (2008) showed that Muslim nurses' views of health and caring blend the scientific basis of the Western biomedical model with the Eastern view that emphasises the whole human being. Rashidi and Rajaram (2001, p. 56) explain that, 'care in the Islamic view is a reflection of the Eastern worldview that emphasises the whole human being and integrates and balances the spirit (*ruh*), body (*badan*) and emotion (*nafs, soul*)'. Muslim nurses' views on disease, illness, healing and death mirrored the Islamic teachings on health and disease and the belief in predestination. The Muslim nurses' spirituality and that of their patients intertwine to create a 'shared spirituality' between nurse and patient, thus supporting the patient's spiritual health (Lovering, 2008, 2012). This blend of caring and shared spirituality depends on the nurse's spirituality, the patient's spirituality and whether the patient expects or accepts spiritual caring from the nurse. This shared spirituality will also depend on the spiritual needs of the patient and the context of caring. The greatest spiritual need in the health experience occurs at the beginning and end of life, and at times of critical illness. Spiritual caring actions by the nurse support the patient during these times of greatest need for spiritual healing.

Meeting patients' spiritual needs

The definition of health as physical, psychological, social and spiritual well-being requires the meeting of spiritual needs as well as physical and psychosocial needs. Muslims believe that humans are judged on the health of their inner being (spirit) and that spiritual disease could lead to physical disease. From this belief, it follows that meeting spiritual needs may have priority over physical and psychosocial needs. The importance of meeting spiritual needs before physical needs emerged as a significant care pattern and central to nurses' caring model (Lovering, 2008). Reading of verses from the Qur'aan, repetition of *hadiths* and use of *ruqyah* (Islamic prayer formulas) have served as a direct source of healing since the beginning of Islam. Different supplications are used in the care of patients, such as during labour and the birth of a baby, to assist in healing, for protection of the patient's health and prior to giving medications, and nearing the time of death. Nurses can support religious healing by providing copies of the Qur'aan, praying for and with patients, and use of supplications. Patients or families may request the use of Zam Zam (Holy) water for medication administration, bathing a patient and flushing a naso-gastric tube (Lovering, 2012). Incorporation of time for daily prayers, and prayer before any procedure or treatment, are important caring actions by nurses. The use of religious words such as *'Bismallah'* (in the name of Allah) before any procedure or treatment, such as venous puncture and giving medications, establishes trust between the nurse and patient, irrespective of whether the nurse and patient share the same religion. These spiritual caring actions support the patient's belief in God as the Ultimate Healer (Mardiyono et al., 2011).

Reflective Activity 8.2

Your child is drowning in a river. On the riverbank are two people who can help – one is a Sheik who can read the Qur'aan, and the other is a strong swimmer. Who would you choose to save your child? Most parents choose the strong swimmer. The doctor says, 'I am the strongest swimmer. Let me take out the eye and save the child. You still need the Sheik to read the Qur'aan, and to pray for your child. Together, we will keep your child safe' (Lovering, 2002, p. 21).

The importance of meeting spiritual needs as well as physical needs as part of the provision of patient care by nurses and doctors is highlighted in the story above, from an ophthalmology hospital. In the paediatric unit, nurses care for families whose children need to have enucleation (removal of the eye) for retinoblastoma (cancer of the retina). Families often do not wish to give consent for an enucleation and seek support from the Sheik (religious healer). In this situation, the medical doctor and religious healer meet spiritual and physical needs jointly. To meet the important spiritual needs while getting support for the physical intervention, the paediatric physicians use the story to assist a family facing the decision to consent to enucleate their child's eye to save child's life.

Blending cultural and religious beliefs about health, illness and healing

For many Muslims, cultural beliefs about health, illness and healing are blended with the teachings of Islam. In some cultures it may be difficult to separate cultural values from religious requirements, and traditions will vary in different social contexts. Many cultures in parts of Europe (Mediterranean), the Middle East, North and West Africa, South and Central Asia and Central America believe that the evil eye causes disease or misfortune. Belief in the evil eye dates to antiquity, and there is reference to the evil eye in the Old Testament and the Qur'aan (113:1–5), placing the evil eye within the spiritual realm mixed with cultural beliefs. Another form of blending religion with cultural beliefs is the belief in the *Jinn* (which are good or bad spirits). The Qur'aan teaches that Allah created humans and the *Jinn* to worship Him. Some believe that the jinn may cause abnormal physical or mental behaviour (Lovering, 2002), such as schizophrenia or epilepsy. Some Muslim patients may believe that the *Jinn* are present within the hospital and request a special religious healer to remove the *Jinn* from their room. The issue of evil eye and *Jinn* is examined in Chapter 12.

The Crescent of Care nursing model

The Crescent of Care nursing model (Figure 8.1) is an outcome of the ethnographic study on Muslim nurses' caring (Lovering, 2008) and was further developed by using collaborative inquiry methodology for application by nurses at the bedside (Lovering, 2012). The development of the nursing model was the outcome of an identified need for a nursing approach to guide the practice of Muslim and non-Muslim nurses in caring for Muslim patients. A number of models were examined including Leininger's theory of culture care (1991, 1995), Watson's theory of human care (1988) and the nursing model developed through Lovering's research (2008). Leininger's theory of culture care (1991, 1995) provided a comprehensive framework for gaining cultural knowledge to enable nurses to provide culturally congruent care with a focus on cultural caring practices. Leininger's transcultural nursing theory lacks the

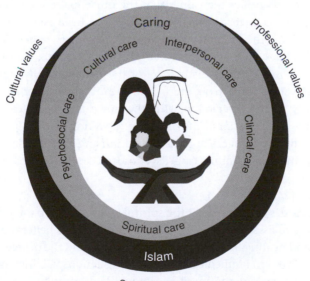

Figure 8.1   Crescent of Care nursing model
Source: Lovering (2012). (Reproduced with permission.)

application of the technical, spiritual and psychosocial aspects of nursing care and its greater applicability in clinical settings.

Watson's theory of human care (1988) is based on an existential-phenomenological philosophy and conceptualises caring as an interpersonal process and a moral ideal to protect, enhance and preserve human dignity. However, Watson's concept of spirituality as an existential transcending experience was inconsistent with the Muslim worldview and lacked the focus on cultural and clinical caring practices. Lovering's (2008) model was based on a patient and family needs-driven approach grounded in the spiritual, cultural and professional values consistent with the patient population and translated well into clinical practice. The Crescent of Care nursing model captures the centrality of Islam in the care of Muslim patients. This holistic nursing model incorporates spiritual, cultural and professional values when caring for Muslim patients to meet their spiritual, cultural, interpersonal, psycho-social and clinical caring needs. The model is applicable in the care of Muslim patients in all cultural contexts, for use by nurses of all faiths.

In the context of this model, health is defined as complete spiritual, psychosocial and physical well-being. In the centre of the Figure are the patient and family as the focus of care; reflecting the importance of family as the primary social unit in Islam. This focus on the family is distinct from most Western-derived nursing models that focus on individual health needs. The outer circle identifies the values that the nurse, patient and family bring to the health experience: Spiritual values (derived from Islam), Cultural values (derived from the cultural worldview of the nurse, patient/family) and Professional values such as professional nursing standards, and the code of ethics that the nurse brings to the care of the patient/family unit. Spiritual and cultural values impact on the health meanings and behaviours of the patient/family in the interaction with the nurse and healthcare team and the provision of professional nursing care (Lovering, 2012). The inner circle captures the components of professional nursing care. These components include: Spiritual care, Cultural care, Psychosocial care, Interpersonal care, and Clinical care.

> **Spiritual care** is action to meet the spiritual needs of the patient and family. The focus of assessment is the patient's and family's beliefs about health, illness and healing from a spiritual perspective; and the degree of blending with the Western biomedical model. Caring actions will include modification of nursing care routines to accommodate reading of the Qur'aan, or providing advance notice of the care plan should the patient wish to pray before treatments or procedures. Spiritual caring actions include recitation of the *Shahadah* (Muslim's profession of faith) by a Muslim for the patient

at end of life as an important caring action. Family members assist in the provision of spiritual care for the patient (Lovering, 2012).

Cultural care is action to meet the cultural needs and support the values, beliefs and traditions of the patient and family. Assessment is focused on traditional beliefs related to health, illness and healing, such as the evil eye and *Jinn*. Skin assessment is important (to identify use of cupping (*hijama*) or other traditional methods that affect skin integrity), as is the use of traditional healing methods and medicines. Some traditional methods such as massaging the skin with oil are not harmful, but others such as the use of honey or herbs to treat wounds may need to be discouraged depending on the patient's condition. Actions to support cultural needs may include the accommodation of traditional or religious healers in the care of the patient. Protection of modesty is a fundamental cultural caring action in all clinical interactions. Family members can assist in guiding the nurse in the provision of cultural caring actions (Lovering, 2012).

Psychosocial care is action to meet the psychological and social needs of the patient and family. Psychosocial care is directed at determining the structure of the family, and the impact of the illness and hospitalisation on the patient's role in the family, and on family roles in the care of the patient. Family members can assist the nurse in assessing and interpreting the patient's psychosocial needs, level of anxiety, stress levels and coping mechanisms. Nurses need to work through the family, in provision of psychosocial care. The obligation to visit is a religious and cultural requirement for family members (close and extended family), and failure to visit a sick relative is considered shameful. This obligation is extended to close neighbours. The family should be in charge of the visitors, and support for the visiting process is a caring action. However, the nurse may need to assist the family to ensure a balance between psychological support through visiting, and the need for rest (Lovering, 2012).

Interpersonal care relates to the relationship between the nurse and patient, including verbal and non-verbal communication. Communication through touch and eye contact is affected by cultural values related to the need to maintain modesty, in particular between different genders. Islamic teachings do not permit unnecessary touching between unrelated male and female adults (Al Shahri, 2002); and this may impact on the use of touch by nurses, in particular male nurses caring for female patients. Some procedures, such as catheterisation, should be done by same gender carers; and male nurses may not provide personal care for female patients. The use of touch by individuals of the same gender is appropriate and can be used as a caring action. The need for modesty also affects eye contact between people of different gender, and needs to be considered when interpreting body language and eye contact in the health interaction.

Clinical care includes the knowledge and skills related to the provision of physical and technical nursing care. Nurses use their scientific knowledge and the nursing process to directly provide technical and physical nursing care. In some cases, the family members will participate in the physical care of the patient in supporting the activities of daily living under the guidance of the nurse. Some aspects of clinical nursing care may need to be modified to accommodate spiritual and cultural needs, such as meeting the needs of fasting patients during Ramadan, or adjusting the care plan to accommodate daily prayer rituals (Lovering, 2012).

The crescent (symbol of medical and nursing care in Islamic societies) surrounds the components of care and symbolises the inseparability of nurses' caring and Islam. In the context of the shared spirituality between nurse and patient, the linking of the crescent of Islam and care components captures the shared spirituality between the nurse and the patient and family. This shared spirituality is fluid, depending on spiritual need. Times of greatest spiritual need include the beginning of life, critical illness and the end of life, requiring great spiritual connectedness between nurse, patient and family. The nurse and patient's spiritual caring may be minimally connected in times of lesser need such as an ambulatory clinic visit for a routine health examination (Lovering, 2008).

Value of the Crescent of Care nursing model

The Crescent of Care nursing model provides a framework to assist the nurse to holistically assess the needs of the Muslim patient: physical, psychosocial, cultural and spiritual. Based on this holistic nursing assessment, caring actions can be planned and the outcomes evaluated against the aim, which is to restore the patient's physical, spiritual, psychological and social well-being. Spiritual and cultural needs are highlighted, as is the impact of spiritual and cultural values on psychosocial, interpersonal and clinical needs. This model assists nurses not familiar with the Muslim patient to prioritise spiritual and cultural needs and place the patient and family at the centre of the model. There is a greater understanding of the centrality of the family in the care of the patient for nurses of all cultures. The Crescent of Care model is valuable to guide the care of Muslim patients within Muslim societies, and immigrant Muslim populations in Western and Eastern cultural contexts. The application of the Crescent of Care model as a framework to guide the care of non-Muslim patient populations is yet to be explored empirically; however, the general concept of meeting patients' spiritual, cultural, psychosocial, interpersonal and clinical needs is applicable cross-culturally. The guiding principle is to first identify the underlying values and beliefs about health, illness and healing and how these belief systems impact on the patients' and nurses' health experience.

Reflective Activity 8.3

Case Study

A middle-aged Muslim male with multiple myeloma was admitted for pain control and end-of-life care. To reduce his severe pain and agitation, large doses of a morphine infusion were given. Psychological and spiritual support was given by the family through reading of the Qur'aan in preparation for death. The family insisted on optimum pain relief measures to keep their loved one in comfort. When death seemed imminent, the family asked for the morphine infusion to be withheld, to enable the patient to communicate his living will (wishes) related to family and business matters. The infusion was stopped for a period, and then restarted later in the day when the family reported that the patient was not alert enough to communicate with them. The patient died peacefully the following day.

- Caring for Muslim patients is based on 'collective care'. What is the role of the family in the caring process?
- How do you meet the following needs:

  (a) Interpersonal needs
  (b) Psychosocial needs
  (c) Spiritual needs.

- Identify some of the conflicting professional and cultural values that may have an impact on nursing care.
- How would you respond when a patient who is in severe pain refuses pain relief medications?
- Compare and contrast this model of care with a Western-oriented model of care.
- How would you apply this caring model to non-Muslim patients?

Comments on Reflective Activity 8.3

This case study demonstrates the application of the Crescent of Care nursing model to guide nursing care. This case was presented by an oncology nurse to an ethics panel during a nursing conference session on 'Ethical Perspectives at the Bedside' (Al-Swailem and Lovering, 2007). The concept of health expressed by the nurse includes spiritual, psychological and physical needs and treating the patient and family as a unit. The psychosocial, cultural, spiritual, interpersonal and clinical needs of the patient are identified. The impact of cultural, spiritual and professional values on the caring experience is shown.

From the beginning of this caring experience, the focus of care is on the patient and the family as an integrated unit. The family is a partner in the care of the patient, and family members make decisions on the patient's care with the healthcare team. In discussing this case, the nurse identified her responsibility to meet the spiritual, clinical, and psychosocial needs of the patient, which is consistent with the definition of health as spiritual, physical and psychosocial well-being. The family members were the key caregivers in meeting the patient's spiritual, cultural and psychological needs. The interpersonal needs of the patient and family were focused on supporting the relationship between the family and patient. However, a conflict occurred, with the family's cultural and social need for the patient to express his living will (his final wishes on family and business matters) taking precedence over the patient's physical and psychological need for pain relief. From the nurse's professional viewpoint, the patient's experience of severe, unnecessary pain meant the nurse believed she did not meet the patient's spiritual, physical and psychological needs when meeting the cultural and social needs of the family unit. In this case, there were conflicting cultural, spiritual and professional values affecting her ability to care ethically for her patient. In this kind of case, the cultural/social and religious aspects that impact on the care of this and similar patients are separated.

In Islamic culture, the family and patient are treated as an integral unit by the healthcare team. The family had a social requirement for the patient to express his wishes concerning family and business issues before his death. From a spiritual/religious point of view, the patient had a right to relief of his pain 'as Allah does not ask us to suffer', and withdrawal of the pain relief caused harm to the patient, which is against Islam. Therefore, spiritual and religious needs must take priority over cultural and social needs. From the nurse's perspective, her professional and religious values directed her to ensure the patient received pain relief for end-of-life care, to prevent the patient's suffering. There are similar cases where a relative or patient makes a request to withhold pain medication for a spiritual need. Some patients wish to pray to Allah with full mental faculties, or believe that pain is endured as a way of becoming closer to Allah.

In summary, achieving health for patients focuses on meeting spiritual, physical and psychosocial needs. This case study shows the impact of culture and Islam on health behaviour and the caring experience and confirms the definition of health as spiritual, physical, and psychosocial well-being. Application of the Crescent of Care model places the patient and family at the centre of caring action, in the provision of psychosocial, interpersonal, cultural, clinical and spiritual care. Identification of the ethical aspects of care highlights the potential conflicts between cultural, spiritual and professional values, and the focus for resolution within the healthcare team.

Conclusion

The Crescent of Care nursing model is a holistic model that captures the blending of Western nursing science with spiritual and cultural caring from the Muslim worldview. At the heart of the model are the patient and family as the focus of care, and caring as an act of shared spirituality between the nurse, patient and family. Spiritual and cultural values about health, illness and healing, of patient, family and nurse, are brought to the health experience. In the Muslim worldview, predestination determines the presence of disease and the effectiveness of medical treatment and other healing. The Western biomedical model of pathology and the science of curing are subject to Allah's will, as is the patient's response to the medical treatment. The nurse assesses the patient's spiritual, cultural, psychosocial, interpersonal and clinical needs, where the focus is to restore the patient to spiritual, psychological, social and physical well-being.

The Crescent of Care model is of value for Muslim and non-Muslim nurses to care for Muslim patients in all cultural contexts. Understanding the centrality of Islam for the patients' well-being enables nurses of all faiths to provide spiritual caring that is supportive of the patient's faith. For Muslim nurses, the shared spirituality between nurse and patient supports the patients' spiritual and religious health and relationship with Allah. Assessment of cultural beliefs about health, illness and healing traditions assists the nurses to identify the unique cultural and religious needs of the patient in the health experience. Beliefs about health, illness and healing are the foundation of nurses' caring models in all cultural contexts. The Crescent of Care nursing model provides a specific focus on the spiritual, cultural, psychosocial, interpersonal and clinical needs of Muslim patients, whether in Muslim societies or immigrant Muslim populations in a Western health context.

References

Al-Jauziyah, Q. (2003) *Healing with the Medicine of the Prophet* (PBUH) (Riyadh, Saudi Arabia: Darussalam Publications).

Al Khayat, M. (1997) *Health: An Islamic Perspective* (Alexandria, Egypt: World Health Organisation Regional Office for the Eastern Mediterranean Region).

Al-Shahri, M. (2002) 'Culturally Sensitive Caring for Saudi Patients', *Journal of Transcultural Nursing* 13, 2, 133–8.

Al-Swailem, A. and Lovering, S. (2007) *Ethical Perspectives at the Bedside*. Building Bridges to the Future, 2nd International Nursing Conference, Jeddah, Saudi Arabia.

Andrews, M. and Boyle, J. (2003) *Transcultural Concepts in Nursing Care* (Philadelphia, PA: Lippincott Williams & Wilkins).

Brooke, D. and Omeri, A. (1999) 'Beliefs about Childhood Immunisation among Lebanese Muslim Immigrants in Australia', *Journal of Transcultural Nursing* 10, 3, 229–36.

Chen, Y. (2001) 'Chinese Values, Health and Nursing', *Journal of Advanced Nursing* 36, 2, 270–3.

Daly, E. (1995) 'Health Meanings of Saudi Women', *Journal of Advanced Nursing* 21, 5, 853–7.

Dawson, P.J. (1997) 'A reply to Goddard's Spirituality as Integrative Energy', *Journal of Advanced Nursing* 25, 2, 282–9.

Dhami, S. and Sheikh, A (2008) 'The Family: Predicament and Promise', in A. Sheikh and A. Gatrad (eds), *Caring for Muslim Patients* (Oxford: Radcliffe Publications).

Emani, A. Benner,P. and Ekman, S.L. (2001) A sociocultural health model for late-in-life immigrants. *Journal of Transcultural Nursing* 12, 1, 15–24.

Fawcett, J. (1984) *Analysis and Evaluation of Conceptual Models of Nursing* (Philadelphia: F.A. Davis).

Fitzgerald, M.H., Mullavey-O'Byrne, C., Clemson, L. et al. (1997) 'Cultural Issues from Practice', *Australian Occupational Therapy Journal* 44, 1–21.

Hedayat, K. and Pirzadeh, R. (2001) 'Issues in Islamic Biomedical Ethics: a Primer for the Pediatrician', *Pediatrics* 108, 4, 965–71.

Holroyd, E., Yue-kuen, C., Sau-wai, C., Fung-shan, L. and Wai-wan, W. (1998) 'A Chinese Cultural Perspective of Nursing Care Behaviours in an Acute Setting', *Journal of Advanced Nursing* 28, 6, 1289–94.

Jones, P. and Meleis, A. (1993) 'Health is Empowerment', *Advances in Nursing Science* 15, 3, 1–14.

Kendall, K. (1992) 'Maternal and Child Care in an Iranian Village', *Journal of Transcultural Nursing* 4, 1, 29–36.

Kleinman, A. (1980) *Patients and Healers in the Context of Culture: An Exploration of the Borderland between Anthropology, Medicine, and Psychiatry* (Berkeley: University of California Press).

Kleinman, A., Eisenberg, L. and Good, B. (1978) 'Clinical Lessons from Anthropologic and Cross-cultural Research', *Annals of Internal Medicine* 88, 2, 251–8.

Leininger, M. (1991) *Culture Care Diversity and Universality: A Theory of Nursing* (New York: National League for Nursing Press).

Leininger, M. (1995) *Transcultural Nursing: Concepts, Theories, Research and Practices* (New York: McGraw-Hill).

Lovering, S. (2002) 'Before the White Spot: Transcultural Ophthalmic Nursing Practice in Saudi Arabia', *International Journal of Ophthalmic nursing* 6, 1, 18–21.

Lovering, S. (2008) *Arab Muslim Nurses' Experiences of the Meaning of Caring*, Doctor of Health Sciences 248 (Sydney, Australia: University of Sydney. Faculty of Health Sciences).

Lovering, S. (2012) 'The Crescent of Care: a Nursing Model to Guide the Care of Arab Muslim Patients', *Diversity and Equality in Health and Care* 9, 171–8.

Luna, L. (1994) 'Care and Cultural Context of Lebanese Muslim Immigrants', *Journal of Transcultural Nursing* 5, 2, 12–20.

Lundberg, P. C. and Boonprasabhai, K. (2001) 'Meanings of Good Nursing Care among Thai Female Last-year Undergraduate Nursing Students', *Journal of Advanced Nursing* 34, 1, 35–42.

Mardiyono, M., Songwathana, P. and Petpichetchian, W. (2011) 'Spiritual-ity Intervention and Outcomes: Cornerstone of Holistic Nursing Practice', *Nurse Media Journal of Nursing* 1, 1, 117–27.

Meleis, A. (1990) 'Being and Becoming Healthy: the Core of Nursing Knowl-edge', *Nursing Science Quarterly* 3, 3, 107–14.

Narayanasamy, A. and Owens, J. (2001) 'A Critical Incident study of Nurses' Responses to the Spiritual Needs of their Patients. *Journal of Advanced Nursing* 33, 4, 446–55.

Nightingale, F. (1992) *Notes on Nursing: What It Is, and What It Is Not* (Philadelphia: J.B. Lippincott).

Padela, A. and Pozo, P.R.D. (2011) 'Muslim Patients and Cross-gender Inter-actions in Medicine: an Islamic Bioethical Perspective', *Journal of Medical Ethics* 37, 1, 40–4.

Rashidi, A. and Rajaram, S. (2001) 'Culture Care Conflicts among Asian-Islamic Immigrant Women in US Hospitals', *Holistic Nursing Practice* 16, 1, 55–64.

Rassool, G. Hussein (2000) 'The Crescent and Islam: Healing, Nursing and the Spiritual Dimension: Some Considerations towards an Understanding of the Islamic Perspectives on Caring', *Journal of Advanced Nursing* 32, 6, 1476–84.

Rassool, G. Hussein (2004) 'Commentary: An Islamic Perspective', *Journal of Advanced Nursing* 46, 3, 281.

Saylor, C. (2003) 'Health Redefined: A Foundation for Teaching Nursing Strategies', *Nurse Educator* 28, 6, 261–5.

Saylor, C. (2004) 'The Circle of Health: a Health Definition Model', *Journal of Holistic Nursing* 22, 3, 98–115.

Sebai, Z. (1982) *Community Health in Saudi Arabia: A Profile of Two Villages in the Qasim Region* (Riyadh, Saudi Arabia: Al Kharj Hospital Program).

Shin, K.R. (2001) 'Developing Perspectives on Korean Nursing Theory: the Influence of Taoism', *Nursing Science Quarterly* 14, 4, 346–53.

Spangler, Z. (1991) 'Culture Care of Philippine and Anglo-American Nurses in a Hospital Context', in M. Leininger (ed.), *Culture Care Diversity and Universality: A Theory of Nursing* (New York: National League for Nursing Press), pp. 119–46.

Struthers, R. and Littlejohn, S. (1999) 'The Essence of Native American Nursing', *Journal of Transcultural Nursing* 10, 2, 131–5.

Thorne, S. (1993) 'Health Belief Systems in Perspective', *Journal of Advanced Nursing* 18, 12, 1931–41.

Tinley, S. and Kinney, A. (2007) 'Three Philosophical Approaches to the Study of Spirituality', *Advances in Nursing Science* 30, 1, 71–80.

VanDan, L. (2004) 'Development of Spiritual Care', in K. Mauk and N. Schmidt (eds), *Spiritual Care in Nursing Practice* (Philadelphia: Lippincott Williams & Wilkins), pp. 39–63.

Watson, J. (1988) 'Some Issues Related to a Science of Caring for Nursing Practice', in M. Leininger (ed.), *Caring, an Essential Human Need* (New York: National League of Nursing), pp. 61–8.

Wehbe-Alamah, H. (2008) 'Bridging Generic and Professional Care Practices for Muslim Patients through Use of Leininger's Culture Care Modes', *Contemporary Nurse* 28, 1–2, 83–97.

Wong, T. and Pang, S. (2000) 'Holism and Caring: Nursing in the Chinese Health Care Setting', *Holistic Nursing Practice* 15, 1, 12–22.

Wong, T.K., Pang, S.M., Wang, C.S. and Zhang, C.J. (2003) 'A Chinese Definition of Nursing', *Nursing Inquiry* 10, 2, 79.

PART
2

Care, Contemporary Issues and Health Concerns

Health Concerns Related to Muslim Communities

9

G. Hussein Rassool

Learning Outcomes:

- Identify the factors that influence the determinants of health.
- Critically evaluate potential health problems in Muslims communities.
- Identify the risk factors for ill-health related to specific Muslim practices.
- Discuss the barriers in the utilisation of health services.
- Discuss heath education activities that may be directed to Muslim patients in relation to lifestyle behaviours.

Reflective Activity 9.1

State whether the following statements are true or false. Give reasons for your answers.

	True	False
1 The determinants of health (things that make people healthy or not) include: income and social status, education, physical environment, employment and working conditions, social support, etc.		
2 The three most common fatal diseases effecting Muslims in Britain are coronary heart disease, diabetes and infectious disease.		
3 The prevalence of coronary heart disease (CHD) is highest among Pakistani men and women.		
4 Family history may also be a significant factor in the development of coronary heart disease.		

	True	False
5 South Asians are being prescribed too many statins and other cardio-protective treatments.		
6 There is evidence to suggest that lack of diabetes-related knowledge has been observed among UK South Asians.		
7 South Asian populations are more prone to develop hypertension.		
8 Obesity is not associated with hypertension.		
9 There seems to be a strong correlation between weight and blood pressure, and between increases in weight and increases in blood pressure.		
10 Consanguinity has been defined as 'a union between a couple related as second cousins or closer'.		
11 The health concern due to consanguinity is related to high levels of mortality, morbidity and congenital defects.		

Introduction

There are many determinants of health and many factors combine together to affect the health of individuals and communities. The determinants of health (things that make people healthy or not), according to the World Health Organisation (2011), are: income and social status, education, physical environment, employment and working conditions, social support networks, culture, customs and traditions, the beliefs of the family, genetics, personal behaviours and coping, access and use of health services, and gender. Muslim communities in the UK and the US are historically, culturally, ethnically and linguistically diverse, including immigrants and the native born (Laird et al., 2007). In the UK, Muslims are mainly ethnic South Asians (Pakistanis, Indians, and Bangladeshis), with smaller percentages of white British, white non-British ethnic and black African Muslims. American Muslims come from various backgrounds, and are one of the most racially diverse religious groups in the United States (Younis, 2009). The three largest ethnic subgroups in the US are of South Asians (Asian Americans are people who live in the United States, but were born in South Asia), or descended from people who were born in South Asia (Bangladeshi, Indian, Nepalese, Pakistani, Sri Lankan and Tamil), and those of Arab and US-born African-American origin. In this chapter the focus will be on the health concerns related to Muslim communities in the UK and US.

Health profile of Muslims

There is a dearth of literature describing the overall health profile of Muslims in the UK. The focus of most research conducted on Muslims, or Muslim groups, has been on specific health-related subject areas such as epilepsy, cancer detection, organ transplantation or mental illness (Choudhury and Hussain, 2008). Many of these studies are attitudinal: they measure and explore attitudes and experiences of Muslims and Muslim communities in relation to a particular illness. The Health Survey findings (Information Centre, 2005) have shown poor health and lifestyle choices of the Asian community in general and the Muslim community in particular. In the UK, in comparison with other religious groups, Muslims have the highest age-standardised rate of reported ill health (13% for males, 16% for females) and disability (24% of females, 21% of males), with widespread poverty and deprivation (National Statistics, 2007). The fact that Muslims have higher proportions of poor health and disability suggests greater need for support from outside formal services (Choudhury and Hussain, 2008). Some of the significant health issues are:

- Bangladeshi and Pakistani men and women were more likely to report bad or very bad health than the general population.
- Pakistani women and Bangladeshi men were more likely than those in the general population to report a limiting longstanding illness.
- Pakistanis and Bangladeshis were up to five times more likely than the general population to have diabetes, and Indian men and women were up to three times as likely.
- Levels of overweight including obesity tended to be higher in Pakistani women.
- Bangladeshi women were significantly more likely to have high blood pressure than women in the general population.
- Higher levels of cigarette smoking were reported by Bangladeshi men.

The three most common fatal diseases affecting Muslims in Britain are coronary heart disease, diabetes and cancer (Muslim Health Network). Other medical problems include hypertension, nutritional deficits, tuberculosis, malaria, dental caries, periodontal disease and sickle cell disease. This is not an exhaustive list, but a list of the most commonly reported conditions.

In contrast, Muslims in the US generally have higher socio-economic status than their UK counterparts, although the range is wide (Bukhari, 2003). However, specific health research data on health problems of Muslims in the US are scant. The findings of a study showed that in comparison to the general population, Arab Americans are apparently less healthy than the majority in terms of cardiovascular disease and its risk factors (Aswad and Hammad, 2001; Hammad and Kysia, 1996). These studies found disproportionately high self-reported levels of hypertension, diabetes, and hypercholesterolemia. In one study, the most common health problems reported during the past year included respiratory infection, cardiovascular disease, diabetes, and hypertension. Other health-related problems were identified, including family stress, difficulty in adjusting to the American culture, handling adolescents, and marital stress (Laffrey et al., 1989). Other identified high risk behaviours include a high rate of smoking; overeating; lack of exercise; less frequent female health screening; and not obtaining health care (Hodge, 2005; Jaber et al., 2003).

From all of these studies, we can tentatively conclude that the Muslim population in the US is at increased risk for several diseases, such as heart disease, diabetes, and cancer (Yosef, 2008). Other health concerns that emerge from epidemiological literature focus on risk factors for morbidities related to specific Muslim practices. There is the exposure of pilgrims to infectious diseases, heat and injury during the annual *Hajj* rites in Mecca, Saudi Arabia (Ahmed et al., 2006; Gatrad and Sheikh, 2005). Fasting, during the month of Ramadan may also complicate drug, diet and sleep regimens important in the management of other chronic illnesses (Laird et al., 2007). There is also concern regarding the high rates of consanguineous marriage, especially among Pakistani immigrant Muslims, and congenital disorders. However, the hypothesis that consanguinity explains the higher rates of perinatal mortality and congenital malformations among the Pakistani population has been refuted, as the epidemiological literature is inconsistent in its findings (Ahmad, 1994).

Obesity has become a serious issue worldwide among Muslims and in many Muslim countries, due to the changes including the increased income from oil revenues and acculturation of Western nutritional habits (Rassool, 2013). The dietary habits of the Islamic World are affected by socio-cultural and economic factors, and the nutritional problems therefore also vary (Musaiger, 1993). According to *The Economist* magazine's world rankings, the countries with the highest obesity rates among women are Muslim countries (data from 1999–2003 show 8 of the top 10 to be Muslim majorities: Qatar, Saudi Arabia, Palestinian territories, Lebanon, Albania, Bahrain, Egypt, and the United Arab Emirates). However, it is stressed that although Muslims are united by their faith, they are culturally different depending on their ethnic group. Hence, these cultural and ethnic differences are reflected in a wide range of eating behaviours, weight, and exercise attitudes among Muslims. The next sections will focus on some of the major lifestyle diseases affecting the Muslim community in general.

Cardiovascular disease

Cardiovascular disease is the most common and yet one of the most preventable causes of death in the Western world (Cappuccio, 1997). South Asian communities are highly susceptible to developing cardiovascular disease. Studies conducted in the UK, South Africa, United States and Canada have demonstrated the prevalence of cardiovascular disease specifically in this group (McKeigue and Sevak, 1994). The incidence rate of myocardial infarction is higher in South Asians than in non-South Asians for both sexes. In the UK, the prevalence of coronary heart disease (CHD) is highest in Indian (6%) and Pakistani (8%) men and a similar pattern is apparent in women (British Heart Foundation, 2010). Bhopal (2002) listed four reasons why this group are more susceptible to this condition: excess exposure to known risk factors, greater susceptibility, new risk factors, and competing causes. The established risk factors commoner in South Asians include low levels of high density lipoprotein cholesterol, diabetes (much commoner in South Asians), and lack of aerobic exercise. When the risk profile is seen in the context of social factors linked to coronary heart disease such as relative poverty, social upheaval after migration, and long working hours, this explanation deserves more consideration (Bhopal, 2002). Bhopal (2002) further establishes a link between coronary heart disease and poverty, migration, long working hours, and genetic differences which are common to many South Asian groups. Family history may also be a significant factor in the development of coronary heart disease.

The majority of Pakistani, Bangladeshi and Indian foods, including curries, chapattis, sweets and rice, is cooked with oil. Eating oily or high levels of saturated fats or fatty food is one of the biggest predictors for developing conditions such as coronary artery disease, hypothyroidism, obesity and diabetes. Although unsaturated fats (olive and canola oils, fish, safflower, sunflower, corn, and soya oils) help to lower blood cholesterol, because they are high in calories they may contribute towards obesity and diabetes if eaten in large quantities. A high concentration of oil or ghee in food contributes to a build-up of plaque (fat, cholesterol, and calcium). The build-up of plaque narrows the arteries and reduces blood flow to the heart, and can cause angina or a heart attack (Labarthe, 1998; Pais et al., 1996).

Diabetes

Diabetes mellitus is a metabolic disorder associated with thirst, frequency in urination and tiredness. There are two main types of diabetes: Type 1 results from the body's failure to produce insulin, and Type 2 is a condition in which the cells fail to use insulin properly (Watkins, 2003). According to the World Health Organisation (WHO, 2002), 170 million people of South Asian origin will develop diabetes by 2025. In the studies conducted in the UK, the risk of Type 2 diabetes in the South Asian populations has increased six-fold compared with the indigenous population (Barnett et al., 2006; Mohanty et al., 2005).

South Asian communities have an increased susceptibility to developing insulin resistance in response to certain environmental factors, including obesity and lifestyle. The condition can cause problems with the kidneys, legs and feet, eyes, heart, nervous system and blood flow. Diabetes is almost four times as prevalent in Bangladeshi men, and almost three times as prevalent in Pakistani and Indian men, as men in the general population. Among women, diabetes is more than five times as likely among Pakistani women, at least three times as likely in Bangladeshi and Black Caribbean women, and two and a half times as likely in Indian women, compared with women in the general population (Information Centre, 2004).

There are a number of cultural and social factors that may be linked to the increased prevalence of Type 2 diabetes in South Asian populations, including lack of knowledge, poor use of health resources, and a different attitude towards chronic diseases (Barnett et al., 2006). There is evidence to suggest that lack of diabetes-related knowledge has been observed among UK South Asians (Rankin and Bhopal, 2001; Vyas et al., 2003). Barnett et al. (2006) suggested that lack of diabetes-related knowledge could result from a communication gap between patients and their care providers, or from problems with literacy. Other social factors that could have a significant influence are the low income of a high number of people from ethnic minority communities and the fact that they live in the most deprived areas in the UK. It is also clear that many people of South Asian extraction are not using health resources adequately and may be less likely to be prescribed statins and other cardio-protective treatments (O'Hare et al., 2004; Ward et al., 2005).

Hypertension

Hypertension is another factor for developing cardiovascular conditions and renal disease. Using current guidelines, hypertension is defined as persistent high readings (>140/90 mmHg) taken at rest, or taking drugs for blood pressure. Risk factors for developing hypertension include lifestyle factors such as poor diet, excess alcohol, smoking, high salt intake and caffeine, and for secondary hypertension, diabetes. It is reported that South Asian populations are more prone to develop hypertension, which in turn increases the likelihood of developing associated conditions such as stroke, cardiovascular problems and diabetes (Gupta et al., 2006). In addition, Indians have higher blood pressure, Pakistanis lower blood pressure, with Bangladeshis having even lower blood pressure than the native white population (Agyemang and Bhopal, 2003).

Stroke

Stroke is a major cause of mortality in the UK, accounting for around 53,000 deaths every year (British Heart Foundation and the Stroke Association, 2009). Within the UK, mortality from stroke is higher among South Asians compared to European whites (Gunarathne et al., 2009). High blood pressure, diabetes and high cholesterol are associated factors that increase the likelihood of stroke; such conditions have been reported to be more prevalent in the South Asian groups. Social inequalities in stroke are persistent and premature death rates in the most deprived areas are around three times higher than in the least deprived (British Heart Foundation and the Stroke Association, 2009).

Obesity

The prevalence of obesity generally across the world has become a concern for many health organisations, with warnings suggesting a financial impact and strain on health services. Obesity is often associated with hypertension, so there seems to be a strong correlation between weight and blood pressure and between increases in weight and increases in blood pressure. Obesity 'doubles the risk of all-cause mortality, coronary heart disease, stroke and type 2 diabetes, and increases the risk of some cancers, musculoskeletal problems and loss of function, and carries negative psychological consequences' (Department of Health, 2004). The prevalence of obesity within South Asian groups has been linked to their lifestyle issues, high levels of saturated fats in their diet, and a lack of exercise. A study by Sidik and Rampal (2009) found risk factors associated with obesity related to socio-demographic factors such as age, ethnicity and religion. Sidik and Rampal (2009) suggested that Muslim groups have the highest levels of obesity, followed by Hindus.

Ethnicity has been reported as a prevalent factor associated with increased body weight, overweight and obesity (Paeratakul et al., 2002). The epidemic of obesity has affected Muslim youth and adults and the high obesity levels among women may be partially due to cultural prohibitions against physical activity. In a study of Pakistani women, Ludwig et al. (2011) found that the women (N = 55) lacked the motivation to address weight gain and were unsure how to do so. There was a limited awareness of the link between weight gain and Type 2 diabetes. Other barriers included the influence of cultural and familial expectations on home cooking, perceptions that weight gain is inevitable (owing to ageing, childbirth or divine predestination) and the prioritisation of family concerns over individual lifestyle changes.

Chronic kidney disease

People from South Asian communities living in the UK are more likely to need a kidney transplant than the rest of the population (NHSBT Organ Donation). This is because people from these communities are more likely to develop diabetes or high blood pressure, both of which are major causes of kidney failure (NHSBT Organ Donation). It is also essential to increase the number of people from these communities who are willing to donate organs after their death as only around 2 per cent of those on the NHS Organ Donor Register (ODR) are Asian. Muslim scholars of the most prestigious academies are unanimous in declaring that organ donation is an act of merit and in certain circumstances can be an obligation (see Chapter 16).

Consanguinity

Consanguinity is sometimes referred to as inbreeding; this means that offspring of such marriages are predicted to inherit copies of identical genes from each parent. The health concern due to consanguinity is related to high levels of mortality, morbidity and congenital defects (Dhami and Sheikh, 2000). Such marriages are much more common among Muslims of South Asian and Arab origin than in the general population. Among Pakistani Muslims, current estimates are that some 75% of couples are in a consanguineous relationship, and approximately 50% are married to first cousins. This represents an increase from the generation of their parents, of whom only 30% are married to first cousins (Darr and Modell, 1988). A study of 4,934 children of different ethnic groups demonstrated a threefold increase in infant and childhood deaths in the offspring of Pakistani parents (Bundey and Alam, 1993). Other possible factors in the birth outcome debate include the high prevalence of deprivation among Muslims, difficulties with access to high-quality genetic and prenatal counselling, and the possible risks associated with culturally insensitive maternity care (Bowler, 1993). However, consanguinity confers many advantages, which, at least in part, explain its continued appeal. For example, it allows a thorough knowledge of the future marriage partner of sons or daughters, a particularly important consideration in Muslim minority communities where the usual social networks that facilitate the search for an appropriate partner may be lacking.

Barriers in service utilisation

Muslim patients seem to be confronted with barriers when using health services. Equal access to health care is a fundamental human right (Vulpiani et al., 2000). Studies on the utilisation of hospital services by South Asian patients in the UK have consistently demonstrated levels of dissatisfaction with care in relation to meeting religious and cultural needs, although there are few studies on minority ethnic patients' utilisation of acute hospital services (Vydelingum, 2000). According to Choudhury and Hussain (2008), some studies have suggested that discrimination and 'Islamophobia' have contributed to health disparities, made worse by 'faith-blind' health policies.

In the US, the barriers faced by the Muslim population in accessing health services include modesty and gender preference, and illness causation misconceptions, which arise out of their cultural beliefs and practices. Other barriers are related to the complexity of the healthcare system and the lack of culturally competent services within this system (Yosef, 2008). There was little research into the experiences of disabled Muslims. However, research has suggested that South Asian families with disabled children experience discrimination and disadvantage in accessing the health and care services needed (Bywaters et al., 2003). Research conducted by Sheridan found that the terrorist attack on 11 September 2001 had a negative impact on the health and well-being of Muslims (Sheridan, 2006). A study by Ahmed (2009) found that Muslim youths do not approach statutory agencies for issues relating to their mental health. According to Ahmed (2009), this is partly because they feel service providers do not understand Muslims, their religion, culture and other norms young Muslims are faced with within their own community structures. This finding has serious implications for public services with a responsibility for mental health.

The potential barriers occurred at three different levels according to Scheppersa et al. (2006). The barriers at patient level were related to the patients' characteristics, such as: demographic variables, social structure variables, health beliefs and attitudes, personal enabling resources, community enabling resources, perceived illness and personal health practices. The barriers at provider level were related to the providers' characteristics, such as skills and attitudes. The barriers at system level were related to the system characteristics: the organisation of the healthcare system. Nonetheless, care providers are often oblivious to these barriers, although they may share to some extent the burden of responsibility for them. Some of the barriers in the utilisation of service provision are presented in Table 9.1.

Table 9.1 Barriers in utilisation of service provision

Language barriers	Differences in language between health service providers and users. Reducing the effectiveness of treatment received. Interpretation of a different set of health beliefs. Use of medical jargon.
Cultural barriers	Religious and cultural restrictions on discussing personal issues. Undressing in front of a member of the opposite sex. Experience or perception of racism or stereotyping.
Access to health information	Some health information is produced only in English. Some ethnic groups are not given literature in their first language.
Lack of awareness of the services	Affects all disadvantaged groups in society, and especially those who do not speak or read English.
Practical barriers	Lack of flexibility of services. Inability to attend appointments during working hours. Fear of racism.

Implications for nursing

The provision of health services and culturally appropriate nursing for Muslim patients should be based on community-based needs assessment, ethnic monitoring, and consultation with local minority ethnic communities. All nurses should receive cultural awareness training, covering religious and dietary needs, naming systems, social customs and, where appropriate, refugee-specific issues, including the need to register asylum seekers as permanent patients. The role of the nurse in helping Muslim patients to lead a healthier lifestyle through the provision of advice on diet, exercise, stopping smoking and other health problems and issues is examined elsewhere.

Reflective Activity 9.2

Case Study

Not long after the end of Ramadan, a 56-year-old man with Type 2 diabetes who had been undertaking a voluntary fast outside the month of Ramadan was admitted urgently through the Accident and Emergency (A&E) department, with severe hypoglycaemia. On arrival at his home, paramedics noted a capillary blood glucose level of 2.2 mmol/l. On admission to hospital, computed tomography of his brain showed evidence of a new right cortical infarct. A working diagnosis was made of acute stroke secondary to hypoglycaemia, complicated by aspiration pneumonia. Intravenous glucose infusion and antibiotics were commenced, with no improvement in consciousness level. He was admitted to the stroke unit, and his condition improved significantly over a period of 10 days. He required rehabilitation on the stroke unit, but was discharged after four weeks with a residual mild left-sided weakness.

Source: Chowdhury, T.S. (2011) 'Severe Hypoglycaemia in a Muslim Patient Fasting during Ramadan', *Diabetic Hypoglycemia* 4, 2, 11–13. Reproduced with permission.

- What are the immediate needs of the patient, Mr Ahmed?
- What may be the cause of the severe hypoglycaemia?
- Mr Ahmed spoke little English. How would you assess his needs?
- How can this risk be prevented?
- What other health education activities may be necessary for Mrs Ahmed and the family?

Comments on Reflective Activity 9.2

The patient will be referred to as Mr Ahmed. This case illustrates the high risk of severe hypoglycaemia in Muslim patients with diabetes who fast outside the month of Ramadan. On a patient's admission to the hospital, the nurse should be observant of the signs and symptoms of hypoglycaemia, including anxiety, irritability, dizziness, diaphoresis, pallor, tachycardia, headache, shakiness, and hunger. During the nursing assessment in this case, the patient mentioned that he had been fasting during the last few days. The nurse completed a health history and physical assessment with the help of a professional interpreter as Mr Ahmed spoke little English. Other collateral information was obtained from the grown-up children of the patient, who spoke fluent English. Several factors put individuals at risk of a hypoglycaemic episode. These include: a mismatch in the timing, amount, or type of insulin given, and in the carbohydrate intake; under nutrition; a history of severe hypoglycaemia; renal failure; liver disorders; glucocorticoid or catecholamine deficiencies; and leukaemia (Tomky, 2005).

In Mr Ahmed's case it was a reduction in his insulin dose to a critical level that prompted the hypoglycaemic episode. When questioned, he stated that he was advised by his diabetes nurse not to fast, but had decided to do so anyway, reducing the insulin dose to what he thought was a safe level.

Although it is recommended that all Muslim patients with diabetes undergo a pre-fasting/Ramadan assessment, and that if deemed to be at high risk they should be advised not to fast, in this case, because it was outside the period of Ramadan, he should have had an assessment to determine his medication regimen during the periods of voluntary fast. Many Muslims with diabetes are very passionate about voluntary fasting on specific dates, such as Monday and Thursday as recommended by the Sunnah. Others fast in order to complete those fasts that they have missed during Ramadan because of ill health or for other valid reasons.

A pre-fasting diabetes assessment is recommended so that patients can be made aware of individual risks, and recommended strategies to minimise these risks or even advised to refrain from full observance due to their current health status. Those who plan to fast despite going against medical advice, will require individualised advice on adjusting their medication regimen whether fasting in or out of Ramadan. It is important for the diabetic nurse to focus on fasting-focused diabetes education for people with diabetes as the role of structured education is well established in the management of diabetes (Hassanein, 2010). An education programme should include standard diabetes education as well as fasting/Ramadan-related issues such as the possible risks of fasting for people with diabetes, the importance of capillary blood glucose monitoring, when to stop the fast, as well as meal planning and physical activity that takes into account the prolonged fasting hours (Hassanein, 2010). The education session should also include advice on possible meal choices to avoid hyperglycaemia or hypoglycaemia.

The management of the patient with diabetes should be individualised to suit each patient's personal needs. This does not suggest that all those who observe fasting as a religious commitment should be grouped together; rather, even in such wider groups, management plans will differ. The importance of monitoring blood sugars regularly should be enforced, especially if fasting patients are on an insulin regime. Pre-dawn and post-evening meals should be tailored, for example carbohydrates can be advised pre-dawn, due to the delay in digestion and absorption. It is important that 'breaking the fast' should be encouraged if the blood sugars drop to 3.9 mmols or below, as there is no assurance that they will not drop any further, causing a hypoglycaemia episode.

Conclusion

Some of the main health components affecting the health of Muslims generally have been presented. Health education and promotion activities can help to address Muslim concerns and improve healthcare quality in this rapidly growing population. It is important for health authorities, through outreach work partnerships with mosques and local cultural centres, to create health awareness campaigns targeting the community. There should be health policy to overcome the potential barriers for Muslims needing access to healthcare facilities. Despite the best efforts of health authorities, many service providers continue to find themselves in a position in which they are unable to understand the religious and cultural patterns of their diverse Muslim communities, and unable to view their clients' culturally specific perceptions of these services.

References

Agyemang, C. and Bhopal, R.S. (2002) 'Is the Blood Pressure of South Asian Adults in the UK Higher or Lower than that in European White Adults? A Review of Cross-sectional Data', *Journal of Human Hypertension* 16, 11, 739–51.

Agyemang, C. and Bhopal, R.S. (2003) 'Hypertension and Coronary Heart Disease in South Asians. The Epidemic of Coronary Heart Disease in South Asian Populations: Causes and Consequences', *South Asian Heart Foundation* 108.

Ahmad, W.I. (1994) 'Reflections on the Consanguinity and Birth Outcome Debate', *Journal of Public Health Medicine* 16, 4, 423–8.

Ahmed, Q.A., Arabi, Y.M. and Memish, Z.A. (2006) 'Health Risks at the Hajj', *Lancet* 367, 9515, 1008–15.

Ahmed, S. (2009) *Seen and Not Heard*, Policy Research Centre, www.policyresearch.org.uk/publications/reports/84-seen-and-not-heard, date accessed 4 August 2013.

Aswad, M. and Hammad, A. (2001) *Health Survey of the Arab, Muslim, and Chaldean American Communities in Michigan*, Michigan Department of Community Health – Division of Family and Community Health. In cooperation with the Arab Community Center for Economic and Social Services (ACCESS) Community Health and Research Center, www.naama.com/pdf/arab-chaldean-muslim-michigan-health-survey.pdf, date accessed 4 August 2013.

Barnett, A.H., Dixon, A.N., Bellary, S., Hanif, M.W., O'Hare, J.P., Raymond, N.T. and Kumar, S. (2006) 'Type 2 Diabetes and Cardiovascular Risk in the UK South Asian Community', *Diabetologia* 49, 10, 2234–46.

Bhopal, R. (2002) 'Epidemic of Cardiovascular Disease in South Asians. Prevention must Start in Childhood', *British Medical Journal* 177, 16, 625–6.

Bowler, I. (1993) ' "They're not the same as us?" Midwives' Stereotype of south Asian Maternity Patients', *Social Health & Illness* 15, 2, 157–78.

British Heart Foundation (2010) *Ethnic Differences in Cardiovascular Disease*, www.bhf.org.uk/publications/view-publication.aspx?ps=1001549, date accessed 4 August 2013.

British Heart Foundation and the Stroke Association (2009) 'Stroke Statistics', British Heart Foundation Statistics, Database, www.heartstats.org, date accessed 4 August 2013.

Bukhari, Z.H. (2003) 'Demography, Identity, Space: Defining American Muslims', in P. Strum and D. Tarantol (eds), *Muslims in the United States* (Washington, DC: Woodrow Wilson International Center for Scholars), pp. 7–21.

Bundey, S. and Alam, H. (1993) 'A Five Year Prospective Study of the Health in Children in Different Ethnic Groups, with Particular Reference to the Effect of Inbreeding', *European Journal of Human Genetics* 1, 3, 206–19.

Bywaters, P., Ali, Z., Fazil, Q., Wallace, L.M. et al. (2003) 'Attitudes towards Disability amongst Pakistani and Bangladeshi Parents of Disabled Children in the UK: Considerations for Service Providers and the Disability Movement', *Health and Social Care in the Community* 11, 6, 502–9.

Cappuccio, F.P. (1997) 'Ethnicity and Cardiovascular Risk: Variations in People of African Ancestry and South Asian Origin', *Journal of Human Hypertension* 11, 9, 571–6.

Cappuccio, F.P., Cook, D.G., Atkinson, R.W. et al. (1998) 'The Wandsworth Heart and Stroke Study. A Population based Survey of Cardiovascular Risk Factors in Different Ethnic Groups: Methods and Baseline Findings', *Nutrition Metabolism Cardiovascular Disease* 8, 3, 371–85.

Choudhury, T. (2007) *Muslims in the EU: Cities Report* (United Kingdom: Open Society Institute, EU Monitoring and Advocacy Program).

Choudhury, T. and Hussain, S. (2008) *Muslims in EU Cities Reports – United Kingdom: Preliminary Research Report and Literature Survey* (Budapest: Open Society Institute).

Chowdhury, T.S. (2011) 'Severe Hypoglycaemia in a Muslim Patient Fasting during Ramadan', *Diabetic Hypoglycemia*, 4, 2, 11–13.

Darr, A. and Modell, B. (1988) 'The Frequency of Consanguineous Marriage among British Pakistanis', *Journal of Medical Genetics* 25, 3, 186–90.

Department of Health (2004) *At Least Five a Week – Evidence on the Impact of Physical Activity and its Relationship to Health – A Report from the Chief Medical Officer* (London: Department of Health).

Dhami, S. and Sheikh, A. (2000) 'The Muslim Family: Predicament and Promise', *Western Journal of Medicine* (November) 173, 5, 352–6.

Economist.com rankings for obesity among women, http://wikiislam.net/wiki/Health_Effects_of_Islamic_Dress#cite_ref-TDCJul12010_18-0, date accessed 4 August 2013.

Gatrad, A.R. and Sheikh, A. (2005) 'Hajj: Journey of a Lifetime', *British Medical Journal* 330, 7483, 133–7.

Gunarathne, A., Patel, J.V., Gammon, B., Gill, P.S., Hughes, E.A. and Lip, G.Y. (2009) 'Ischemic Stroke in South Asians: a Review of the Epidemiology, Pathophysiology, and Ethnicity-related Clinical Features', *Stroke* 40, 6, e415–23. Epub 2009 Apr 23.

Gupta, M., Singh, N. and Verma, S. (2006) 'South Asians and Cardiovascular Risk', *What Clinicians Should Know* 113: e924–e929.

Hammad, A. and Kysia, R. (1996) *Arab-American Primary Care and Health Needs Assessment Survey* (Dearborn, MI: ACCESS).

Hassanein, M.M. (2010) 'Diabetes and Ramadan: How to Achieve a Safer Fast for Muslims with Diabetes', *British Journal of Diabetes & Vascular Disease* 10, 5, 246–50.

Hodge, D.R. (2005) 'Social Work and the House of Islam: Orienting Practitioners to the Beliefs and Values of Muslims in the US', *Social Work* 50, 2, 162–73.

Information Centre (2005) 'The Health of Minority Ethnic Groups', *The Health Survey for England 2004*; www.ic.nhs.uk, date accessed 4 August 2013.

Jaber, L., Brown, M., Hammad, Q., Zhu, Q. and Herman, W. (2003) 'Lack of Acculturation is a Risk Factor for Diabetes in Arab Immigrants in the US', *Diabetes Care* 26, 7, 2010–14.

Labarthe, D. (1998) *Epidemiology and Prevention of Cardiovascular Disease: A Global Challenge* (Gaithersburg, MD: Aspen Publishers).

Laffrey, S.C., Meleis, A.I., Lipson, J.G., Solomon, M. and Omidian, P.A. (1989) 'Assessing Arab-American Health Care Needs', *Social Science & Medicine* 29, 7, 877–83.

Laird, L.D., Amer, M.M., Barnett, E.D. and Barnes, L.L. (2007) 'Muslim Patients and Health Disparities in the UK and the US', *Archives of Disease in Childhood* 92, 10, 922–6.

Ludwig, A.F., Cox, P. and Ellahi, B. (2011) 'Social and Cultural Construction of Obesity among Pakistani Muslim Women in North West England', *Public Health and Nutrition* 14, 10, 1842–50. Epub 2011 Jan 4.

McKeigue, P.M. and Sevak, L. (1994) *Coronary Heart Disease in South Asian Communities* (London: Health Education Authority).

Mohanty, S.A., Woolhandler, S., Himmelstein, D.U. et al. (2005) 'Diabetes and Cardiovascular Disease among Asian Indians in the United States', *Journal of General Internal Medicine* 20, 5, 474–88.

Musaiger, A.O. (1993) 'Socio-cultural and Economic Factors Affecting Food Consumption Patterns in the Arab Countries', *Journal of the Royal Society of Health* 113, 2, 68–74.

Muslim Health Network, www.muslimhealthnetwork.org/, date accessed 4 August 2013.

National Statistics (2007) Focus on Religion,. www.statistics.gov.uk/focuson/religion, date accessed 4 August 2013.

NHSBT Organ Donation, www.uktransplant.org.uk/ukt/how_to_become_a_donor/black_and_other_minority_ethnic_communities/black_and_other_minority_ethnic_communities.jsp, date accessed 4 August 2013.

O'Hare, J.P., Raymond, N.T., Mughal, S. et al. (2004) 'Evaluation of Delivery of Enhanced Diabetes Care to Patients of South Asian Ethnicity: the United Kingdom Asian Diabetes Study (UKADS)', *Diabetic Medicine* 21, 12, 1357–65.

Paeratakul, S., White, M.A., Williamson, D.A., Ryan, D.H. and Bray, G.A. (2002) 'Sex, Race/Ethnicity, Socioeconomic Status, and BMI in Relation to Self-Perception of Overweight', *Obesity Research* 10, 5, 345–50.

Pais, P., Pogue, J., Gerstein H. et al. (1996) 'Risk Factors for Acute Myocardial Infarction in Indians: a Case-control Study', *Lancet* 10, 348 (9024), 358–63.

Rankin, J. and Bhopal, R. (2001) 'Understanding of Heart Disease and Diabetes in a South Asian Community: Cross-sectional Study Testing the 'Snowball' Sample Method', *Public Health* 115, 4, 253–60.

Rassool, G. Hussein (2014) 'Nutrition: Obesity and Overweight', in G. Hussein Rassool (ed.), *Health Psychology from an Islamic Perspective: A Guide for Health Professionals* (Riyadh, Saudi Arabia: International Islamic Publication House, in press).

Scheppersa, E., van Dongenb, E., Dekkerc, J., Geertzend, J. and Dekkere, J. (2006) 'Potential Barriers to the Use of Health Services among Ethnic Minorities: a Review', *Family Practice* 23, 3, 325–48.

Sheridan, L. (2006) 'Islamophobia Pre- and Post-September 11th, 2001', *Journal of Interpersonal Violence* 21, 3, 317–36.

Sidik, S.M. and Rampal, L. (2009) 'The Prevalence and Factors Associated with Obesity among Adult Women in Selangor, Malaysia', *Asia Pacific Family Medicine* 8, 1, 2.

Tomky, D. (2005) 'Detection, Prevention, and Treatment of Hypoglycemia in the Hospital', *Diabetes Spectrum* (January) 18, 1, 39–44.

Vulpiani, P., Comelles, J.M. and Dongen, van E. (eds) (2000) *Health for All, All in Health: European Experiences on Health Care for Migrants* (Perugia: Cidis/Alise).

Vyas, A., Haider, A.Z., Wiles, P.G., Gill, S., Roberts, C. and Cruickshank, J.K. (2003) 'A Pilot Randomized Trial in Primary Care to Investigate and Improve Knowledge, Awareness and Self-management among South Asians with Diabetes in Manchester', *Diabetic Medicine* 20, 12, 1022–6.

Vydelingum, V. (2000) 'South Asian Patients' Lived Experience of Acute Care in an English Hospital: a Phenomenological Study', *Journal of Advanced Nursing* (July) 32, 1, 100–7.

Ward, P.R., Noyce, P.R. and St Leger, A.S. (2005) 'Multivariate Regression Analysis of Associations between General Practitioner Prescribing Rates for Coronary Heart Disease Drugs and Healthcare Needs Indicators', *Journal of Epidemiology and Community Health* 59, 1, 86.

Watkins, P.J. (2003) *ABC of Diabetes*, 5th edn (London: BMJ Publishing).

World Health Organisation (2011) The determinants of health, www.who.int/hia/evidence/doh/en/, date accessed 4 August 2013.

World Health Organisation (2002) *The World Health Report 2002 – Reducing Risks, Promoting Healthy Life*, www.who.int/whr/2002/en/, date accessed 4 August 2013.

Younis, M. (2009) *Muslim Americans Exemplify Diversity, Potential*. Key findings from a new report by the Gallup Center for Muslim Studies, www.gallup.com/poll/116260/Muslim-Americans-Exemplify-Diversity-Potential.aspx, date accessed 4 August 2013.

Yosef, A.R.O. (2008) 'Health Beliefs, Practice, and Priorities for Health Care of Arab Muslims in the United States: Implications for Nursing Care', *Journal of Transcultural Nursing*, published online 29 April 2008, http://tcn.sagepub.com/content/early/2008/04/29/1043659608317450, date accessed 4 August 2013.

10 Fasting and Health Care

G. Hussein Rassool

Learning Outcomes:

- Have an understanding of the importance of Ramadan for Muslim patients.
- Discuss the benefits and virtues of fasting during the month of Ramadan.
- Describe the physiological and psychological changes during the fast.
- Identify good practices in nutrition during Ramadan.
- Examine the potential health complications that may develop during the month of Ramadan.
- Identify the behaviours that may invalidate a fast.
- Identify the risks associated with fasting and be able to advise people with diabetes on how to fast safely during Ramadan.
- Discuss the role of the nurse in relation to health education/health promotion activities before the start of Ramadan.

Reflective Activity 10.1

State whether the following statements are true or false. Give reasons for your answers.

	True	False
1 For Muslims, fasting is complete abstinence from food and drink between dawn and dusk.		
2 No one is exempted from fasting.		
3 Fasting has a number of biopsychosocial and spiritual benefits.		

	True	False
4 Technically, the fasting state starts eight hours or so after the last meal.		
5 In Ramadan, weight loss does not result in better control of diabetes and reduction in blood pressure.		
6 A diabetic, diagnosed as insulin dependent, does not need to adjust their drug treatment.		
7 Fasting results in higher levels of certain hormones appearing in the blood (endorphins), resulting in a better level of alertness and an overall feeling of general mental well-being.		
8 It is recommended to break the fast by eating some ripe dates or dry dates, or with some water.		
9 Patients requiring multiple oral/injected medications during the day are able to fast.		
10 There are no concessions for women during menstruation, post-natal bleeding, pregnancy or breastfeeding, allowing them not to fast.		
11 Unintentional vomiting does not invalidate the fast.		

Introduction

Ramadan is the period of fasting for Muslims all over the world to fulfil the fourth pillar of Islam. Fasting is complete abstinence from food and drink between dawn and dusk. Muslims are obliged to fast during a whole month except for those who can't afford to practise it because they have a valid excuse or medical/psychological reasons. All those who are ill or frail, pregnant or menstruating women, breastfeeding mothers, and travellers are exempted. But they are required to make up the number of days missed at a later date or give a fixed sum to charity. The rulings of fasting for Ramadan are established in the Qur'aan, the Prophetic traditions, and the consensus of Muslim scholars. The Noble Qur'aan states that (interpretation of the meaning):

☐   *O you who believe! Observing As-Saum (the fasting) is prescribed for you as it was prescribed for those before you, that you may become Al-Muttaqun (the pious). (Al-Baqara [The Cow] 2:183)*

Allah, Exalted be He, also refers to (interpretation of the meaning):

☐ *The month of Ramadan in which was revealed the Qur'aan, a guidance for mankind and clear proofs for the guidance and the criterion (between right and wrong).* (Al-Baqara [The Cow] 2:185)

Thus, fasting is 'decreed' for all healthy Muslims. The aims of this chapter are to examine the potential benefits of fasting, the physiological and psychological changes that occur, things that invalidate fasting, the provision of healthy food during fasting and the potential medical problems and solutions.

Benefits and virtues of fasting

Fasting, according to Islamic law, means abstaining from certain behaviours and activities such as eating, drinking, having sexual intercourse, or committing immoralities (Sheikh Al-Fawzan, 2009). From an Islamic perspective, fasting has a number of biopsychosocial and spiritual benefits. It enables the purification of the soul, the renouncing of worldly pleasures and desires, and empathy with the poor and those suffering hardship or hunger, and promotes worship. A summary of the spiritual benefits of fasting is presented in Table 10.1.

Table 10.1 Spiritual benefits and gains from fasting

Heightened consciousness of God	• Reflecting on spiritual matters rather than being preoccupied with physical appetites. • It enables a person to develop sustained consciousness of God (*Taqwa*).
Healthy lifestyle	• Appreciating the value of food. • Control and discipline in abstaining from food during the fast. • Helps a person to choose a healthier lifestyle by making changes to their nutritional intake.
Compassion and charity	• Empathy with the poor and needy.

(Continued)

Table 10.1 Continued

	• The Prophet Muhammad described Ramadan as 'the month of mercy'. His companions observed: 'The Prophet (Muhammad) was the most generous of people, but he would be his most generous during Ramadan . . .' (Bukhari).
Community spirit	• Ramadan has significant importance as a medium for the building and consolidation of unity amongst the *Ummah* (community).
	• Promotes the well-being of the community.
A fast without the spirit is empty of blessing	• Ramadan is an ideal time to break bad habits, to reflect on your personality and to improve your character.
	• The blessed Prophet said that fasting is not merely 'abstention from eating and drinking, but also from vain speech and foul language' (Bukhari).

Source: Adapted from Community in Action (2007) Ramadhan Health Guide. © Crown Copyright 2007. Reproduced under the Open Government Licence v.2.0.

Physiological and psychological changes during the fast

Technically, the fasting state starts eight hours or so after the last meal, when the gut finishes absorption of nutrients from the food. In normal circumstances the body glucose, stored in the liver and muscles, is the main source of energy. However, during a fast, this store of glucose is used up first to provide energy. Later in the fast, once the stores of glucose run out, fat becomes the next stored source of energy for the body. Only in cases of 'starvation' or a prolonged fast of days and weeks, does the body eventually turn to protein for energy. This involves protein being released through the breakdown of muscle, which is why people who starve look 'anorexic', emaciated, and become very weak. This health condition does not happen during the normal fast of Ramadan. This is because the fast only extends from dawn till dusk, so the body can store the required energy during the pre-dawn and dusk meals. The replenishment of food during the break of the fast prevents the body from using glucose or fat as the main source of energy, and prevents the breakdown of muscle for protein. The use of fat for energy aids weight loss, preserving the muscles, and in the long run reduces cholesterol levels. In addition, weight loss results in better control of diabetes and reduces blood pressure (Community in Action, 2007). On a physiological level, there are no changes in the oesophagus and spleen. The liver releases glucose, and acids in the stomach are reduced. The gall bladder collects bile ready for the next meal intake. In the pancreas, insulin production is shut down. In the small intestines, the digestive juices are shut down, with contractions of the small intestine once every 4 hours. The large intestine performs the following functions: it reabsorbs water and maintains the fluid balance of the body, absorbs certain vitamins, processes undigested material (fibres) and stores waste before it is eliminated.

A detoxification process also seems to occur. Many toxins, stored in the fatty tissue, dramatically enter into the bloodstream at a rapid rate. The toxins are dissolved and removed from the body. It has been suggested that after a few days of the fast, higher levels of certain hormones appear in the blood (endorphins), resulting in a better level of alertness and an overall feeling of general mental well-being (Community in Action, 2007). The findings of a study on Ramadan fasting among Muslims suggest that a high-fat diet, providing around 36 percent of energy through fat (including poly-unsaturated fat), may be beneficial in preventing elevation of blood cholesterol or uric acid levels and better retention of protein in the body (Nomani, 1997).

Psychological effects on the individual are also significant during the fasting, and maybe the post-fasting, period. According to Athar (1998) there is peace and tranquillity for those who fast during the month of Ramadan, and personal hostility is at a minimum. Muslims take advice from the Prophet who said, 'If one slanders you or aggresses against you, say "I am fasting"' (Hakim). This psychological improvement could be related to better stabilisation of blood glucose during fasting, as hypoglycaemia after eating aggravates behavioural changes. Similarly, recitation of the Qur'aan not only produces a tranquillity of heart and mind, but improves the memory (Athar, 1998). The physical and psychological benefits of fasting are presented in Table 10.2.

Table 10.2 Physical and psychological benefits of fasting

- Self-control (good manners, good speech, and good habits).
- Detoxification process – removal of toxins from the body.
- Lowering of blood sugar.
- Self-regulation.

(Continued)

Table 10.2   Continued

- Self-training.
- Weight loss (control of diabetes, control of blood pressure).
- Reducing cholesterol levels.
- High level of awareness.
- General mental well-being.
- Maintaining tranqulity and peace of mind.
- Decrease in anger.
- Reduces hostility.

Good practice in nutrition

The prescribed time for daily fasting begins at daybreak and lasts until sunset. It is permissible to eat and drink until dawn, indicating the desirability of having a pre-dawn meal (*Suhoor*) during Ramadan. The Prophet said: 'Take the early pre-dawn meal, for indeed there is a blessing (*Barakah*) in the pre-dawn meal' (Bukhari and Muslim [a]). It is desirable to delay the pre-dawn meal and have it shortly before dawn (Sheikh Al-Fawzan, 2009). The pre-dawn meal should be wholesome, moderate, slowly digested foods that are filling and provide enough energy for many hours. It is also desirable to hasten breaking the fast by hearing the call to prayer (Sheikh Al-Fawzan, 2009). It is an act of prophetic tradition (Sunnah) to break the fast by eating some ripe dates or dry dates, or with some water (Abu Dawud). A review or the nutritional and functional constituents of dates and their seeds are described in Al-Farsi and Lee (2008). The flesh of the date is found to be low in fat and protein but rich in sugars, mainly fructose and glucose' and in minerals including selenium, copper, potassium, and magnesium; the major vitamins are the vitamin B-complex and vitamin C. It is high in dietary fibres 8.0g per 100g. Dates are a good source of antioxidants, mainly carotenoids and phenolics' and are a high source of energy, as 100g of flesh can provide an average of 314 kcal.

Maintaining a well-balanced food and fluid intake is important between fasts. The meals should contain adequate levels of 'energy food' such as some fat and carbohydrates. Hence, a balanced diet with adequate quantities of nutrients, salts and water is vital. Ramadan is a month of self-regulation and self-training, with the hope that this training will last beyond the end of Ramadan (Athar, 1998). Not only can overeating during the period of Ramadan harm the body but it is thought also to interfere with a person's spiritual growth during the month (Community in Action, 2007). It has been advocated that the faithful indulging in overeating during the Holy Month should remember that Ramadan is a month of austerity and of exercising self-restraint (Sheikh Abdus Salam Al Basuni, 2009). Moreover, the exhaustive culinary preparations for Ramadan that most Muslims engage in are contrary to Allah's orders and contradict the true spirit of Ramadan. They are also unhealthy and uneconomical (Sheikh Muhammad al-Hamad). Ibn al-Qayyim (cited in Sheikh Muhammad al-Hamad) stated that:

> Overeating leads to all sorts of evil consequences. How many are the sins that have come about as a result of satiation and overeating. How many are the good deeds that have failed to materialize on account of it. Whoever safeguards himself from the evil of his stomach has indeed saved himself from a great evil. When a soul is satiated, it becomes restless and goes about seeking opportunities for indulgence. When it is hungry, it becomes tranquil and shows humility and submissiveness.

For the main post-fast meal, some guidelines on the foods that benefit and foods that harm are presented in Table 10.3. The Noble Qur'aan and the Prophetic traditions have not only stated the permissible and impermissible

Table 10.3 Food that benefits and food that harms

Food that benefits	Examples
Complex carbohydrates are foods that will help release energy slowly during the long hours of fasting.	Barley, wheat, oats, millets, semolina, beans, lentils, wholemeal flour, basmati rice, etc.
Fibre-rich foods are also digested slowly.	Bran, cereals, whole wheat, grains and seeds, potatoes with the skin, vegetables such as green beans, and almost all fruit, including apricots, prunes, figs, etc.
Food that harms	**Alternative foods**
Deep-fried foods, e.g. pakoras, samosas, fried dumplings.	Whole grains, e.g. chickpeas (plain, or with potato, in yoghurt, with different Indian spices), samosas baked instead of fried, and boiled dumplings.

(Continued)

Table 10.3   Continued

High-sugar/high-fat foods, e.g. Indian sweets such as ghulab jamun, rasgulla, balushahi, baklawa.	Milk-based sweets and puddings, e.g. rasmalai, barfee.
High-fat cooked foods, e.g. parathas, oily curries, greasy pastries.	Alternate with chapattis made without oil, and baked or grilled meat and chicken. Try to make pastry at home and use a single layer.
Cooking methods to avoid	**Alternative cooking methods**
Deep frying	Shallow frying – usually there is very little difference in taste.
Frying	Grilling or baking is healthier and helps retain the taste and original flavour of the food, especially chicken and fish.
Curries with excessive oil	Start with measuring the oil used in curry and try to bring the oil content down gradually, e.g. reducing five tablespoons to four. This is a good way of reducing oil without noticing much difference in the taste. A useful tip is to use more onions and tomatoes in the bulk of the curry.

Source: Adapted from Community in Action (2007) Ramadan Health Guide. © Crown Copyright 2007. Reproduced under the Open Government Licence v.2.0.

foods but go to the extent of giving useful tips regarding a balanced diet. This also corresponds to modern guidelines on a healthy diet and will help to maintain balanced, healthy meals during Ramadan (Community in Action, 2007). The foods most commonly consumed by Prophet Muhammad include milk, dates, lamb/mutton and oats. Healthy foods mentioned in the Noble Qur'aan are fruit and vegetables, such as olives, onions, cucumber, figs, dates, grapes, as well as pulses such as lentils. The encouragement of eating fish can be seen in the fact that Islamic law spares fish from any specific slaughter requirements, making it easy to incorporate fish in a meal (Community in Action, 2007).

Light exercise is also recommended for everyone, and specifically those who have sedentary jobs. Light exercise includes stretching or walking. It is important to follow good time management practices for prayers and other religious activities, and for sleep, studies, job, and physical activities or exercise (islamic-world.net).

Food and drinks: total avoidance

It is important during Ramadan and post-Ramadan to avoid the heavily-processed, fast-burning foods that contain refined carbohydrates in the form of sugar and white flour, or too much fatty food. The intake of fried and high-fat cooked foods such as parathas, oily curries, greasy pastries and deep-fried foods such as pakoras, samosas, and fried dumplings should be avoided if possible, or consumed minimally. It is also desirable to avoid caffeine drinks such as coffee, cola, or tea. Caffeine is a diuretic and stimulates faster water loss through urination. Three days to five days before Ramadan, gradually reduce the intake of these drinks. A sudden decrease in caffeine prompts headaches, mood swings and irritability. Smoking is a health risk factor in many diseases as well as being unacceptable. If you cannot give up smoking, cut down gradually starting a few weeks before Ramadan. Smoking has a negative effect on utilisation of various vitamins, metabolites and enzyme systems in the body.

Potential health complications

There are potential health complications that may develop during the month of Ramadan. If someone has either high or low blood pressure, it is recommended that they see their medical practitioner before the start of Ramadan for possible review of medications. For those with low blood pressure, it is recommended that they ask for advice on their intake of fluids and salts. Table 10.4 presents some of the potential health complications during Ramadan and their management.

There are certain behaviours that invalidate the fast – that is, abstaining from food, liquids and sexual activity from dawn to sunset. The intention to fast must be made every day before dawn. The intention (*niyyah*) may be made at night before going to sleep or it can also be made at the time of the pre-fast meal (*Suhoor*) before dawn. Some of the behaviours that invalidate the fast are presented in Table 10.5.

Table 10.4   Potential health complications and interventions

Potential health complications	Interventions
Headache, mood swings and irritability	• Avoid caffeinated drinks such as cola, coffee or tea. • Avoid smoking.
Muscle cramps	• Increase intake of vegetables, fruit, meat or dairy products in the diet.
Dehydration	• Drink lots of water.
Constipation	• Maintain good hydration (drink water). • Eat lots of fruit and vegetables. • Increase the fibre content of your diet (e.g. eat bran). • Light activity.
Stress	• Correct for causes such as lack of food or water, changes in routine, disturbed sleeping pattern.
Heartburn, indegestion	• Medication for indegestion: antacids (e.g. Gaviscon), antihistamines (e.g. Zantac) or proton pump inhibitors (e.g. Losec, Zoton or Nexium). • Dietary fibre helps reduce gastric acidity.
Control of heartburn or belching/colic	• Avoid spicy, oily, deep-fried food. • Stop smoking. • Reduce caffeine intake. • Peppermint oil may help reduce belching or colic. • Sleep with your head raised on a few pillows. • Long-term weight loss.
Peptic ulcer	• Avoid spicy foods and consult a doctor for appropriate medicine and diet.
Diabetes (Type 1) on insulin	• Advised not to fast.
Diabetes (Type 2)	• Visit general practitionner before Ramadan to review medications, if appropriate. • Regular self-monitoring of blood glucose.

(Continued)

Table 10.4 Continued

Potential health complications	Interventions
	• Low blood sugar levels (hypoglycaemia) are dangerous, and if untreated may lead to fainting or fits.
	• People with complications such as angina or heart failure, stroke, retinopathy (eye disease), nephropathy (kidney disease) or neuropathy should seek medical advice.

Source: Adapted from Community in Action (2007) Ramadan Health Guide. © Crown Copyright 2007. Reproduced under the Open Government Licence v.2.0.

Table 10.5 Behaviours that invalidate the fast

Smoking	Tobacco and smokeless tobacco.
Blood transfusion	For those who are fasting.
Gastroscopy	If the gastroscope is inserted into the stomach without introducing any other substances, then it does not break the fast, but if some greasy substance or anything else is introduced with it then it does invalidate the fast.
Water	Slipping down the throat while making *wudu* (performing ablution) even if not done deliberately.
Nutrient injections	
Vomiting	Intentional vomiting nullifies one's fasting.
Deliberate drinking and eating	These would nullify the fast but if an individual forgets that he is fasting and unconsciously has an intake of food or drink, the validity of his fast is not affected.
Ejaculation	Ejaculation nullifies fasting when it results from kissing, touching, masturbating or lustful gazing. There is no expiation but the individual is obliged to make up for it. Wet dream is excluded from this.

(*Continued*)

Table 10.5 Continued

Sexual intercourse	If a man has sexual intercourse with his wife, his fasting is not valid. He is obliged to make up for that day. In addition, the individual will have to expiate for it. The acts of expiation include fasting for two months consecutively, and if unable to fast due to a legal excuse, he should feed sixty poor persons.
Sublingual medication	Medicines that are placed under the tongue to treat angina pectoris and other problems, do not invalidate the fast, so long as one avoids swallowing anything that reaches the throat.
Medication-injections, inhalers	Taking tablets invalidates the fast. Injections, inhalers, patches, ear drops etc. that are not comparable to food and drink do not break the fast. (It is advisable to avoid these if possible, due to the difference of opinion among Muslim jurists.)
Asthma	Muslim jurists differ on this issue. Using an asthma inhaler is not classified as eating or drinking- and is regarded as permissible by some. Others argue that as the inhaler provides small amounts of liquid medicine to the lungs, it breaks the fast. However, the strongest opinion is that it is permissible for an asthma patient to use an inhaler during Ramadan.

However, there are some behaviours that do not invalidate the fast. These include:

- Forgetting that one is fasting. Anyone who forgets that they are fasting and eats or drinks should complete the fast, for it is only Allah who has fed them and given them drink. (Muslim)
- Unintentional vomiting.
- Breastfeeding a baby.
- Swallowing things that it is not possible to avoid, such as one's saliva, street dust, smoke, etc.
- Ejaculation of semen during sleep.
- Brushing the teeth. When using powder or paste to clean the teeth, if anything of these substances slips down the throat, the fast is nullified.

- Using a *miswak* to clean the teeth, even if the *miswak* is fresh and has a taste.
- Injection or intra-venous drips which are solely medical and not nutritional.

Implications for nursing

Nurses have an important preventative role to play during the month of Ramadan. Ramadan provides a window of opportunity for nurses to promote health improvement among Muslims by offering healthy lifestyle advice on topics such as nutrition, diet, alcohol, drug use and smoking cessation. However, nurses and other healthcare professionals must be aware that Muslim communities in the Western world are a heterogeneous group with varying attitudes towards lifestyles and health behaviours. Fasting during Ramadan is intended as a discipline and requires total abstinence from dawn to dusk for a month. This includes food, water and smoking. Fasting is a requirement after puberty for all able-bodied Muslims of sound mind and good health, but there are concessions for old people, those who are on a journey or who are ill, as well as for women during menstruation, post-natal bleeding, pregnancy or breastfeeding.

Fasting may have an impact on diseases affecting the cardiovascular, renal and gastrointestinal systems, such as hypertension, renal impairment and peptic ulcers. In elderly people, fasting may not be well tolerated physiologically due to those chronic conditions. It is important that the nurse or healthcare professional monitor the patients' condition in case of detrimental consequences. However, for people with chronic conditions (for example, ophthalmic, dermatological, or neurological problems), fasting may have no impact and can continue as normal. If oral medication is required, fasting can be facilitated by reducing the dose to once or twice daily. Sheikh Ibn Baaz was asked about the ruling on a person who has blood taken when he is fasting in Ramadan for the purpose of testing. He replied: 'A test of this nature does not affect the fast, rather it is excused, because it is something needed, and it is not like the things that are known to break the fast according to shari'ah' (Sheikh Ibn Baaz, 15/274).

During pregnancy and breastfeeding, the mother's nutrition and hydration are paramount and, while fasting is permissible, it is medically better for the mother to utilise the concession and compensate for or make up the missed fasts at a later time (Community in Action, 2007). Or if she fears for herself or for the baby, she can break the fast and pay the 'ransom', in which case she does not have to make up the days missed (Sabiq, 1991). It is clear that physical examinations do not invalidate the fast, but for patients who require clinical investigations such as blood tests, or those requiring intravenous access or oral contrast, these would preclude the fast during those particular days. However, where there is a high risk of complications for the patient, investigations should clearly not be delayed.

In relation to Muslims with diabetes, there is evidence to suggest that management of their condition before, during and after the month of Ramadan is vital to ensure that patients with diabetes who wish to fast do so safely (Omar and Motala, 1997; Sulimani, 1997). It is important that diabetics adjust their drug treatments, particularly those patients diagnosed with insulin dependent diabetes mellitus. There are three important factors: drug regimen adjustment, diet control and daily activity – the 'Ramadan 3D Triangle' (Azizi and Siahkolah, 1998). The monitoring of blood glucose is an important prerequisite in the management of patients whose diabetes whether it is treated with insulin or without insulin (Azizi and Siahkolah, 1998). This observation would enable the review of, and adjustments to, the insulin dose required by the patient. Khodabaccus (2009) suggested that clinic-based blood tests should also be performed and records made of any hypoglycaemic and hyperglycaemic attacks so that patients may be advised to discontinue fasting if necessary. According to Khodabaccus (2009), patients should also be educated so that they understand:

- How and when to check their urine for acetone
- The warning symptoms of dehydration, hypoglycaemia and hyperglycaemia
- The need to break their fast as soon as any complication or harmful condition occurs
- The importance of seeking immediate medical help if they have concerns regarding the management of their diabetes.

These educational programmes should commence before the fasting month so that patients are well prepared. For the management of addictive behaviour problems such as alcohol or drug use, see Chapters 13 and 14.

It has been stated that fasting during Ramadan is prescribed for every healthy, adult Muslim whereas the weak, the sick, children, travellers and menstruating women are among those exempt. The Qur'aan specifically exempts the sick from fasting (2:183–5), especially if fasting might lead to harmful consequences for the individual. But if the sickness is temporary, such as a cough or headache, then the missed fasts must be made up later. An individual who is suffering from a chronic illness and has no hope of recovery, and elderly people who are unable to fast, should feed a poor person some of the staple food of his country (equivalent to one and a half kilograms of rice) for every day that has been missed. It is permissible to do this all at once, on one day at the end of the month, or to feed one poor person every day. It has to be done by giving actual food and cannot be done by giving money to the poor (Sheikh Muhammed Salih Al-Munajjid).

In general, patients with Type 1 diabetes, especially if their diabetes is poorly controlled, are at very high risk of developing severe complications and should be strongly advised not to fast during Ramadan. In addition, patients who are unwilling or unable to monitor their blood glucose levels numerous times daily are at high risk and should be advised not to fast (Al-Arouj et al., 2005). It is stated that 'Patients with Type 1 diabetes who have a history of recurrent hypoglycaemia or hypoglycaemia unawareness, or who are poorly controlled, are at very high risk for developing severe hypoglycaemia. On the other hand, an excessive reduction in the insulin dosage in these patients (to prevent hypoglycaemia) may place them at risk for hyperglycaemia and diabetic ketoacidosis' (Al-Arouj et al., 2005). However, the dilemma arises for health professionals when a Muslim patient wants to fast during Ramadan, but doing so will compromise their health.

Reflective Activity 10.2

Case Study 1

A 65-year-old female with diabetes Type 2 and a long-standing hypertension was non-compliant with her prescribed treatment regimen. She was unable to control her weight and had several episodes of hospital admissions due to complications of her diabetes and hypertension. She was on diabetic, anti-hypertensive and diuretics medications. She wants to fast for Ramadan despite recommendations from her General Practitioner (medical doctor) not to fast during Ramadan.

Case Study 2

A 27-year-old South Asian man has a five-year history of Type 1 diabetes, which was diagnosed when he presented with diabetic ketoacidosis. His initial insulin treatment was complicated by poor glycaemia control, frequent hypoglycaemia, and weight gain. He was admitted to hospital recently due to an episode of angina, and denied the implications of his disorders. He is a devout Muslim and wants to fast during the month of Ramadan.

- How would be you approach these situations?
- How are you going to convince the patient that fasting would be detrimental to their health?

- Who would you involve in 'counselling' the patient?
- What health education activities could be implemented to ensure Muslim patients are prepared for Ramadan?

Comments on Reflective Activity 10.2

The patient's decision to fast during Ramadan should be made after ample discussion with his or her doctor or physician concerning the risks involved. Their doctors and diabetes care specialists should assess whether they increase their health risk by doing so (Al-Arouj et al., 2005). In the above cases, these patients are at high risk and should be advised not to fast as it can lead to worsening diabetes control. But if they continue to insist on fasting, going against medical advice, the decision maker in the family, or a significant person or the local *Imam* (religious preacher), should be involved in persuading the patient not to fast. If the patient insists in fasting for Ramadan, some general good practice guidelines include:

- Be aware of customs that show respect. This will help to establish a strong rapport with the patient, their family and their friends.
- Ensure clear communication about the high risks of doing the Ramadan fast, because of their medical conditions.
- Although people with a moderate comprehension of English may appear to understand discussions, use a professional interpreter to communicate complex medical information.
- Use written material, if appropriate, to help disseminate information to all family members and others about the risks of fasting with the existing medical conditions.
- Consider a family meeting.
- The significant person or the key decision maker may not be the partner or the primary caregiver.
- Be aware of family dynamics.
- Offer the family the opportunity to have a religious advisor in attendance.
- Ensure the family and the patient understand the risks of doing Ramadan.
- Invite them to ask questions.
- Keep a written record of all communications.

Some patients, for example those with diabetes Type 1 on insulin medications, may be able to fast. For those patients, a pre-Ramadan assessment is required and they should receive a complete physical examination with their doctor. This can ensure good health, along with necessary education related to physical activity, meal planning, glucose monitoring, dosage and timing of medications. Hui et al. (2010) suggest that if patients choose to fast despite medical advice, it will help if they are familiar with carbohydrate counting. They suggest that the patients reduce their background insulin by 20% and omit the midday rapid-acting insulin if their capillary blood glucose concentration is ≤7 mmol/l. If their blood glucose concentration is >7 mmol/l, patients will need to calculate their insulin correction dose as determined by their specialists. However, whether the patient is being treated or monitored in a hospital or a community setting, the care management plan must be highly individualised, based on the needs of the patient. There should be close monitoring, and follow-up is essential to reduce the risk of developing complications.

Primarily, the religious sanction should take precedence when medical advice is being given not to fast. If the patient insists on fasting, he or she will be going against the clear guidance given in the Qur'aan (interpretation of the meaning):

☐ *But if any of you is ill, or on a journey, the prescribed number (of Ramadan days) should be made up from days later. For those who cannot do this except with hardship there is a ransom: the feeding of one that is indigent. ... Allah intends every ease for you; He does not want to put you to difficulties...* (Al-Baqara [The Cow] 2:184–5)

That is, not to fast if sick because sickness would adversely affect the patient's well-being during the fasting period. A sick Muslim who fasts would jeopardise his health further, thus ultimately will benefit neither himself nor his role in society and he should be discouraged from observing the fast (Akhtar). The ultimate decision remains with the patient. It is important to remember that it is unlikely that a healthcare professional will be legitimately criticised if a competent patient has made an informed decision to pursue a particular course of action.

Conclusion

This chapter has made an attempt to illustrate that there is Islamic guidance to ensure that fasting is not prejudicial to a patient's health. Islamic fasting is different from total fasting or crash diet plans because in Ramadan fasting, there is no malnutrition, selected food exclusion or inadequate calorie intake. Fasting during the entire month of Ramadan is reserved usually for healthy Muslims. However, people with stable chronic diseases (of the heart, lung, liver, etc.) may fast; but they should consult their medical practitioner on the potential risk. Generally, people requiring multiple oral/injected medications during the day should not fast. Islam places the responsibility for practising religion on the individual and, as a result, it is important that nurses or other healthcare professionals discuss religious observance needs with each patient. Since not all fasting Muslim patients will mention their religious practices during Ramadan, healthcare providers may want to offer a discussion of how to fast safely and successfully. Good communication and open dialogue are the key to providing culturally sensitive care.

References

Abu Dawud – Book 13, Hadith 2349.

Akhtar, S. *Fasting during Ramadan: a Muslim pharmacist's perspective*, www.deenislam.co.uk/dua/Ramadan/10.htm, date accessed 4 August 2013.

Al-Arouj, M., Bouguerra, R., Buse, J., Hafez, S., Hassanein, M., Ibrahim, M.A. et al. (2005) 'American Diabetes Association Recommendations for Management of Diabetes during Ramadan', *Diabetes Care* 28, 9, 2305–11.

Al-Farsi, M.A. and Lee, C.Y. (2008) 'Nutritional and Functional Properties of Dates: A Review,. *Critical Review in Food Science and Nutrition* 48, 10, 877–87.

Aroura, A. (1982) Community Health in Islamic Perspectives, Paper entitled *'Islamic Perspectives on Philosophy and Policy of Health'*, presented at the Second International Meeting on Islamic Medicine, Islamic Medical Organisation, Kuwait, www.islamset.com/hip/ahmed_aroua.html, date accessed 4 August 2013.

Athar, S. (1998) *Ramadan Fasting*, www.islamic-world.net/sister/h24.htm, date accessed 4 August 2013.

Azizi, F. and Siahkolah, B. (1998) 'Ramadan Fasting and Diabetes Mellitus', *International Journal of Ramadan Fasting Research* 2, 8–17.

Bukhari no. 1923, cited in www.islamlecture.com/books/ramadaan%201434%20A%20H/Ahaadeeth%20%28al-Bukhaaree%20and%20Muslim%29/1-The%20Excellence%20of%20Taking%20the%20Sahoor.pdf, date accessed 4 August 2013.

Communities in Action (2007) *Ramadan Health Guide – A Guide to Healthy Fasting*, www.dh.gov.uk/prod_consum_dh/groups/dh_digitalassets/@dh/@en/documents/digitalasset/dh_078408.pdf, date accessed 4 August 2013.

Hakim, cited in www.islaminfocentre.org.uk/articles/51-happy-ramadan.html, date accessed 4 August 2013.

Hui, E., Bravis, V., Hassanein, M., Hanif, W., Malik, R., Chowdhury, T.A., Suliman, M. and Devendra, D. (2010) 'Management of People with Diabetes Wanting to Fast during Ramadan', *British Medical Journal* 340: c3053, www.bmj.com/content/340/bmj.c3053.full?ijkey=RhP6 GwQb5TAzfiq&keytype=ref, date accessed 4 August 2013.

Kalantan, cited in Khodabukus, R. (2009) 'Advising Patients with Diabetes about Fasting during Ramadan', *Nursing Times* 99, 28, 26.

Khodabukus, R. (2009) 'Advising Patients with Diabetes about Fasting during Ramadan', *Nursing Times* 99, 28, 26–7.

Muslim [a] 2544, 4/406. Sahih Muslim – Book 04 – *The Book of Prayers, Kitab Al-Salat*, www.docstoc.com/docs/14981232/Sahih-Muslim—Book-04—The-Book-of-Prayers-_Kitab-Al-Salat, date accessed 4 August 2013.

Muslim [b], http://sunnah.org/ibadaat/fasting/sawm.html.

Nomani, M.Z.A. (1997) 'Dietary Fat, Blood Cholesterol and Uric Acid Levels during Ramadan Fasting', *International Journal of Ramadan Fasting Research* 1, 1, 1–6.

Nomani, M.Z.A. *Diet during Ramadan*, www.islamic-world.net/, date accessed 4 August 2013.

Muslim, no. 2412, cited in www.islamlecture.com/books/ramadaan% 201434%20A%20H/Ahaadeeth%20%28al-Bukhaaree%20and%20Muslim %29/1-The%20Excellence%20of%20Taking%20the%20Sahoor.pdf, date accessed 4 August 2013.

Omar, M. and Motala, A. (1997) 'Fasting in Ramadan and the Diabetic Patient', *Diabetes Care* 20, 38, 1925–6.

Rassool, G. Hussein (1995) 'The Health Status and Health Care of Ethno-Cultural Minorities in the United Kingdom: an Agenda for Action', *Journal of Advanced Nursing* 21, 2, 199–201.

Sabiq, A.S. (1991) *Fiqh us-Sunnah*, Vol. III (Washington: American Trust Publications).

Sheikh Abdus Salam Al Basuni (2009) *Avoid Overeating during Ramadan*, www. arabianbusiness.com/avoid-overeating-during-ramadan-islamic-scholar-14466.html, date accessed 4 August 2013.

Sheikh Al-Fawzan, S. (2009) *A Summary of Islamic Jurisprudence*, Volume 1 (Riyadh, Saudi Arabia: Al-Mainman Publishing House).

Sheikh Ibn Baaz. Majmoo' Fataawa Ibn Baaz, 15/274, cited in http://islamqa. info/en/50406, date accessed 23 October 2013.

Sheikh Muhammad al-Hamad. *'Eat and drink, but be not excessive'*, http://en.islamtoday.net/artshow-267-3155.htm, date accessed 4 August 2013.

Sheikh Muhammed Salih Al-Munajjid (Fataawa al-Lajnah al-Daa'imah, 10/198).

Al-Siyaam 70 Matters Related to Fasting, www.islam-qa.com/en/ref/books/105, date accessed 4 August 2013.

Sulimani, R.A. (1997) 'Management of Typical 2 Diabetes with Oral Agent during Ramadan', in *The Congress of the Diabetes Mellitus During the Holy Month of Ramadan* (Cairo, Egypt), p. 8 (Abstract).

Sulimani, R.A, Laajam, M., Al-Attas, O. et al. (1999) 'The Effect of Ramadan Fasting on Diabetes Control Type II Diabetic Patients', *Nutrition Research* 11, 23, 261–4.

11 Pilgrimage (*Hajj*) and Health Considerations

G. Hussein Rassool

Learning Outcomes:

- Have an understanding of Islamic beliefs and the importance of *Hajj*.
- Identify the health and safety risks associated with *Hajj*.
- Provide advice and guidance on how to ensure patients are prepared for the journey of *Hajj*.
- Examine the specific factors for poor diabetic control during *Hajj*.
- Describe the practical considerations and management of people with diabetes intending to perform the *Hajj*.

Reflective Activity 11.1

State whether the following statements are true or false. Give reasons for your answers.

	True	False
1 *Hajj* refers to the pilgrimage to Makkah.		
2 According to Islam, every physically able Muslim must undertake the *Hajj* more than once in his or her lifetime.		
3 Makkah is also the setting for a smaller ritual called *Umrah*, performed year-round.		
4 The holy object within the square shrine of the Kaa'ba is a black meteorite.		
5 Face-masks cannot be used during the *Hajj*, to reduce the airborne transmission of disease.		
6 All pilgrims and local at-risk populations must now be given the quadrivalent polysaccharide vaccine.		

	True	False
7 Food poisoning is another important cause of diarrhoea and vomiting during the *Hajj*.		
8 Cardiovascular disease is the most common cause (43%) of death during the *Hajj*.		
9 It has been suggested that those who are not accustomed to high temperatures are not more liable to sunstroke than the residents of tropical regions.		
10 The symptoms of heatstroke can develop over several days in vulnerable people, such as the elderly and those with long-term health problems.		
11 *Id al-Adha* is the Day of Sacrifice during the month of the *Hajj*, when an animal is sacrificed to recall the submission of Abraham.		
12 Muslim women complete the *Hajj* by shaving their heads.		
13 The *Hajj* pilgrimage includes long rituals involving standing and walking coupled with heat, sweating, and obesity, which contribute to the risk of skin infections.		
14 Diabetes is common among Muslims and has been reported as a rising leading cause of morbidity and mortality during *Hajj*.		
15 It is not permissible for the Muslim woman to wear any women's clothes she pleases.		
16 There is no problem of hypoglycaemia even if the insulin in Saudi Arabia is different from that of the patient's country of origin.		
17 Diabetics with neuropathy have developed deep burns that involved the entire weight-bearing area of the sole.		

Introduction

One of the pillars of the Islamic faith and a major act of Islam is the pilgrimage (*Hajj*) to Makkah, in Saudi Arabia. In the Qur'aan, Allah stated that (interpretation of meaning):

☐ *In it are clear signs [such as] the standing place of Abraham. And whoever enters it shall be safe. And [due] to Allah from the people is a pilgrimage to the*

> *House – for whoever is able to find thereto a way. But whoever disbelieves – then indeed, Allah is free from need of the worlds.* ('Āli 'Imrān [The Family of Imran] 3:97)

It is therefore obligatory for all adult Muslims who can afford to undertake the journey and are in good health. The main purpose of *Hajj* and *Umrah* (lesser pilgrimage) is to worship Allah in the places he commanded us to worship Him (Sheikh Al-Fawzan, 2009). It is stated that the Prophet said: 'Perform *Hajj* only once and whoever performs it more than that, it is a voluntary act for Him' (Muslim). According to Sheikh Al-Fawzan (2009, p. 405), there are five conditions that must be fulfilled as prerequisites in the performance of *Hajj*: to be a Muslim; to be sane; to have reached puberty; to be free; and to be able to perform it (physically and financially). Those who meet these requirements are obliged, without delay, to perform *Hajj*, and those who defer it without a valid excuse are deemed sinful. However, if a person can afford *Hajj* financially but is in poor health, or has a chronic disease or is disabled, in this case, that person may assign someone to perform *Hajj* on their behalf. Many Muslims from all over the world will make the journey to perform *Hajj* and the lesser pilgrimage on one or more occasions. Mass gatherings such as the *Hajj* are associated with unique health risks including problems of infectious diseases, heat and injury. This chapter examines briefly the rites and significance of *Hajj* and the health risks associated with it, and the appropriate preventive actions that need to be taken to reduce the risk and harm.

The spiritual journey

Hajj lasts for five days, and, as the Islamic calendar is lunar, the precise Gregorian calendar dates of the *Hajj* season will vary each year (Gatrad and Sheikh, 2005). The *Hajj* is performed on the eighth, ninth and tenth of the month of *Dhu al-Ḥijjah* (the twelfth and final month in the Islamic calendar). This spiritual journey starts with the intention that the performance of *Hajj* is only for the sake of Allah. It is stated that an individual who intends to perform *Hajj* should repent of all sins; ask the forgiveness of those who have been wronged; repay all trusts, loans and debts; and ensure that the money used for the expenses of the pilgrimage is lawfully obtained (Sheikh Al-Fawzan, 2009, p. 416). During the *Hajj* rites, a pilgrim should also treat people with kindness and good manners, avoid quarrelling or annoying others, or backbiting, and safeguard his tongue against insult (Sheikh Al-Fawzan, p. 416). It is narrated that the Prophet Muhammad, Allah's final messenger, said: 'Perform *Hajj* and *Umrah* (lesser pilgrimage) making them follow each other, for they remove poverty and sins as a blacksmith's bellows removes impurities from iron, gold and silver. And an accepted *Hajj* gets no reward less than Paradise' (Tirmidhî [a] et al.).

It is important to note that an accepted performance of *Hajj* is the completion of all the rites, unblemished by ill deeds, and is also that which is worthy of being accepted by Allah (Sheikh Al-Fawzan, p. 416). Before the performance of *Hajj* or the lesser pilgrimage, an individual must enter the state of *Ihram* (derived from the Arabic word *haram* – forbidden or prohibited). This state involves the declaration of the intention to perform the rites of *Hajj* or *Umrah*; the wearing of the two pieces of cloth worn by male pilgrims; and the state of consecration in which the pilgrims are, during *Hajj* or *Umrah*. There are restrictions regarding men's footwear as these should not cover the toes and ankles (socks and shoes are prohibited). For women there are no restrictions. There are specific places where a pilgrim must enter the state of *Ihram* before heading for Makkah. Once a pilgrim assumes the state of *Ihram*, he or she should recite the *Talbiyah*, meaning:

☐ *'Here I am at Your service, O Allah, here I am at Your service. Here I am at Your Service, You have no partner, here I am at Your service. Verily, all praise, blessings, and dominion are Yours. You have no partner.'*

After arriving in Makkah, pilgrims go to the Grand Mosque, which contains the Kaa'ba, the most sacred site in Islam, and perform a circumambulation (*tawaaf*), circling the Kaa'ba seven times counter-clockwise. A single circumambulation can take hours, especially before or after the compulsory prayers. In addition to *tawaaf*, pilgrims perform *sa'i*, walking or running seven times between the hills of Safa and Marwah (now enclosed by the Grand Mosque). On the morning of *Dhul-Hijjah* 8, the pilgrims are recommended to move to Mina where they spend the rest of the day and the night, performing five prayers there. After the sun rises on *Dhul-Hijjah* 9, pilgrims leave Mina and proceed to Arafat. *Hajj* culminates on the Plain of Arafat, where pilgrims spend the day in supplication, praying and reading the Qur'aan; it is the pinnacle of most pilgrims' spiritual lives. The Prophet said, 'The *Hajj* is Arafat' (Tirmidhî [b]). After sunset, the pilgrims leave for Muzdalifah and spend the night in an open area. Afterwards the pilgrims head for Mina shortly before sunrise for the symbolic ritual of stoning the devil at Jamaraat. After Jamaraat, pilgrims traditionally sacrificed an animal to symbolise the ram that the Prophet Abraham sacrificed instead of his son. 'Eid al-Adha', the 'Festival of the Sacrifice', begins on the tenth day and ends on the thirteenth of that month. After a final *tawaaf*, pilgrims leave Makkah, ending the *Hajj*. Many pilgrims go to Madina to visit the Mosque of the Prophet before leaving Saudi Arabia. All the different rituals and practices are physically demanding and require the pilgrims to be in a state of optimum health.

Health risks of pilgrims

There are many health risks associated with *Hajj*, and pilgrims should be made aware of the potential risks and given appropriate prevention health education. In the Kingdom of Saudi Arabia, the temperature may range between 44°C and 50°C during the *Hajj* season and heat exhaustion and heatstroke are leading causes of illness. Sunburn is a significant risk for those pilgrims who are light skinned, who come from mainly the Northern Hemisphere. It has been suggested that those who are not accustomed to high temperatures are more liable to sunstroke than the residents of tropical regions (Al-Khateeb). In addition, pilgrims who are aged, frail, obese, or have high blood pressure, diabetes or heart failure, are easily susceptible to this condition. The use of an appropriate strength sun block is important to minimise the risk of burning, with its associated risk of malignant melanomas (Sheikh and Gatrad, 2008). Some of the symptoms of sunburn include: red, sore skin, skin that is warm and tender to the touch, and flaking and peeling skin after a number of days (usually 4 to 7 days after exposure). The symptoms of sunburn usually begin 3 to 5 hours after exposure to the sun's rays and peak between 12 and 24 hours after being in the sun. Severe sunburn is a medical emergency.

Heat exhaustion and heatstroke are common amongst pilgrims. The symptoms of heatstroke can develop over several days in vulnerable people, such as the elderly and those with long-term health problems. The symptoms of heat exhaustion include: confusion, dark-coloured urine (a sign of dehydration), dizziness, fainting, fatigue, headache, muscle cramps, nausea, pale skin, profuse sweating and rapid heartbeat. The extreme heat that causes heatstroke also affects the nervous system, which can cause other symptoms such as mental confusion, fits (seizures), restlessness or anxiety, problems understanding or speaking to others, hallucinations and loss of consciousness. Heatstroke is a medical emergency and should be treated as such. Pilgrims should be advised to take precautions such as using an umbrella, seeking shade as much as possible, drinking plenty of water (bottled) (to avoid dehydration), wearing sunscreen, and having adequate rest. Some of the rituals can be performed at night to avoid daytime heat.

Infectious diseases

Mass gatherings such as the *Hajj*, where millions of people share crowded spaces and experience extreme heat and exhaustion, wearing down their immune systems, create an ideal environment for spreading infectious diseases. Among the communicable diseases recorded at *Hajj* in the past are meningitis, tuberculosis, polio and zoonotic diseases (any disease or infection that is naturally transmissible from vertebrate animals to humans and vice-versa) (Tomasulo, 2011). The '*Hajj* cough" is the most common complaint of pilgrims. It is reported that the severity and clinical spectrum of disease varies, from mild inconvenience to severe pneumonia leading to hospitalisation and even death (Madani et al., 2006). However, Saudi Arabia provides free health care to all pilgrims during the *Hajj* and also implements stringent infection control measures (Memish, 2010). Because outbreaks of meningococcal disease used to be a problem during the *Hajj*, the Saudi Ministry of Health now requires all pilgrims to receive the meningococcal vaccine, and a medical certificate confirming vaccination is now required before visas will be issued. A change of the *Hajj* pilgrimage requirements from bivalent to quadrivalent (A, C, Y, W 135) meningococcal polysaccharide vaccine has eliminated future meningococcal outbreaks (Borrow, 2009). *Hajj* pilgrims must have had the meningococcal vaccine less than 3 years and more than 10 days before arriving in Saudi Arabia.

Hepatitis A and B and typhoid vaccines are also recommended. Although a requirement for polio vaccine does not include pilgrims from some countries, it is best to ensure full vaccination against polio or to receive an adult booster before travel. Current vaccination requirements are available from the website of the Saudi Arabian Ministry of Health (www.moh.gov. sa). A yellow fever vaccination certificate showing that the person was vaccinated at least 10 days previously and not more than 10 years before arrival is a requirement for all travellers arriving from countries or areas at risk of yellow fever transmission. All visitors aged under 15 years travelling to Saudi Arabia from countries re-infected with poliomyelitis, should be vaccinated against poliomyelitis with the oral polio vaccine (OPV), with proof of vaccination (Editorial, 2010). It is reported that respiratory tract infections are common during *Hajj*, and the most common cause of hospital admission is pneumonia. There are recommendations for pneumococcal polysaccharide vaccine for pilgrims aged ≥65 years and for younger pilgrims with comorbidities (Ahmed and Balaban, 2012). Seasonal influenza vaccine is recommended for all pilgrims.

Other health and safety risks

Diarrhoeal disease is common during *Hajj*, and pilgrims should be educated on the usual prevention measures and self-treatment. Food poisoning is another important cause of diarrhoea and vomiting during the *Hajj* (Al-Mazrou, 2004). Prevention of diarrhoeal diseases includes education of the pilgrims regarding hand hygiene, avoidance of street vendor food (including ice), and avoidance of foods made with fresh eggs (Ahmed et al., 2006). Pilgrims should also take with them oral rehydration therapy and self-treatment for diarrhoea. An anti-motility agent (such as loperamide) can be carried and an antibiotic (Ciprofloxacin, 500mg twice daily for up to three days, in the absence of contraindications) should be considered, especially for those travellers who have an underlying medical condition (www.nathnac.org/travel). Advice should also be provided to potential pilgrims on the importance of eating only food that is cooked and served hot, and of drinking only beverages from sealed containers.

There is a need to remind pilgrims of the importance of seeking medical attention for any unexpected symptoms, such as fever, diarrhoea or jaundice, or a high fever on their return (Sheikh and Gatrad, 2008). The *Hajj* pilgrimage includes long rituals of standing and walking, which, when coupled with heat, sweating, and obesity, contribute to the risk of skin infections. Pilgrims should be advised to keep skin dry, use talcum powder, and be aware of any pain or soreness caused by garments or belts (or by a strip of fabric torn from *Ihram* material) (Ahmed and Balaban, 2012). In addition, any sores or blisters that develop should be disinfected and kept covered.

At the end of *Hajj*, one of the rites for Muslim men is to shave their heads, although cutting the hair short is acceptable. As for the female pilgrim, she should only shorten her hair by cutting the tips. For men who shave their heads, the use of unclean blades can transmit blood-borne infections such as hepatitis B, hepatitis C, and HIV. Licensed barbers are tested for these blood-borne pathogens and are required to use disposable, single-use blades (Ahmed and Balaban, 2012). Male pilgrims should be advised to be shaved only at officially designated barbers. Alternatively, pilgrims can consider taking with them a disposable razor for personal use during this rite.

Trauma

Trauma is a major cause of injury and death during *Hajj*. Pilgrims may walk long distances through or near dense traffic. Motor vehicle accidents are inevitable, and contribute to casualties and deaths during the *Hajj* (Ahmed et al., 2006). Those patients with trauma presenting to surgical departments and intensive care are orthopaedic and neurosurgical (Al-Harthi and Al-Harbi, 2001). Stampede is perhaps the most feared trauma hazard because of the spreading of panic through the crowds, contributing to casualties and in some cases fatalities. This type of hazard has been reduced through enlargement of the sites where large crowds gather, and with more effective crowd management. However, pilgrims should try to avoid the most densely crowded areas during *Hajj* and, when options exist, perform rituals at non-peak hours (Ahmed et al., 2006).

Non-communicable diseases

Cardiovascular diseases

Cardiovascular disease is the most common cause (43%) of death during the *Hajj* (Health Statistics, 2005). Cardiovascular diseases have now replaced infectious diseases as a leading cause of both intensive care unit admission and death (Al-Shimemeri, 2012). Even for healthy adults, *Hajj* is demanding and those with pre-existing cardiac disease, the physical stress can easily precipitate ischaemia (Ahmed et al., 2006). It is deduced that cardiovascular diseases coupled with age and the physical strain associated with the performance of *Hajj* offer a valid explanation for the recent emergence of cardiovascular diseases as the most important cause of death during *Hajj* (Al-Shimemeri, 2012). Cardiac patients planning for the *Hajj* should consult with their doctors before the journey. However, if their cardiac status is risky, the onus is on the pilgrim to avoid the *Hajj*. Despite the encouragement of this preventative stance, most cardiac patients would insist on undertaking the pilgrimage and would, ultimately, like to die and be buried in the Holy places.

Diabetes

Diabetes, common among Muslims, has been reported as a rising leading cause of morbidity and mortality during *Hajj* (Ahmed, 2002; Madani et al., 2007). The specific risk factors for poor diabetes control during *Hajj* include travel to an unaccustomed environment, changes in the weather, frequent short-term movement between Makkah and surrounding places, intermittent illnesses, particularly respiratory infection, heatstroke, and diarrhoea with dehydration and electrolyte imbalance (Beshyah and Sherif, 2008). In addition, many pilgrims have failed to have a pre-medical review of their medications prior to travel, have an inadequate supply of medication and/or monitoring instruments, and have limited access to specialist medical care facilities. During *Hajj*, problems of hyperglycaemia and hypoglycaemia can occur. The second of these is more common as a result of increased physical activity, smaller meals, changes in the usual food intake, and different timing of meals from normal (Beshyah and Sherif, 2008; Khan et al., 2002). Hypoglycaemia may also occur if the insulin in Saudi Arabia is different from that of the patient's country of origin (Gatrad and Sheikh, 2005). Diabetics with neuropathy need to take special precautions regarding the use of quality footwear. Care needs to be taken to avoid wearing uncomfortable shoes or walking barefoot as this may result in foot burns and risks of infection (both fungal and bacterial). Diabetics with neuropathy have developed deep burns that involved the entire weight-bearing area of the sole (Beshyah and Sherif, 2008).

It has been suggested that a diabetic should carry a diabetic card in Arabic and in English, detailing his or her medical status, and a diabetic emergency kit. It is also important for anyone accompanying a person with diabetes to be aware of the symptoms of hypoglycaemia and hyperglycaemia. Table 11.1 presents the practical considerations and management of people with diabetes intending to perform *Hajj*.

In the UK, several diabetes units are now holding pre-*Hajj* education seminars for diabetics going to perform the *Hajj* (Figueira, 2003). There has been a suggestion that future global pre-*Hajj* advice for diabetics will include a consultation with a diabetologist, a nurse specialised in therapeutic education for diabetics, and a consultation with a specialist in travel medicine. Information about glucose control, insulin or oral anti-diabetic medications, nutrition, hydration, prevention of diabetic foot ulcers, information about physical measures aiming to prevent gastro-intestinal and pulmonary infections, and vaccinations, will be provided (Botelho-Nevers et al., 2011).

Women's issues

Hajj is prescribed for every adult Muslim, male and female. However, there are specific issues related to women. For a more comprehensive account, see *A Woman's Guide To Hajj* (Alshareef, www.performhajj.com/women_guide_to_hajj.php). It is permissible for the Muslim woman to wear any women's clothes she pleases which are neither attractive nor resemble the clothes of men. She is not allowed to wear a *burka* (a veil that covers the face and has two holes for the eyes, to permit vision) (Sheikh Al-Fawzan, 2009). So, a woman in *Hajj* should not cover her face or wear gloves, just as a male should not cover his head. There is a clear statement of the Prophet saying that: 'The *Muhrimah* (a female in *Ihram*) should not cover her face, nor should she wear gloves' (Bukhari). However, it is permissible for her to cover her face if she fears the gaze of non-*Mahram* men upon her. There is a great deal of concern regarding menstruation, for women who are going to perform the *Hajj*. It is permissible for a woman to use pills or daily progesterone to delay menstruation, to enable her to perform the rituals of *Hajj*, subject to the condition that this will not cause her harm (islamqa.info/en/ref/36619). It is also permissible for a menstruating woman to enter *Ihram* and do everything that other pilgrims do, performing all the rites of *Hajj*, apart from circumambulation (*tawaaf*) around the Kaa'ba. She should delay *tawaaf* until she becomes pure (for example, until her period ends) (islamqa.info/en/ref/36619). Women who are menstruating or bleeding following childbirth do not have to do the farewell circumambulation (*tawaaf*).

Table 11.1   Practical considerations and management of people with diabetes intending to perform *Hajj*

Pre-travel consultation	Vaccination (mandatory and recommended).
Medical examination	Physical examination. Review of medication. Assessment of pre-travel blood glucose. ECG – asymptomatic coronary artery disease.
Medication	Obtain enough medications, needles, pens, and monitoring instruments (in proper containers). Control blood pressure if hypertensive (adjust the antihypertensive dose accordingly). Reduce morning dose of oral hypoglycaemic agent or insulin (due to exercising the equivalent of 2 hours or more). Insulin should be refrigerated, but not in the freezer compartment, during the stay in Saudi Arabia.
Meal	Taking mid-morning snacks (during the days of travel between Makkah–Madina–Mount Arafat).
Emergency kit	Should contain a small jar of honey and glucagon for ready use in insulin treated patients.
Diabetic-neuropathy	Drink two or more litres of water daily (depending on the weather). Avoid dehydration and carry water bottles. Avoid walking barefoot. Get a waiver to do some parts of *Hajj* wearing protective shoes.
Diarrhoea/vomiting	Attend a health facility. Do not self-medicate.
Chest pain/ shortness of breath or palpitations	Attend a health facility.
Health education	Learn about symptoms and signs of hypoglycaemia and how it should be treated. Person accompanying the diabetic should be able to recognise and provide prompt management of any diabetes problems.

(Continued)

Table 11.1   Continued

Carry a diabetic card	In Arabic and English, containing a detailed diagnosis of the patient's state, medication, dosage, address and telephone number and the telephone number of one of his or her relatives. The following sentence is to be written on the back of the card: 'If found unconscious, please give me some medication via mouth or injection and take me to the nearest hospital' (Al-Khateeb).
Medical record	Carry a brief medical record and a signed statement from their doctor indicating their treatment.
Other considerations	Wear identifying wristbands. Face-mask use. Sunscreen. Seek shade. Perform rituals at night if possible. Avoid severe crowds. Hand hygiene.
After the *Hajj*	Medical follow-up. Early medical help if required.

A pregnant woman should be prevented from doing *Hajj*, following medical recommendations, if it will pose a risk to her or her baby (islamqa.info/en/ref/2983). This is indicated by the words of the Prophet (peace and blessings be upon him), 'There should be no harming nor reciprocating harm' (Ibn Majah). In addition, it is stated that some doctors differentiate between early pregnancy, when there may be a risk to the foetus, and late pregnancy when such fears are groundless (islamqa.info/en/ref/2983). However, there are a few considerations pregnant women should take into account before embarking on this journey, including: having pre-natal medical examinations; getting fully immunised; paying extra attention to the diet and intake of fluids; and stopping to rest when feeling tired or faint during the *Hajj*. Pregnant women who choose to go to the *Hajj* must be fully immunised in order not to expose the unborn child to diseases that may have lifelong effects.

Pre- and post-*Hajj* travel: health education, advice and practical management

Hajj presents a unique challenge that has an impacts on international public health. Nurses and other clinicians must be aware of potential risks of disease transmission and health-related problems associated with *Hajj*; they should provide health education and suggest appropriate strategies and practical management in dealing with the health risks described above and potential health problems. All potential pilgrims must now be protected against meningococcal disease, and other vaccinations are now also mandatory for specified regions or countries. Specific health education and advice should be tailored to the needs of those who are potential pilgrims to *Hajj*. During these classes advice on footwear, medications, food, dehydration, drug doses, and immunisations should be discussed. It has been suggested that all pilgrims should take a basic medical kit that includes simple analgesia (pain killers), plasters, and oral rehydration treatment (www.nathnac.org/travel). Pilgrims who take regular medication should ensure they have an adequate supply and carry a copy of their prescription.

Nurses and other clinicians must also be aware of the risks presented by the returning pilgrims, and be alert to the possibility of post-*Hajj* illness. They should be observant, looking for signs of diseases including meningitis, tuberculosis, hydatid (parasitic infection) disease, malaria, and hepatitis. Fever, rash, jaundice, pyoderma, foot ulcers, diarrhoea or vomiting should alert a healthcare professional to the possibility of an infection having been acquired during *Hajj* (Sheikh and Gartrad, 2008). In many countries local health organisations, travel organisations and local Mosques are now holding pre-*Hajj* education seminars. The contents may include: introduction and misconceptions about *Hajj*; a guide to *Hajj* and *Umrah*; health advice and information; medical advice; nutrition; hand hygiene; the use of face-masks and disposable handkerchiefs; women's issues; *Ihram* demonstration; and flight/hotel information. There is usually an audio-visual presentation. Pilgrims should also seek advice about the health risks for any travel that may be undertaken either before or following *Hajj* or *Umrah*. Information on health risks for other destinations throughout the world can be found on the NaTHNaC Saudi Arabia Country Information page. Table 11.2 presents some general health education and advice regarding *Hajj* and *Umrah*.

Conclusion

Hajj is one of the pillars of Islam and every adult Muslim, physically and financially able, is obliged to perform it. Health risks associated with Hajj are significant due to large crowds, high temperatures and extensive walking. The risk factors include heat exhaustion, heatstroke, sunburn, and infectious diseases. Children, the elderly and those with certain health problems (such as heart disease or diabetes) are at even higher risk. Pilgrims are well advised to have pre- and post-Hajj medical examinations, counselling, and screening for illnesses before and after Hajj. Nurses and other health clinicians should

Table 11.2 General health education and advice regarding *Hajj* and *Umrah*

Pre-*Hajj* travel	Vaccinations	Meningococcal vaccine. Seasonal influenza (those with pre-existing conditions; the elderly, those with chronic chest or heart diseases or cardiac, hepatic or renal failure). Polio vaccine – specific countries. Recommended for travel: vaccinations against influenza, hepatitis A, hepatitis B, typhoid. Routine vaccines. Physical fitness: begin walking for 10–15 minutes, 3–5 days per week. Rest and Sleep.
	Health	Physical check-up (those who have pre-existing medical conditions, or who are frail, or elderly). Review of medications. Screening. Counselling. Carry a copy of prescriptions.
	Safety tips	Make a photocopy of your passport to carry with you at all times. Designate meeting points in case of separation from your travelling companions.
	Basic medical kit	Simple analgesia (pain killers), plasters, and oral rehydration treatment. Pack medications in carry-on bag, not in suitcase.
During *Hajj*	Drinking/fluids	Drink plenty of water to prevent dehydration. Drink only beverages that have been bottled and sealed. Avoid tap water, fountain drinks and ice cubes. Increase dietary salt intake or use salt tablets.
	Food	Eat only food that is cooked and served hot. Avoid buying exposed foods prone to contamination. Ensure washing of fruits and vegetables thoroughly before cooking or eating.

(Continued)

Table 11.2   Continued

	Storing cooked food for more than 2 hours at room temperature or in buses causes growth of germs leading to food poisoning.
Heat exposure	Wear sunscreen (at least SPF 15) to prevent sunburn, and wear sunglasses with UV protection to protect your eyes. Cover your head, when possible, to reduce heat exposure. Use an umbrella. Some rituals can be performed at night to avoid daytime heat.
Heat injuries	*Tawaf* (circumambulation of the Kaa'ba), avoid especially in the middle of the day. *Sa'i* (walking between Safa and Marwa), especially in cases of crowding and high temperature. Avoid Arafat in the middle of the day.
Sunburn	Cover up the affected areas of skin. Stay in the shade until the sunburn has healed. Apply a moisturising lotion or after-sun cream. Use a non-steroidal anti-inflammatory drug (NSAID) to relieve pain, reduce inflammation and lower a high temperature.
Footwear	You are likely to be doing a lot of walking: invest in a sturdy, hard-wearing pair of sandals (easy to slip on and off but can also be secured at the back for more stability).
Swollen feet	Keep feet elevated at night time. Massage your legs in a one-way direction, from toes upwards only, and not down. Avoid tight-fitting socks.
Eye protection	Use sunglasses. Do not use contact lenses except after referring to your oculist. Use moisturising eye drops after referring to your oculist.

(Continued)

Table 11.2 Continued

	General hygiene	Use a face-mask.
		Wash your hands often with soap and water, especially after coughing or sneezing.
		Cover your nose and mouth with a tissue when you cough or sneeze. Throw the tissue in the trash after you use it.
		Avoid close contact with sick people.
		If you are sick, limit contact with others as much as possible to keep from infecting them.
		Avoid sharing sharp objects, such as razors, with others.
	Dermatological diseases: exfoliation (between thighs).	Maintain personal hygiene and regular bathing.
		Use powder and other moisturising cream when needed.
		Walk in strides to avoid exfoliation as much as possible.
		Keep the area in-between the thighs clean and dry.
	General safety instructions	Adhere to the schedules designated for you by your *Hajj/Umrah* organiser.
		Avoid crowded places.
Post-*Hajj* travel		Restore your body by drinking extra fluids.
		If you do not feel well after you return from your trip, you should get medical attention and mention that you have recently travelled.
		Have a post-travel medical check-up.

be aware of the health risks associated with the Hajj pilgrimage and provide health education on ways in which pilgrims can protect their health. It has been suggested that 'a multi-pronged approach involving awareness programmes for pilgrims and their health advisers, supported by rapid diagnosis, timely treatment, prevention by vaccine, community measures, infection prevention and control practices are necessary' (Shafia et al., 2008).

Reflective Activity 11.2

Case Study

Nadia, a 24-year-old Moroccan, is about 12 weeks pregnant. She wants to perform the *Hajj* (pilgrimage) with her husband for the first time, in the next few weeks. She speaks French but has a little understanding of English.

- How would you communicate with her?
- What are the risks involved if she attends the *Hajj* pilgrimage at this stage of her pregnancy?
- What advice would you give to her in relation to:

  (a) Pre-natal medical examination?
  (b) Immunisation and vaccination?
  (c) Physical demands of *Hajj*?
  (d) Risks of obstetric emergency?

- What other health advice should nurses give to Muslims who have the intention to attend the *Hajj* pilgrimage?

References

Ahmed, A.M. (2002) 'Care of Diabetic Patients on the *Hajj*', *Diabetes International* 12, 8–9. 7.

Ahmed, Q.A., Arabi, Y.M. and Memish, Z.A. (2006) 'Health Risks at the *Hajj*', *Lancet* 367, 9515, 1008–15.

Ahmed, Q. and Balaban, V. (2012) *Hajj Pilgrimage*, Saudi Arabia, Centers for Disease Control and Prevention, wwwnc.cdc.gov/travel/yellowbook/2012/chapter-4-select-destinations/hajj-pilgrimage-saudi-arabia.htm, date accessed 4 August 2013.

Al-Harthi, A.S. and Al-Harbi, M. (2001) 'Accidental Injuries during Muslim Pilgrimage', *Saudi Medical Journal* 22, 6, 523–5.

Al-Khateeb, M. *Sunstroke and Hajj Rituals*, Faculty of Medicine, Al-Azhar University, www.onislam.net/content/english/hajj/health/01.shtml, date accessed 4 August 2013.

Al-Mazrou, Y.Y. (2004) 'Food Poisoning in Saudi Arabia. Potential for Prevention?' *Saudi Medical Journal* 25, 1, 11–14.

Alshareef, M. *A Woman's Guide To Hajj*, www.performhajj.com/women_guide_to_hajj.php, date accessed 4 August 2013.

Al-Shimemeri, A. (2012) 'Cardiovascular Disease in *Hajj* Pilgrims', *Journal of the Saudi Heart Association* 24, 2, 123–7.

Beshyah, S.A. and Sherif, I.H. (2008) 'Care for People with Diabetes during the Moslem Pilgrimage (*Hajj*) An Overview', *Libyan Journal of Medicine* 3, 1, 39–41.

Borrow, R. (2009) 'Meningococcal Disease and Prevention at the *Hajj*', *Travel Medicine and Infectious Disease* 7, 4, 219–25.

Botelho-Nevers, E., Aubry, C., Atlan, C. and Gautret, P. (2011) 'The *Hajj*', *British Medical Journal* 343. Doi: d5593.

Bukhari 3/55, No. 1838, Darus-Salam Edition, Sahih by Sheik Al-Albani.

Editorial (2010) 'Health Conditions for Travellers to KSA for *Hajj* 1431H/2010', *Journal of Infection and Public Health* 3, 3, 93–4, www.moh.gov.sa/en/HealthAwareness/EducationalContent/HealthTips/Pages/Tips-2010-10-12-001.aspx, date accessed 4 August 2013.

Figueira E. (2003) 'Diabetes and the Pilgrimage of Hajj: Piloting of an Education Programme for Muslim Patients with Diabetes', *Diabetes Today* 6, 41–2.

Gatrad, A.R. and Sheikh, A. (2005) '*Hajj*: Journey of a Lifetime', *British Medical Journal* (15 January) 330, 7483, 133–7.

Health Statistics (2005) Saudi Ministry of Health. Cited in Ahmed, Q.A., Arabi, Y.M. and Memish, Z.A. (2006) 'Health Risks at the *Hajj*', *Lancet* 367, 9515, 1008–15.

Ibn Majah, 2340. See Jaami' al-'Uloom wa'l-Hikam, by Ibn Rajab, 1/302.

islamqa.info/en/ref/2983, *Can a Pregnant Woman Perform Hajj?* http://islamqa. info/en/ref/2983, date accessed 4 August 2013.

islamqa.info/en/ref/36619, *Rulings that Apply Only to Women during Hajj*, http://islamqa.info/en/ref/36619/WOMEN%20MENSTRUATION%20IN% 20HAJJ, date accessed 4 August 2013.

Khan, S.A., Bhat, A.R. and Khan, L.A. (2002) 'Hypoglycaemia in Diabetics during *Hajj*', *Saudi Medical Journal* 23, 12, 1548.

Madani, T.A., Ghabrah, T.M., Albarrak, A.M., Alhazmi, M.A., Alazraqi, T.A., Althaqafi, A.O. and Ishaq, A. (2007) 'Causes of Admission to Intensive Care Units in the *Hajj* Period of the Islamic Year 1424 (2004)', *Annals of Saudi Medicine* 27, 2, 101–5.

Madani, T.A., Ghabrah, T.M., Al-Hedaithy, M.A., Alhazmi, M.A., Alazraqi, T.A., Albarrak, A.M. et al. (2006) 'Causes of Hospitalization of Pilgrims in the *Hajj* Season of the Islamic Year 1423 (2003)', *Annals of Saudi Medicine* 26, 5, 346—51.

Memish, Z.A. (2006) 'Health Risks at the *Hajj*', *Lancet* 367, 9515, 1008–15.

Memish, Z.A. (2010) 'The *Hajj*: Communicable and Non-communicable Health Hazards and Current Guidance for Pilgrims', *Eurosurveillance* 15, 39: pii=19671, www.eurosurveillance.org/ViewArticle.aspx?ArticleId= 19671, date accessed 4 August 2013.

Muslim 3257, 5/112.

NaTHNaC. Saudi Arabia Country Information page, www.nathnac.org/travel/factsheets/Hajj_Umrah.htm, date accessed 4 August 2013.

Saudi Arabian Ministry of Health, www.moh.gov.sa/en/Pages/Default.aspx, date accessed 4 August 2013.

Shafia, S., Booy R., Haworth, E., Rashid, H. and Memish Z.A. (2008) '*Hajj*: Health Lessons for Mass Gatherings', *Journal of Infection and Public Health* 1, 1, 27—32.

Sheikh Al-Fawzan, S. (2009) *A Summary of Islamic Jurisprudence*, Volume 1 (Riyadh, Saudi Arabia: Al-Maiman Publishing House), p. 405.

Sheikh, A. and Gatrad, A.R. (2008) '*Hajj*: Journey of a Lifetime', in A. Sheikh and A.R. Gatrad (eds), *Caring for Muslim Patients*, 2nd edition (Oxford: Radcliffe Publications), p. 92.

Tirmidhî [a], 809, 3/175; An Nasai 2630, 3/122; Ibn Majah 2887, 3/407 and 288, 3/407; cited in S. Sheikh Al-Fawzan (2009), A *Summary of Islamic Jurisprudence*, Volume 1 (Riyadh, Saudi Arabia: Al-Maiman Publishing House), p. 415.

Tirmidhî, [b] 2975.

Tomasulo, A. (2011) Infectious Disease and *Hajj*, http://healthmap.org/news/infectious-disease-and-hajj, date accessed 4 August 2013.

www.nathnac.org/travel/factsheets/Hajj_Umrah.htm, date accessed 4 August 2013.

www.onislam.net/content/english/hajj/step_by_step/05.shtml, date accessed 4 August 2013 'All About Ihram).

12 Mental Health: Cultural and Religious Influences

G. Hussein Rassool and E.M. Gemaey

Learning Outcomes:

- Discuss the perception of Muslim patients towards mental health problems.
- Identify the problems of mental health in Muslim communities.
- Discuss the principles of assessment of Muslims patients with mental health problems.
- Have an understanding of the concepts of evil eye (*nazar*), *jinn*, and spirit possession.
- Discuss how cultural and religious factors have an influence in the presentation of mental health problems.
- Discuss the non-pharmacological treatment interventions for those with mental health problems.
- Discuss the rationale of why Western-oriented counselling may not be appropriate for Muslim patients.

Reflective Activity 12.1

State whether the following statements are true or false. Give reasons for your answers.

	True	False
1 Culture-bound syndromes associated with various cultures may be mistaken for psychiatric symptoms.		

		True	False
2	Misunderstandings of cultural and religious influence have no effect on ethical dilemmas, practice problems, and problems in communication.		
3	The suicide rate is high in Muslim countries.		
4	The lack of understanding of the interplay between religious influences on health or sickness behaviours can have a significant effect upon delivery of nursing practice.		
5	Traditionally, Islam links all mental health problems to supernatural causes.		
6	Islamic teachings explain mental health problem in a variety of ways: as a defective relationship with God, as a punishment from God, or, simply, as the imponderable result of God's will.		
7	Muslims' mental health problems are identified by mainstream mental health services.		
8	Supernatural causes of illnesses are widely acknowledged and are considered very real within Islam.		
9	Islam does not regard a mental health problem as a condition that results from an unbalanced lifestyle or an unbalanced body.		
10	'Evil eye' and 'spirit possession' may be regarded as universal phenomena.		
11	Trance or possession disorders are not accepted or classified as a form of psychological disorder.		
12	Being possessed by an evil spirit could be a delusion or a culturally sanctioned experience of an altered state of consciousness.		
13	Most people are content to utilise biomedical treatments without giving up traditional explanations of illness.		
14	There is increasing acceptance that the biomedical model is adequate in accounting for the differences in mental health indicators across ethnic groups.		
15	Generally, members of the Muslim population seek spiritual advice from traditional faith healers for psychiatric and related problems.		

Introduction

Muslim religious beliefs have an impact on the mental health of individuals, families and communities, and are considered a central component of their identity (Nasser-McMillan and Hakim-Larson, 2003). The lack of understanding of the interplay between religious influences on health or sickness behaviours can have a significant effect upon delivery of nursing practice. Misunderstandings can develop easily and can lead to ethical dilemmas, practice problems, and problems in communication (Catlin and Boffman, 1998). The Muslim community is experiencing social exclusion (social exclusion correlates with mental health problems) related to their cultural and religious identity. Often, Muslim individuals are stigmatised and families are rejected and isolated for their association with mental health problems, addiction and suicide (Pridmore and Pasha, 2004). There are indicators that Muslims experience mental ill health but that they either are unidentified by mainstream mental health services or present late to the services (Ali and Milstein, 2012; Maynard, 2008). This chapter examines the religious and cultural influences on mental health beliefs of Muslims.

Muslims and mental health problems

Muslims in the United States and in European countries are a minority group who face increasing religious, cultural, and ethnic discrimination (Ali et al., 2005; Triandafyllidou, 2012). There are no large-scale epidemiological reports on the prevalence and incidence rates of mental health problems amongst Muslims in the 57 Islamic states who are members of the Organisation of the Islamic Conference. In fact, there is no satisfactory single description of mental health services possible, and only limited English-language information is available (Pridmore and Pasha, 2004). A review (Al-Issa and Al-Junun, 2000) of the existing international epidemiological data on several disorders and conditions concludes that the rate of schizophrenia in Muslims is similar to that of non-Muslims. There is no difference in the prevalent rate of anxiety disorders between Muslims and non-Muslims. In a study by Abu-Ras and Abu-Bader (2008) on the effects of the 9/11 attacks on the mental health of American Arabs, the findings showed an increase in worrying about the future, feelings of anxiety, fear of hate crimes, stigmatisation, and the break-up of communities, leading to isolation. However, high rates of Post-Traumatic Syndrome Disorder were found in both Muslim men and women facing post-9/11-related trauma and discrimination in the US (Abu-Ras and Abu-Bader, 2009). Higher rates of depression in women than in men are also seen in Muslim populations. It has been found that Muslims from the US, Canada and Australia reported more stress following 9/11 (Barkdull et al., 2011). A British Muslim sample (Sheridan, 2006) suggested that more than one-third of its British Muslim participants had high scores on a depression scale, which indicated poor mental health.

Suicide is strictly forbidden in Islam because it is an affront to God. In relation to suicide or self-harm, it appears as if the rates are low or almost non-existent in Muslim countries (WHO, 2007). International studies in Pakistan and Malaysia showed a low prevalence of suicide (Murty et al., 2008; Zakiullah et al., 2008). In Saudi Arabia, suicides have been estimated to occur at a rate of 1.1/100 000 population per annum, and to be most common among men, people aged 30 to 39 years, and immigrants (Al-Khathami, 2001). Elderly suicide rates were among the lowest only in the five Middle Eastern Islamic countries in a cross-national study of 87 countries (Shah et al., 2007). While low rates of completed suicides are reported in Muslim countries, ideation and attempts are relatively high, particularly in young women experiencing intergenerational conflict (Ali et al., 2009). In a recent cross-national study on the relationship between suicide and Islam, the findings of Shah and Chandia's study (2010) showed a significant negative relationship between suicide rates and adherents of Islam and rejected the notion that modernisation has weakened this relationship. However, advocates of Islam do commit suicide, and nurses and other healthcare professionals should carefully assess the potential risk of suicide in all depressed Muslim patients.

In the UK, it is suggested that a sense of always being under attack, hostility and lack of understanding are creating increasing anxiety and high levels of depression and stress among Muslims (Dunning, 2011). In addition, there are growing reports of stress within the Bangladeshi, Pakistani and Somali communities, driven by deprivation and concerns over the media's and politicians' characterisation of some Muslims as radicalised (House of Commons Communities and Local Government Committee, 2010). It is argued that 'exclusion and discrimination are known to be key causative factors in mental health problems, and there is little doubt that these processes have detrimentally affected British Muslim mental health, raising the question of the link between mental health problems and young Muslims' vulnerability to identity crisis' (Ahmed, 2009). In summary, the common mental health problems reported by respondents in England included: anxiety and depression, ADHD (Attention Deficit Hyperactivity Disorder) and apparent conduct disorders, substance misuse, alcoholism and gambling, issues regarding identity, relationships and psychosexual problems, domestic violence (in relation to both the perpetration and the experience of it) and religious delusional behaviour (Maynard, 2008).

Muslims' understanding of mental health problems

Research has identified that religion and religious belief are absolutely central to the way Muslims interpret the cause and development of mental health problems (Nada, 2007). According to Rassool (2000), Muslims believe an illness is not something to be viewed negatively, but should be seen, rather, as a positive event that purifies the body. The Prophet Muhammad said: 'There is no affliction which befalls a Muslim but that Allah expiates some of his wrong actions by it, even when a thorn which pricks him' (Bukhari). Muslims perceive mental health problems as part of human suffering and a way of atoning for sins, or as trials and tests from Allah. Believing illness is punishment from God for some wrongdoing influences some Muslims to take a passive attitude towards dealing with afflictions (Ali et al., 2009). For this reason, many Muslims do not seek help, as they believe illness can and will purify the body (Rassool, 2000).

Traditional Islamic teachings explain mental health problem in a variety of ways: as a defective relationship with God, as a punishment from God, or, simply, as the imponderable result of God's will (Al-Krenawi and Graham, 1999). The defective relationship with God entails a weakness of *Imaan* (right creed) and the sufferers' weak belief in predestination. This leads them to feel fearful, pessimistic, with a loss of hope and unable to accept their fate (predestination). The findings of a survey (Abu-Ras and Abu-Bader, 2009) showed that 98% of survey respondents, when asked about their perceptions of mental health problems, agreed that the stresses of life are a test of one's faith; 84% of respondents believed in devil possession of mentally ill persons. It is also perceived that when *jinns* (spirits, mentioned in the Qur'aan and Islamic theology, who inhabit an unseen world) possess individuals, hallucinations, delusional beliefs and disorganised behaviour may result. Other professed supernatural causes are black magic and the evil eye (Abu-Ras and Abu-Bader, 2009). It is important to note that traditionally, supernatural causes of illnesses are widely acknowledged and are considered very real within Islam (Mrana, 2009). However, not all mental health problems are associated with supernatural causes (Rahman, 1998). One of the early Muslim scholars in psychiatric health care, Ibn Sina, rejected the popular notion that mental health problems originated from evil spirits (Pridmore and Pasha, 2004).

Historically, Islamic law protects people who are 'insane' and they are cared for and supported. Allah says in the Qur'aan (interpretation of the meaning):

☐ *And give not unto the foolish your property which Allah has made a means of support for you, but feed and clothe them therewith, and speak to them words of kindness and justice.* (An-Nisâ' [The Women] 4:5)

This Qur'aanic verse summarises Islam's attitudes towards those with mental health problems, who were considered unfit to manage property but must be treated humanely and kept under the care of a guardian, according to Islamic law (Paladin, 1998). An insane person has no right of disposal over property, and a guardian is appointed to protect such an individual's property. Although the person is considered to be a Muslim if his or her family is Muslim, he or she is not obligated to fulfil the pillars of the faith (for example, five daily prayers) (Dols, 2007). For instance, obligatory prayers, fasting or pilgrimage are not required. In the first instance the family, if any, is responsible for the patient. If this is not possible, his or her care becomes the responsibility of the State. For those who are insane, committing self-harm or suicide would not be regarding as a major sin. A Muslim may have a mental or physical illness that affects his psychological health to such a great extent that he does not know what he is saying or doing. If this results in him killing himself, he will not be placed with the sinners who have fallen into the major sin of suicide. Rather he will be excused because there was an impediment to his being accountable, namely his loss of reason (islamqa, Fatwa 146375).

The Prophet said: 'The Pen has been lifted from three: from the sleeper until he awakens, from the child until he reaches puberty and from the insane person until he comes to his senses' (Abu Dawud). However, there is wide consensus amongst Muslim scholars that mental or psychological disorders are legitimate medical conditions, that is, distinct from illnesses of a supernatural nature. This belief has paved the way for Muslims to accept the existence of mental or psychological disorders and to seek treatment, with more community support and less stigma associated with their diagnoses. A study by Inayat (2005) examined barriers to utilisation of mental health services by Muslim clients and suggested that therapists need to take care when interpreting client distress in a multicultural setting. The author highlights six areas of functioning which contribute to the under utilisation of mental health services by Muslim clients. These include: mistrust of service providers, fear of treatment, fear of racism and discrimination, language barriers, differences in communication, and issues of culture.

Possession of the soul

The concepts of 'evil eye' and 'spirit possession' are reported in so many cultures that they may be regarded as universal phenomena (Spooner, 2004). Evil eye represents a fear of evil influence through other people. Belief in it is defined as a 'belief that the envy elicited by the good luck of fortunate people may result in their misfortune' (Webster's-online-dictionary). In most cultures, the primary victims are thought to be babies and young children, because they are so often praised and commented upon by strangers or by childless women. Belief in the evil eye started in antiquity. Nowadays, this phenomenon is strongest in the Middle East, East and West Africa, South Asia, Central Asia, and Europe, especially the Mediterranean region. The Asian term for evil eye is '*nazar*'. Belief in the evil eye is found in the Noble Qur'aan, based on the following verse (interpretation of the meaning):

☐ *And from the evil of the envier when he envies.* (Al-Falaq [The Daybreak] 113:5)

The Messenger of Allah stated that: 'The influence of an evil eye is a fact, if anything would precede the destiny it would be the influence of an evil eye, and when you are asked to take bath (as a cure) from the influence of an evil eye, you should take bath' (Muslim [a]). 'Spirit possession', on the other hand, refers to the belief that a spirit can enter a living person, possess them, and control what they say and do. The belief in 'spirit possession' or 'evil eye' is common within the Muslim and Asian communities, particularly where the Western diagnosis would be of depression and psychological illness. The concept of depression is not commonly found in Muslim cultures. It is more usual for people to say that 'the person's soul has been possessed, by a bad spirit'. The idea of another person making someone ill by the use of 'witchcraft or voodoo' is also common. These two concepts of 'soul possession' and 'witchcraft' should be considered when understanding the influence of culture on health, as many ethnic minorities from the Indian subcontinent, Africa and the Middle East, in the UK and elsewhere, strongly believe that these can affect their health.

There are numerous references to *jinn* in the Qur'aan and Hadith. According to Islamic writings, *jinn* live alongside other creatures but form a world other than that of mankind. Though they see us, they cannot be seen. Characteristics they share with human beings are intellect, and freedom to choose between right and wrong and between good and bad (Al-Ashqar, 2003). However, according to the Qur'aan the origin of the *jinn* is different from that of man (interpretation of the meaning):

☐ *And indeed, We created man from sounding clay of altered black smooth mud. And the jinn, We created aforetime from the smokeless flame of fire.* (Al-Ĥijr [The Rocky Tract] 15:26–7)

In Islamic writings true *jinn* possession can cause a person to have seizures and to speak in an incomprehensible language (Al-Ashqar, 2003). The possessed is unable to think or speak of his own free will. However, according to Aziz (2001), such cases are greatly outnumbered by those of physical or psychological origin, and he castigates faith healers for taking money for treatment of the latter. The belief that an individual has been entered by an alien spirit is encountered in many cultures.

Differential diagnosis: *jinn* or mental health problems?

In the case of mental health problems, most Muslims believe that *jinn* have the power to possess the minds of people. Both good *jinn* and bad *jinn* exist. Bad *jinn* can cause mental health problems through possession. However, they also believe that certain prayers over the ill person can exorcise the *jinn* and purify the environment from the bad *jinn* (Muhaimin, 2009). Some Western practitioners may be surprised to find 'possession state' as a diagnostic entity within the Diagnostic Statistical Manual IV (DSM-IV) (American Psychiatric Association, 2000) and the International Classification of Disease, Version 10 (ICD-10) (WHO, 2001). The criteria in these two documents are similar, apart from the marked distress and impairment in social or occupational functioning included in DSM-IV. In ICD-10, trance or possession disorders are classified under dissociative (conversion) disorders – disorders in which there is a temporary loss of the sense of personal identity and of full awareness of the surroundings. Possession or trance has to be involuntary and to occur outside religious or culturally accepted situations. This classification excludes states associated with psychotic disorders, affective disorders, organic personality disorder, post-concussion syndrome and psychoactive substance intoxication. It is reported that the most common psychological symptoms caused by evil eye, magic, or *jinn* possession include anxiety, insomnia, estrangement, hyperactivity, psychotic disturbances, altered consciousness, abnormal movements, somatic complaints, obsessions and fear of developing disease (Al-Habeeb, 2003).

Cultural factors also have a significant influence on the presentation of mental health problems. The DSM Manual IV (American Psychiatric Association, 2000) identifies behaviours (culture-bound syndromes) associated with various cultures that may be mistaken for psychiatric symptoms. However, there is a need for close collaboration between faith healers and mental health workers in order to achieve a culturally sensitive healthcare system (Rashid et al., 2011).

Guidelines for the assessment and treatment of Muslim patients

At the initial interview, it is important to assess the patient's preferred language in case the patient does not share the same language as the nurse.

The use of a professional translator may be necessary. Issues of confidentiality should be discussed with the patient and the family. The nurse needs to be aware of the beliefs about the patient's illness, its causes, and when and from whom to seek care as this may have a significant influence on the presentation of illness or sickness behaviours. Muslim patients are not a homogeneous group, so it is important for the nurse or healthcare professional to enquire about a patient's individual customs and preferred practices. During the process of engagement and the development of the therapeutic relationship the nurse will be in a better position to explore the patient's religious and spiritual beliefs. Religious affiliation can be a defining feature of a patient's cultural identity (Rahiem and Hamid, 2012). A spiritual religious assessment can be separated into a brief assessment and a longer more in-depth assessment. The brief assessment may explore such issues as the patient's religious practices, beliefs, special celebrations and religious support network. That is to assist the patient by putting them in touch with their religious network. The support network or religious group may be a source of support or of a religiously oriented coping mechanism.

Expressions of symptoms may differ between the different Muslim communities because cultural influences on presentation of symptoms need to be considered. It has been observed that due to the lesser stigma of physical symptoms and the language used, mental health problems are often expressed as physical symptoms (El-Islam, 2008). Mood symptoms such as a sense of hopelessness, self-deprecatory thoughts, and feelings of worthlessness are uncommon. It is stated that women who are diagnosed with depression 'frequently first present with "conversion" disorders and no self-recognition of psychological distress or sadness' (Al-Krenawi and Graham, 2000). Expressions of symptoms from African Muslims may differ from those from South-East Asia. For example, clinicians should be aware of the presence of visual rather than auditory hallucination in persons with schizophrenia (Bhui, 2001). Paranoia and a religious content to beliefs are more common among West Indians and West Africans (Littlewood and Lipsedge, 1988). It is believed that when *jinns* possess individuals, hallucinations, delusional beliefs and disorganised behaviour may result (Ali et al., 2009; Blom et al., 2010). However, 'the existence of *jinn* (evil spirits) may be confused with delusions of possession and control, and may prevent patients and family members from recognizing medical or psychiatric problems' (El-Islam, 2008).

When assessing a Muslim patient and constructing a cultural formulation it is important to examine the patient's cultural and religious identity, the patient's explanatory model of their problem or illness, cultural factors related to the psychosocial environment, the nurse–patient therapeutic relationship, and treatment interventions. This kind of assessment enables patients to understand their 'illness' and health-related needs (physical/medical, psychosocial and spiritual needs), avoids stereotyping or mislabelling, and provides information on what interventions are required.

The maintenance of rapport, empathy, genuineness and being non-judgemental are critical in the process of assessment. The following questions have been adapted from the model proposed by Kleinman et al. (1978) to be directed to the patient:

- What do you think has caused your current problem?
- Why do you think it started when it did?
- What do you think your illness does to you?
- What do you fear most about your illness?
- What are the main problems that have affected you?
- How severe is your problem?
- What kind of treatment are you receiving from your own culture?
- What kind of treatment do you think you should receive?
- What are your expectations of the treatment?

The wording of questions will vary depending on the characteristics or personality of the patient, the problem presented, and the setting. Questions should be asked sensitively and the patient should be given plenty of time to consider their responses. The expressions used in presenting symptoms may differ amongst Muslims. Some cultures use terms like 'nerves', 'wind', 'cold' or 'hot' to explain or describe symptoms. Different terminology often results in poor assessment of problems and needs, and subsequently leads to misdiagnosis. A Muslim patient may be reluctant or feel shame in openly discussing his/her problems because of cultural and religious expectations. In traditionally Muslim families, there may be reluctance to share family issues or to express negative feelings with a nurse or doctor. The issues of suicide, sexual behaviours and alcohol and drug use may provide some uneasiness in both the nurse or clinician and the patient. These are taboo subjects in the Muslim community. Sensitivity must be applied when making an assessment concerning suicidal thoughts, and this may require special phrasing (for example, 'Have you been wishing that God would allow you to die somehow?') (Ali et al., 2009). It is important to examine the family dynamics and the psychosocial stressors emanating from the family. A lack of cultural competence may influence the assessment process and the subsequent quality of care and interventions. The principles of assessment of Muslim patients with mental health problems are presented in Table 12.1.

Table 12.1   Principles of assessment of Muslim patients with mental health problems

---

- A holistic assessment of a patient includes assessment of culture and religious beliefs, presenting problems, and collateral information from significant others.
- Inquire about patients' cultural identity to determine their ethnic or racial background.
- Identify language ability and the patient's preferred method of communication. Make necessary arrangements if translators are needed.
- Identify the cultural or religious beliefs the patient holds about his or her illness.
- Identify the personal and social meaning the patient attaches to his or her psychological state.
- Examine the expectations of the patient about his or her problem.
- Examine the patient's (and significant others') therapeutic goals or what their expectations are of the healthcare interventions.
- Identify their degree of religious conservatism as reflected in their choices of clothing; eating and drinking habits; and many traditions, customs, and beliefs.
- Consider cultural factors related to the psychosocial environment and levels of functioning.
- This assessment includes culturally relevant interpretations of social stressors, available support, and levels of functioning, as well as the patient's disability (Lopez and Guarnaccia, 2000).
- Identify the patient's major support and family configurations and include the family in the assessment process and treatments.

Therapy: orthodox or spiritual?

Different societies have different patterns of help-seeking, and some countries involve traditional healers in their healthcare systems (Goldberg, 1999). Contrary to a Western therapeutic emphasis on the individual, all interventions with Muslim patients need to be embedded in the context of the family and of the extended family or community. The uses of pharmacological and non-pharmacological interventions in the management of mental health problems are acceptable to Muslim patients. Abu-Ras and Abu-Bader (2008) found that 80 per cent of Muslim patients believe in use of medication for the treatment of the mentally ill. Non-pharmacological interventions include individual, group, or family and marital therapy, counselling, psychotherapy, cognitive behaviour therapy, solution-focused therapy and relapse prevention. It has been suggested that patients from collective cultures may be more interested in family therapy, which could involve the extended family as well; and patients from individualistic societies may be more amenable to individual psychotherapy (Caraballo et al., 2006; Rahiem and Hamid, 2012). Most studies suggest that for major mental health disorders, a treatment approach involving both drugs and psychotherapy is more effective than either treatment method used alone (Doebbeling, 2007). Combined use of Qur'aanic healing and Western psychotherapy is the preferred method of treatment for Muslims (Abu-Ras and Abu-Bader, 2008). It is worth noting that Muslim patients have expectations that mental health treatment will be similar to physical or medical treatment in its timeliness and in its lack of demand for patient contribution (Al-Krenawi and Graham, 2000).

Use of religious and spiritual interventions

The use of religious and spiritual interventions is sometimes combined with modern orthodox treatment for mental disorders. Muslims believe that religious and spiritual interventions, and community rehabilitation, are an essential part of supporting someone with mental illness (Khan, 2006) or during traumatic times (Ai et al., 2005). This is supported by the finding from Abu-Ras and Abu-Bader's (2008) study that 95 per cent of the respondents believed that an emotionally disturbed person could be cured by studying the Qur'aan and Hadith. To promote healing, excessive ritual acts of devotion, such as prayer, fasting, repentance, and recitation of the Qur'aan are adopted (Abu-Ras and Abu-Bader, 2008). Prayer has also been found as a regular source of support and comfort (Khan, 2006). The findings of a study by Cinnirella and Loewenthal (1999) showed that prayer is perceived by Muslims as a treatment for depression and schizophrenia.

Muslims often seek guidance for mental health problems from *Imams* (religious leaders). *Imams* report that their congregants come to them for a full range of emotional problems, marital and family problems, and psychological and social concerns (Ali et al., 2005). However, a major barrier for the preference for *Imams* is that they are not trained to act as agents of referral to mental health professionals (Ali et al., 2009). It has been suggested that encouraging collaboration and communication between mental health professionals and Muslim religious leaders has the potential to facilitate proper referrals and improve access to culturally appropriate mental health services (Ali et al., 2009). The findings of a study showed that Muslim attitudes toward seeking formal mental health services are most likely to be affected by cultural and traditional beliefs about mental health problems, knowledge of and familiarity with formal services, perceived societal stigma, and the use of informal indigenous resources (Alouda and Rathurb, 2009).

In cases where Muslim patients are deemed to have a medical or psychiatric disorder but are not receptive to medical explanations, it would be appropriate to encourage patients to take the prescribed treatment while they continue with spiritual therapy with an *Imam*. This double strategy may be the best hope of securing adherence to prescribed treatments. There may also be the additional very important benefit that patients and their families may be willing to enter into discussion about the other therapies that are being tried. However, where medical and psychosocial interventions do not produce a positive outcome for the patient, there is concern that, in desperation, some families may turn to exorcists who inflict physical harm in an attempt to free the individual from possession – sometimes with catastrophic consequences. It is very important, therefore, to establish channels of communication with the patient, the family and any spiritual practitioner whose help is being sought. Lastly, there is a need for humility since, despite all our scientific developments, the symptoms and experiences of patients commonly remain medically unexplained.

There is evidence to suggest that religious commitment and spirituality are associated with many positive outcomes including, but not limited to, improved ability to cope with stress, reduced incidence of depression and anxiety, reduced risk of suicide and criminal behaviour, and decreased use of tobacco, drugs, and alcohol (Gartner, 1996; Larson et al., 1992; McCullough and Larson, 1999). Several studies have found that a form of religious psychotherapy may be effective with Muslim clients who suffer from anxiety, depression, and/or bereavement (Azhar et al., 1994; Azhar and Varma, 1995a, 1995b; Razali et al., 1998). The findings of these studies showed that patients in religious psychotherapy groups responded significantly faster than those receiving standard treatment. In this approach, unproductive beliefs are identified and modified, or replaced with beliefs derived from Islam, as a variation of cognitive therapy making use of religious themes (Azhar et al., 1994; Azhar & Varma 1995b).

Management of evil eye and *jinn* possession

There is a recognition by mental health professionals that some symptoms commonly seen in mental health problems, such as delusions or hallucinations, could represent a culturally appropriate behaviour. For example, being possessed by an evil spirit could be a delusion, or a culturally sanctioned experience of an altered state of consciousness. It is important to be cautious so as not to judge individual cultural variations as psychopathology.

Table 12.2 Signs of symptoms of *jinn* possession and evil eye

Jinn possession	Evil eye
Turning away and reacting strongly when hearing the *adhaan* or Qur'aan.	Headaches that move from one part of the head to another.
Fainting, seizures and falling when the Qur'aan is read over him/her.	Yellow pallor in the face.
	Sweating and urinating a great deal.
A lot of disturbing dreams or nightmares.	Weak appetite.
	Tingling, heat or cold in the limbs.
Being alone, keeping away from people and behaving strangely.	Palpitations in the heart.
	Pain in the lower back and shoulders.
The devil who is dwelling in him may speak when the Qur'aan is read over him/her.	Sadness and anxiety.
	Sleeplessness at night.
	Strong reactions due to abnormal fears.
	A lot of burping, yawning and sighing.
	Withdrawal and love of solitude.
	Apathy and laziness.
	Health problems with no known medical cause.

Source: Adapted from Fatwa No. 125543; Islam Q&A. Evil Eye – Shaykh 'Abd al-'Azeez al-Sadhaan, www.islam-qa.com/en/ref/125543, date accessed 17 February 2013.

It is helpful to consult with other nurses or healthcare providers from diverse cultural or ethnic groups to understand these behaviours. There are some signs and symptoms that may indicate whether a person has been possessed by the *jinn* or affected by the evil eye. These are not an exhaustive list, as definitive symptoms may vary amongst individuals. A list of signs and symptoms is presented in Table 12.2.

So, what refutes the evil eye? Quite simply, it is the Holy Qur'aan. There are specific verses in the Qur'aan, such as the Surah An-Nas and Al-Falaq, which are especially effective for this, as well as Surah Al-Fatihah and Ayatal Kursi. Sheikh al-Fawzan stated that 'If the one who may cause harm with the evil eye fears that he may harm the thing he is looking at, then he should say: *Allaahumma baarik 'alayhi* (O Allah, bless it). Similarly it is *mustahabb* [recommended] for him to say: *Ma sha Allah laa quwwata illa Billaah* (As Allah wills, there is no power except with Allah).'

The unorthodox therapies most frequently prescribed by faith healers to the patients with evil eye, *jinn* possession, and magic are: *Ruqyah* (reading specific verses from the Holy Qur'aan), soothing sayings by the Prophet Muhammad, regular performance of prayers, exorcism (of *jinn* and other devious supernatural spirits), physical punishment, temporary strangulation, cautery, *saaout* (snuff – inhalation of a herb powder), local application of a paste made of different types of herbs, drinking water mixed with herbs, water mixed with paper on which are written Qur'aanic verses, and local application and/or drinking of some oils. *Saaout* may also imply the use of herbal nasal drops, or a similar material mixed with oil or an oily substance, used as a nasal spray (Al-Habeeb, 2003). However, some of the therapies are not acceptable Islamic practices.

In any case of alleged *jinn* possession, underlying organic disorders should be excluded by physical examination and by such investigations as are necessary. Any underlying mental health problem should be treated by the usual psychiatric methods, but the clinician should respect the cultural issues and avoid directly contradicting statements from the patient or relatives about the reality of possession. Most people are content to utilise biomedical treatments without giving up traditional explanations of illness (Dein, 2002). Therefore, there may be a strong case for involving an *Imam* in the management of these cases (Khalifa and Hardie, 2005). It is recommended not to have a conversation with the *jinn* as they are liars. For a more comprehensive account on how to provide religio-culturally competent care to Muslim clients, see (Ahmed and Amer, 2012). The management of these patients is presented in Table 12.3.

Counselling the Muslim patient

☐ *Help you one another in virtue, righteousness and piety; but do not help one another in sin and transgression.* (Surah Al-Mā'idah [The Table Spread] 5:2)

In the above verse of the Qur'aan (interpretation of the meaning), Allah commands His believing servants to help one another to perform righteous, good deeds and to avoid sins. Allah forbids His servants from helping one another in sin and overstepping the limits. That is, one should consult one's fellows, advise them, and cooperate with them. Islamic counselling emphasises spiritual solutions, based on love and fear of Allah and the duty to fulfil our responsibility as the servants of Allah (Imam Magid). Moreover, the Messenger of Allah stated that: 'The religion (Islam) is sincere counselling and good advice' (Muslim [b]). The Noble Qur'aan also reminds us that in any form of counselling, or in one-to-one interaction, Allah is present and hears what we

Table 12.3 Management of evil eye and *jinn* possession

	Nursing interventions
Attitude	Be non-judgemental and non-punitive. No condemnation of their cultural and spiritual beliefs.
Communication	Examine and listen to the patient, recognise their way of being, be culturally sensitive.
Assessment	Questionnaire: age, gender, marital status, employment, country of birth, language. Results are a condensate sample.
Expectations	Patients will expect medications for pain relief. Family involvement in care.
Religious leaders	Healthcare professionals should work with religious leaders in supporting the patient.

are saying, and that in counselling we need to help others to be righteous and to be obedient to Allah (Al-Mujādila [The Pleading Woman] 58:7–8).

In recent years, there has been a greater focus on counselling with ethnic minorities, especially with the development and implementation of multicultural counselling competencies (Sue and Sue, 2008). However, it is absolutely clear that some culture-bound forms of Western psychotherapy have limited use with Muslim clients and can at times be harmful (Badri, 2009). Muslims coming from the Arab and South Asian cultures anticipate qualities in a therapist that may be quite opposite to the expectations one may have in Western cultures (Haque, 2004). There are inherent conflicts when patients and therapists differ in their religious beliefs because the inclusion of spiritual/religious narrative in counselling is perceived as less important by the therapists than by their patients (Bergin and Jensen, 1990). Muslim patients report fear that their values will be undermined by secular counselling (Jafari, 1993). In fact, many Muslim patients who do seek mental health care prefer a counsellor with an understanding of Islam (Kelly et al., 1996).

During the past few years there has been an emergence of Islamic counselling as a form of therapy for Muslim patients. Islamic counseling can be tentatively defined as a form of counselling which incorporates spirituality into the therapeutic process and has a faith-based perspective. The principles of Islamic counselling, according to Imam Magid, include the following: confidentiality, trust, respect, recognising the difference between arbitration and counselling, loving what is good for other people, making peace between people, concern about Muslim affairs, good listening habits, understanding others' cultures, the partnership between *Imams* and professionals, awareness of the law of the land, and the ultimate goal of connecting people with Allah and offering spiritual solutions to them.

Haque (2004) stated that the Muslim counsellor plays an advisory and a teacher's role and the client is a learner or a disciple, thus the client may not challenge what the therapist has to say. In contrast to Western psychotherapy, Islamic counselling uses a more directive approach as most Muslims come to clinicians seeking advice or the offer of an approach to deal with their issues (Abdullah, 2007). It has been suggested that simple advice-giving by a counsellor may not be as useful as facilitating a process whereby the patient may gain insight into their own experiential process (Keshavarzi and Haque, 2013). In addition, the therapist may also describe personal situations, problems, and anecdotes, from which the client is supposed to learn and adapt to new positive behaviours. There are also problems regarding the counsellors being different in gender from the Muslim clients. To complicate matters further, both male and female Muslim clients cannot make direct eye contact with counsellors of the opposite sex – this is common in many Muslim families – thus counsellors may wrongly assume that the client is 'lying' or has poor self-esteem (Carter and Rashidi, 2004, p. 153).

Muslim clients may require a basic explanation about the nature of counselling or psychotherapy, the nature and scope of treatment interventions, expectations, and the roles of the therapist and patient in the therapeutic process. In addition, a central role of the counsellor is in helping guide the process toward self-actualisation and instilling a willingness to be introspective (Keshavarzi and Haque, 2013). Counselling Muslim patients must incorporate 'their ideological beliefs, cultural traditions, family support systems, and personal experiences. It must also include the cultural conflict that may not be recognised by the patients themselves' (Kobeisy, 2004, p. 71). Thus the counsellor needs to be aware of the social, political and cultural context of Muslim clients, particularly as they relate to issues surrounding relationship preferences and practices, extended family history, and modifications of traditional therapy (Ali et al., 2009). An ethical practitioner must also recognise the limitations of one's ability to help Muslim clients and to make appropriate referrals, while identifying their personal boundaries and serving the best interests of the patient (Keshavarzi and Haque, 2013). The confidential nature of therapy, and agreement on protection of information from family members, should be discussed because of the Islamic prohibition on expressing negative thoughts or emotions towards one's family (Ali et al., 2009). According to Al-Issa and Al-Junun (2000), the Muslim therapist needs to be assertive in telling a client what the problem is, unlike Western cultures where the choice to do something may be offered by the therapist but the client is not obligated to do it. According to Hamdan (2008), there are several significant cognitions (the mental process of knowing, including aspects such as awareness, perception, reasoning, and judgement) from the Islamic faith that can be incorporated into the counselling process with Muslim patients.

- Understanding the Temporal Reality of This World
- Focusing on the Hereafter
- Recalling the Purpose and Effects of Distress and Afflictions
- Trusting and Relying on Allah (*Tawakkul*)
- Understanding that After Hardship There will be Ease
- Focusing on the Blessings of Allah
- Remembering Allah and Reading Qur'aan
- Supplication (*Du'ah*).

Reflective Activity 12.2

Case Study 1

Mrs Salma Amin, a 49-year-old married Somali housewife, was admitted to a local hospital following episodes of severe neglect, apathy, and abnormal, disinhibited behaviour, low mood and delusional ideas. She had previously been given a diagnosis of schizophrenia but had not taken any of her regular neuroleptic medications for several months. During her brief admission, she repeatedly expressed the belief that she was possessed by *jinn*, having thought-insertion, and claimed to have supernatural power to heal. Her extended family also thought that she was possessed by *jinn* and discharged her from the psychiatric unit, against medical advice. She was taken to a local faith healer, who reinforced their views and treated her in the traditional African way. However, her condition deteriorated over the next few weeks and she was readmitted to hospital.

Case Study 2

A 25-year-old woman with no previous psychiatric history gradually withdrew from other people, became uncommunicative and stopped eating and drinking. The patient had reported prior to her breakdown that: 'Since I have got married, I frequently have very frightening dreams about my husband and others I love. Before marriage I never had frightening dreams as I always make my prayers at bedtime. Sometimes I see that there are *jinns* inside other people and I am trying to fight them by reciting "*Ayatul-Kursi*", but they are stopping me from doing so. I cannot sleep at night and wake up several times. A friend suggested to me that it may be the evil eye brought on by others who are jealous.'

Comments on Reflective Activity 12.2

Comments on Case Study 1

It is debatable whether this lady did in fact have *jinn* possession or whether she was a highly suggestible person with a possible dissociative state. However, it is clear that her lapse and relapse are due to her not adhering to her course of psychotropic therapy. Her complaining of hearing voices or thought-insertion did not disappear after having traditional healing treatment from the faith healer. In fact, her condition became unmanageable after seeing the traditional faith healer. There is a difference between psychotic state episodes and religious experiences. In psychosis, these include, according to Dein (2004): experiences that are often very personal, their details exceeding conventional expressions of belief; in many cases, the only distinguishing feature is the intensity of the belief, with the patient thinking of nothing else, and the onset of the beliefs and behaviours marks a change in the patient's life, with a deterioration of social skills and personal hygiene.

Comments on Case Study 2

The evil eye is a mental or physical condition of instability that overpowers the person affected. This can be caused by another human or by a *jinn*. When a patient or their family or friends believe that *jinn* are the cause of symptoms or unusual behaviour, the first and most important step is to

- Elicit, in an open and non-judgemental manner, the patient's (and if appropriate, the family's) ideas, concerns and expectations.
- Recognise that symptoms attributed to possession by *jinn* are commonly manifestations of a mental health disorder that may benefit from medical treatment.
- Appreciate that, although it may be obvious that the patient and relatives have interpreted symptoms incorrectly, beliefs that are strongly held (and often socially convenient) will be hard to alter at a time when anxiety is running high.

Conclusion

The above cases illustrate the difficult interactions between cultural and religious beliefs and conventional medicine. Clearly, in any case of alleged *jinn* possession, underlying organic disorders should be excluded by physical examination and investigations. Any underlying mental health problems should be treated by the usual psychiatric methods, but the clinician should respect the religious and cultural issues and avoid directly contradicting statements from the patient or relatives about the reality of possession. When medicine invites conflict with culture and religion, the therapeutic alliance suffers (Khalifa and Hardie, 2005). Most people are content to utilise biomedical treatments without giving up traditional explanations of illness (Dein, 2002; Luckmann, 1999); therefore there may be a strong case for involving an *Imam* or religious leader in the management of these cases.

From an Islamic perspective, there is no doubt that genuine belief in God can be the best cure for most of our psychological disturbances. It is worth noting that Sheikh 'Abd al-'Azeez ibn Baaz said: 'Although it is permissible to use physical medicine, the sick person should also look for spiritual remedies as prescribed in Islam, in which Allah has put the cure for both physical and mental health problems, such as *Ruqya* as prescribed in Islam, in which Qur'aan or words narrated in the Sunnah are recited' (Sheikh 'Abd al-'Azeez Ibn Baaz, Fatwa69766, 3/274). Sheikh Ibn 'Uthaymeen was asked: 'Can a believer become mentally ill? What is the treatment for that according to Shariah?' He replied: 'Undoubtedly a person may suffer from psychological or mental diseases, such as anxiety about the future and regret for the past. Psychological diseases affect the body more than physical diseases affect it. Treating these diseases by means of the things prescribed in Shariah – for example, *Ruqya* – is more effective than treating them with physical medicines, as is well known.'

Islamic institutions can play a most effective and vital role in the promotion of mental health and the prevention of chronic mental health problems. Hospital-based psychiatric nurses and community psychiatric nurses could collaborate with *Imams* through outreach services to help fulfil a potentially vital role in improving access to appropriate mental health and social services for minority Muslim communities where there currently appear to be unmet psychosocial needs (Ali et al., 2005). Above all, there is a need to foster communication and trust between Muslim religious leaders and mental health professionals to improve access to religiously and culturally appropriate psychiatric services. Multicultural counselling methods are imperative if we are to ensure that our students of counselling are well prepared to work with diverse families, particularly those from Muslim backgrounds (Khaja and Frederick, 2008). However, although most training programmes and workshops place an emphasis on being culturally sensitive, there has been limited attention paid to how to go beyond being sensitive, to providing culturally integrative and efficacious care (Keshavarzi and Haque, 2013).

References

Abdullah, S. (2007) 'Islam and Counseling: Models of Practice in Muslim Communal Life', *Journal of Pastoral Counseling* 42, 42–55.

Abu Dawud. 4403, cited in http://islamqa.info/en/ref/146375, date accessed 4 August 2013.

Abu-Ras, W. and Abu-Bader, S.H. (2008) 'The Impact of the September 11, 2001, Attacks on the Well-being of Arab Americans in New York City', *Journal of Muslim Mental Health* 3, 217–39.

Abu-Ras, W. and Abu-Bader, S. (2009) 'Risk Factors for Posttraumatic Stress Disorder (PTSD): the Case of Arab- and Muslim-Americans, post-9/11', *Journal of Immigrant & Refugee Studies* 7, 4, 393–418.

Ahmed, N. (2009) *Memorandum from the Institute for Policy Research & Development* (PVE 19), Executive Summary (London: Institute for Policy Research & Development) (www.iprd.org.uk).

Ahmed, S. and Amer, M.N. (2012) *Counselling Muslims. Handbook of Mental Health Issues and Interventions* (New York: Routledge).

Ai, A.T., Tice, T.N., Huang, B. and Ishisaka, A. (2005) 'Wartime Faith-based Reactions among Traumatized Kosovar and Bosnian Refugees in the United States', *Mental Health, Religion & Culture* 8, 4, 291–308 (18).

Al-Ashqar, Umar S. (2003) *The World of the Jinn and Devils in the Light of the Qur'an and Sunnah* (Riyadh, Saudi Arabia: International Islamic Publishing House).

Al-Habeeb, T.A. (2003) 'A Pilot Study of Faith Healers' Views on Evil Eye, *Jinn* Possession, and Magic, Al-Qassim Region, Saudi Arabia', *Saudi Society, Family and Community Medicine*, 10, 3, 31–8.

Ali, O.M. and Milstein, G. (2012) 'Mental Illness Recognition and Referral Practice among *Imams* in the United States', *Journal of Muslim Mental Health* VI, 2, 3–13, http://hdl.handle.net/2027/spo.10381607.0006.202, date accessed 30 October 2013.

Ali, O.M., Milstein, G. and Marzuk, P.M. (2005) 'The *Imam*'s Role in Meeting the Counseling Needs of Muslim Communities in the United States', *Psychiatric Services* 56, 2, 202–5.

Ali, O., Abu-Ras, W. and Hamid, H. (2009) *Muslim Americans*, http://ssrdqst.rfmh.org/cecc/index.php?q=node/25, date accessed 6 August 2013.

Al-Issa, I. and Al-Junun (2000) 'Mental Health Problems in the Islamic World' (International Universities Press; 1st edition), www.ssfcm.org/english/index.php?fuseaction=content.main&mainsection=0000000543, date accessed 6 August 2013.

Al-Khathami, A. (2001) *The Implementation and Evaluation of Educational Program for PHC Physicians to Improve their Recognition of Mental Health Problem, in the Eastern Province of Saudi Arabia* [Dissertation] (Saudi Arabia: AL Khobar, King Faisal University).

Al-Khathami, A.D. and Ogbeide, D.O. (2002) 'Prevalence of Mental Health Problem among Saudi Adult Primary-care Patients in Central Saudi Arabia', *Saudi Medical Journal* 23, 6, 721–4.

Al-Krenawi, A. and Graham, J.R. (1999) 'Social Work and Koranic Mental Health Healers', International Social Work (January) 42, 1, 53–65.

Al-Krenawi, A. and Graham, J.R (2000) 'Culturally Sensitive Social Work Practice with Arab Clients in Mental Health Settings, 2000', National Association of Social Workers, www.socialworkers.org/pressroom/events/911/alkrenawi.asp?print=1, date accessed 6 August 2013.

Alouda, N. and Rathurb, A. (2009) 'Factors Affecting Attitudes toward Seeking and Using Formal Mental Health and Psychological Services among Arab Muslim Populations', *Journal of Muslim Mental Health* 4, 2, 79–103.

American Psychiatric *Rrevision (TR)* (Washington, DC: American Psychiatric Association) (DSM-IV-TR).

Azhar, M.Z. and Varma, S.L. (1995a) 'Religious Psychotherapy in Depressive Patients', *Psychotherapy and Psychosomatics* 63, 3–4, 165–8.

Azhar, M.Z. and Varma, S.L. (1995b) 'Religious Psychotherapy as Management of Bereavement', *Acta Psychiatrica Scandinavia* 91, 4, 233–5.

Azhar, M.Z., Varma, S.L. and Dharap, A.S. (1994) 'Religious Psychotherapy in Anxiety Disorder Patients', *Acta Psychiatrica Scandinavia* 90, 1, 1–3.

Aziz, S. (2001) 'Do Souls of the Dead Return Back to the World?' *As-Sunnah Newsletter. 2001*, issue 13, www.ahya.org/amm/modules. php?name=Sections&op=viewarticle&artid=160, date accessed 6 August 2013.

Badri, M. (2009) *Can the Psychotherapy of Muslim Patients be of Real Help to Them Without being Islamized?* www.zeriislam.com/artikulli.php?id=987, date accessed 6 August 2013.

Barkdull, C., Khaja, K., Queiro-Tajalli, I., Swart, A., Cunningham, D. and Dennis, S. (2011) 'Experiences of Muslims in Four Western Countries post–9/11', *Journal of Women & Social Work* 26, 2, 139–53.

Bergin, E. and Jensen, J.P. (1990) 'Religiosity and Psychotherapists: a National Survey', *Psychotherapy* 27, 1, 3–7.

Bhui, K. (2001) 'Epidemiology and Social Issues in Psychiatry', in D. Bhugra and R. Cochrane (eds), *Multicultural Britain* (London: Gaskell), pp. 49–74.

Blom J.D., Eker, H., Basalan, H., Aouaj, Y. and Hoek, H.W. (2010) 'Hallucinations Attributed to Djinns', Nederlands Tijdschrift voor Geneeskunde 154: A973.

Bukhari, Chapter 78. The Book of Patients, no. 5137, The Sahih Collection of al-Bukhari, www.sunnipath.com/library/Hadith/H0002P0078.aspx, date accessed 5 August 2013.

Caraballo, A., Hamid, H., Lee, J.R., McQuery, J.D., Rho, Y., Kramer, E.J., Lim, R.F. and Lu, F.G. (2006) 'A Resident's Guide to the Cultural Formulation', in R.F. Lim (ed.), *Clinical Manual of Cultural Psychiatry* (Arlington, VA: American Psychiatric Publication), pp. 243–65.

Carter, J.D. and Rashidi, A. (2004) 'East Meets West: Integrating Psychotherapy Approaches for Muslim Women, *Holistic Nursing Practice*, May–June, 152–9.

Catlin, A.J. and Boffman J.H. (1998) 'When Cultures Clash: Review of Anne Fadiman, *The Spirits Catch You and You Fall Down'*, *Pediatric Nursing* 24, 2, 170–3.

Cinnirella, M. and Loewenthal, K.M. (1999) 'Religious and Ethnic Group Influences on Beliefs about Mental Health Problems: a Qualitative Interview Study', *British Journal of Medical Psychology* 72, 4, 505–24.

Dein, S. (2002) 'Transcultural Psychiatry', *British Journal of Psychiatry* 181, 6, 535–6.

Dein, S. (2004) 'Working with Patients with Religious Beliefs', Advances in Psychiatric Treatment 10, 4, 287–94

Doebbeling, C.C. (2007) Treatment of Mental Health Problems, www.merckmanuals.com/home/mental_health_disorders/overview_of_mental_health_care/treatment_of_mental_illness.html, date accessed 6 August 2013.

Dols, M.W. (2007) 'Historical Perspective: Insanity in Islamic Law', *Journal of Muslim Mental Health* 2, 1, 81–99.

Dunning, J. (2011) 'Using Faith to Help Muslims Face Mental Health Problems', *Community Care.co.uk*, www.communitycare.co.uk/Articles/02/03/2011/116342/using-faith-to-help-muslims-face-mental-health-problems.htm, date accessed 6 August 2013.

El-Islam, M.F. (2008) 'Arab Culture and Mental Health Care', *Transcultural Psychiatry* 45, 671–82, http://dx.doi.org/10.1177/1363461508100788, date accessed 6 August 2013.

Gartner, J. (1996) 'Religious Commitment, Mental Health, and Prosocial Behavior: a Review of the EmpiricalLliterature', in E.P. Shafranske (ed.), *Religion and the Clinical Practice of Psychology* (Washington, DC: American Psychological Association), pp. 187–214.

Goldberg, D. (1999) 'Cultural Aspects of Mental Disorder in Primary Care', in D. Bhugra and V. Bahl (eds), *Ethnicity: An Agenda for Mental Health* (London: Gaskell), pp. 23–8.

Hamdan, A. (2008) 'Cognitive Restructuring: an Islamic Perspective', *Journal of Muslim Mental Health* 3, 1, 99–116.

Haque, A. (2004) 'Religion and Mental Health: the Case of American Muslims', *Journal of Religion and Health* 43, 1, 45–58.

House of Commons Communities and Local Government Committee (2010) 'Preventing Violent Extremism'. Sixth Report of Session 2009–10. 2010 House of Commons (London: The Stationery Office), www.publications. parliament.uk/pa/cm200910/cmselect/cmcomloc/65/65.pdf, date accessed 6 August 2013.

Imam Magid. *Islamic Perspective of Counseling*, www.isna.net/Resources/ articles/community/Islamic-Perspective-of-Counseling.aspx, date accessed 6 August 2013.

Inayat, Q. (2005) 'Psychotherapy in a Multi-ethnic Society', *Psychotherapist* 26, 7.

islamqa, Fatwa 146375, http://islamqa.info/en/ref/146375, date accessed 5 August 2013.

Jafari, M.E. (1993) 'Counselling Values and Objectives: a Comparison of Western and Islamic Perspectives', *American Journal of Islamic Social Studies* 10, 3, 326–39.

Kelly, E.W., Aridi, A. and Bakhtiar, L. (1996) 'Muslims in the United States: an Exploratory Study of Universal and Mental Health Values', *Counseling and Values* 40, 3, 206–18.

Keshavarzi, H. and Haque, A. (2013) 'Outlining a Psychotherapy Model for Enhancing Muslim Mental Health within an Islamic Context', International Journal for the Psychology of Religion 23, 3. DOI: 10.1080/10508619.2012.712000.

Khaja, K. and Frederick, C. (2008) 'Reflection on Teaching Effective Social Work Practice for Working with Muslim Communities', *Advances in Social Work* 9, 1, 1–7.

Khalifa, N. and Hardie, T. (2005) 'Possession and *Jinn*', *Journal of the Royal Society of Medicine* 98, 8, 351–3.

Khan, Z. (2006) 'Attitudes toward Counseling and Alternative Support among Muslims in Toledo, Ohio', Journal of Muslim Mental Health 1, 1, 21–42.

Kleinman, A., Eisenberg, L. and Good, B. (1978) Culture, Illness, and Care: Clinical Lessons from Anthropologic and Cross-cultural Research, Annals of Internal Medicine 88, 2, 251–8.

Kobeisy, A.N. (2004) Counseling American Muslims: Understanding the Faith and Helping the People (Wesport, CT: Greenwood Publishing Group).

Larson, D.B., Sherrill, K.A., Lyons, J.S., Craigie, F.C., Thielman, S. B., Greenwold, M.A. et al. (1992) 'Associations between Dimensions of Religious Commitment and Mental Health Reported in the *American Journal of Psychiatry* and Archives of General Psychiatry: 1978–1989', *American Journal of Psychiatry* 149, 557–9.

Littlewood, R. and Lipsedge, M. (1988) 'Psychiatric Illness among British Afro-Caribbeans' (editorial), *British Medical Journal* 296, 6627, 950–1.

Lopez, S.R. and Guarnaccia, P.J.J. (2000) 'Cultural Psychopathology: Uncovering the Social World of Mental Illness', *Annual Review of Psychology* 51, 571–98.

Luckmann, J. (1999) *Transcultural Communication in Nursing* (Albany, NY: Delmar Publishers).

Maynard, S. (2008) *Muslim Mental Health. A Scoping Paper on Theoretical Models, Practice and Related Mental Health Concerns in Muslim Communities*, Stephen Maynard & Associates, www.signposts.org.uk/Assets/downloads/bme/Muslim%20Mental%20Health%20-%20Stephen%20Maynard.pdf, date accessed 6 August 2013.

McCullough, M.E. and Larson, D.B. (1999) 'Religion and Depression: a Review of the Literature', *Twin Research* 2, 2, 126–36.

Mrana (2009) *Mental Health Problem and Islam*, www.smilecan.org/mental-illness-and-islam, date accessed 6 August 2013.

Muhaimin, A.N. (2009) personal communication, 28 November, cited in Nursesaida's Blog, Module 3 – Religion and Muslim Culture on Health Beliefs, http://nursesaida.wordpress.com/about/, date accessed 30 October 2013.

Murty, O.P., Cheh, L.B., Bakit, P.A., Hui, F.J., Ibrahim, Z.B. and Jusoh, N.B. (2008) 'Suicide and Ethnicity in Malaysia', *American Journal of Forensic Medicine and Pathology* 29, 1, 19–22.

Muslim [a], Sahih Muslim Hadith 5427, www.islamhelpline.com/node/966, date accessed 5 August 2013.

Muslim [b], Hadith 7: The Religion is *Naseehah* (Sincere Advice), www.islaam.net/main/display.php?id=136&category=24, date accessed 6 August 2013.

Nada, E. (2007) *Perceptions of Mental Health Problems in Islam: a Textual and Experimental Analysis* (PhD Thesis, University of Western Australia), http://repository.uwa.edu.au:80/R/-?func=dbin-jump-full&object_id=9033&silo_library=GEN01, date accessed 6 August 2013.

Nassar-McMillan, S.C. and Hakim-Larson, J. (2003) 'Counseling Considerations among Arab Americans', *Journal of Counseling & Development* 81, 2, 150–9.

Paladin, A.V. (1998) 'Ethics and Neurology in the Islamic World: Continuity and Change', *Italian Journal of Neurological Science* 19, 4, 255–8.

Pritchard, C. and Amanullah, S. (2007) 'An Analysis of Suicide and Undetermined Deaths in 17 Predominantly Islamic Countries Contrasted with the UK', *Psychological Medicine* 37, 3, 421–340.

Pridmore, S. and Pasha, M.I. (2004) 'Religion and Spirituality: Psychiatry and Islam', *Australasian Psychiatry* 12, 4, 380–5.

Rahiem, F.T. and Hamid, H. (2012) 'Mental Health Interview and Cultural Formulation', in S. Ahmed and M. Amer (eds), *Counselling Muslims: Handbook of Mental Health Issues and Interventions* (New York: Routledge), pp. 52–66.

Rahman, F. (1998) *Health and Medicine in the Islamic Tradition* (Chicago: ABC International Group).

Rashid, S., Copello, A. and Birchwood, M. (2011) 'Muslim Faith Healers' Views on Substance Misuse and Psychosis', *Journal of Mental Health, Religion & Culture* 0, 0, 1–21.

Rassool, G. Hussein (2000) 'The Crescent and Islam: Healing, Nursing and Spiritual Dimensions: Some Considerations towards an Understanding of the Islamic Perspectives on Caring', *Journal of Advanced Nursing* 32, 2, 1476–84.

Razali, S.M., Hasanah, C.I., Aminah, K. and Subramaniam, M. (1998). 'Religious Sociocultural Psychotherapy in Patients with Anxiety and Depression', *Australian and New Zealand Journal of Psychiatry* 32, 6, 867–72.

Shah, A. and Chandia, M. (2010) 'The Relationship between Suicide and Islam: a Cross-national Study', *Journal of Injury and Violence Research* 2, 2, 93–7.

Shah, A., Bhat, R., MacKenzie, S. and Koen, C. (2007) 'Elderly Suicide Rates: Cross-national Comparisons and Association with Sex and Elderly Age-bands', *Medical Science and the Law* 47, 3, 244–52.

Sheikh 'Abd al-'Azeez ibn Baaz, Fatwa-69766. Majmoo' Fataawa al-Sheikh Ibn Baaz, 3/274, http://islamqa.info/en/ref/69766/mental%20illness, date accessed 6 August 2013.

Sheikh Al-Fawzan: al-Muntaqa (1) question no. 87, www.islam-qa.com/en/ref/89604, date accessed 6 August 2013.

Sheikh Ibn 'Uthaymeen Fataawa Islamiyyah, 4/465, 466, http://islamqa.info/en/ref/21677/mental%20illness, date accessed 6 August 2013.

Sheridan, L.P. (2006) 'Islamophobia pre- and post-September 11th, 2001', *Journal of Interpersonal Violence* 21, 3, 317–36.

Spooner, B. (2004) 'The Evil Eye in the Middle East', in M. Douglas (ed.), *Witchcraft, Confession and Accusation* (London: Routledge), pp. 311–20.

Sue, D.W. and Sue, D. (2008) *Counseling the Culturally Diverse: Theory and Practice*, 5th edn (New York, NY: Wiley).

Triandafyllidou, A. (2012) *Addressing Cultural, Ethnic and Religious Diversity Challenges in Europe. A Comparative Overview of 15 European Countries* (San Domenico de Fiesole, Italy: European University Institute, Robert Schuman Centre for Advanced Studies).

Websters-online-dictionary, www.websters-online-dictionary.org/definitions/Evil+eye, date accessed 6 August 2013.

World Health Organisation (WHO) (2001) *ICD-10 Classification of Mental and Behavioral Disorders*, www.who.int/classifications/icd/en/bluebook.pdf, date accessed 6 August 2013.

World Health Organisation (WHO) (2007) *SUPRE Prevention of Suicidal Behaviours: A Task for All* (Geneva: World Health Organisation).

Zakiullah, N., Saleem, S., Sadiq, S., Sani, N., Shahpurwala, M., Shamim, A., Yousuf, A., Khan, M.M. and Nayani, P. (2008) 'Deliberate Self-harm: Characteristics of Patients Presenting to a Tertiary Care Hospital in Karachi, Pakistan', *Crisis: Journal of Crisis Intervention & Suicide* 29, 1, 32–7.

Addictive Behaviours: Drug Use and Gambling from an Islamic Perspective

13

G. Hussein Rassool

Learning Outcomes:

- Examine the nature and extent of drug use and gambling in Muslim communities.
- Identify measures of prevention and public health from an Islamic perspective.
- Discuss the Islamic perspective on addiction and addictive behaviours.
- Examine Muslim responses to addictive behaviours.
- Discuss nursing interventions in the care of a patient with addiction problem.

Reflective Activity 13.1

State whether the following statements are true or false. Give reasons for your answers.

	True	False
1 The range of addictive behaviours includes both pharmacological and non-pharmacological addictions.		
2 Many Muslim countries are not protected from HIV/AIDS because of religious and cultural norms.		
3 The public health problem related to addictive behaviours is only confined to illicit drugs.		

	True	*False*
4 The consequences of addiction affect not only the individuals user but also their families, communities and the entire society and economy.		
5 Tobacco use kills fewer people every year than HIV/AIDS, tuberculosis and malaria combined.		
6 Heroin is the world's most widely used illicit substance, followed by amphetamine-type stimulants.		
7 Gambling, now recognised as a psychiatric disorder, has become a growing concern in public health policy.		
8 In Islam, gambling is not only customary but also taken to be a cause of pride, nobility and honour.		
9 Muslim scholars are unanimous on the prohibition of drugs including tobacco, cannabis, opiates and other psychoactive substances.		
10 The assessment of drug problems should focus on the current pattern of drug use, the quantities, and associated problems.		
11 The treatment interventions for problem gamblers include only pharmacological therapies.		
12 The 'lesser of the two evils' principles are used to justify the permissibility of harm reduction approaches, as drug use and HIV pertain to matters of life and death.		
13 Nurses should provide health information about the prevention of blood-borne viruses (such as HIV and hepatitis B and C), including reducing risky injecting and sexual behaviours.		
14 Islamic rules and values prohibit adultery, homosexuality, and intravenous drug use.		
15 Safer sex can be practised outside legal marriage.		
16 All Islamic countries include harm reduction as part of their national policies on HIV and drugs.		
17 Harm reduction approaches have been advocated in dealing with both the use of drugs and injecting behaviour and the control of HIV.		

Introduction

Our society has an appetite for seeking the next novel experience of enjoyment and instant gratification through activities, food and pharmacological substances. Our constant exposure to, and the accessibility of, both addictive substances and addictive activities have created new social and cultural norms that have influenced people and made them more susceptible to addictions (Rassool, 2011). The range of addictive behaviours include both pharmacological and non-pharmacological addictions: eating, alcohol drinking, drug use, gambling, work, exercise and sexuality. In addition, there is an increase in the prescription and use of antidepressants, pain killers and sleeping tablets. Addictions to psychoactive substances continue to be a major concern for society and are now regarded as a public health problem. The consequences of addiction do not only affect the individual users but also their families, communities and the entire society and economy. Addictive behaviour problems can affect every one of us regardless of age, sex, race, marital status, place of residence, income level, or lifestyle. From an Islamic perspective, the 'War on Drugs' and other addictive behaviours began 14 centuries ago (Philips). This chapter will focus on addictive behaviours related to drug misuse, gambling addiction and associated problems from an Islamic perspective. For a more comprehensive account of addictive behaviours such as Internet addiction, eating disorders and sexual addictions, see Rassool (2011).

Addictive behaviours: nature and extent

UNODC (2012) estimates that around 5 per cent of the world's adult population (aged 15 to 64) have used an illicit drug. Cannabis is the world's most widely used illicit substance followed by amphetamine-type stimulants, cocaine and opiates. However, the use of synthetic drugs is feared to be increasing in the developing world. New psychoactive substances are now being pushed as 'legal highs' and substitutes for other illicit stimulants, such as cocaine or ecstasy. These formulations include 'spice', which mimics the effects of cannabis; mephedrone and MDPV, which are often sold as 'bath salts' or 'plant food'; and piperazine. Tobacco use kills more than 5 million people every year – more than HIV/AIDS, tuberculosis and malaria combined (WHO, 2009). In addition to its direct health effects, it is reported that tobacco leads to malnutrition, increased healthcare costs and premature death (WHO, 2004). It also contributes to a higher illiteracy rate, since money that could have been used for education is spent on tobacco-related problems instead. Recent studies have shown that the more young people are exposed to tobacco advertising, the more likely they are to start smoking. Despite this, only 5% of the world's population is covered by comprehensive bans on tobacco advertising, promotion and sponsorship (WHO, 2008). Tobacco companies, meanwhile, continue targeting young people by falsely associating the use of tobacco products with qualities such as glamour, energy, and sex appeal.

Gambling, now recognised as a psychiatric disorder, has become a growing concern in public health policy as there has been a rapid increase in the proliferation and accessibility of legalised gambling in many parts of the world. According to American statistics of the National Council, 3 million adults are addicted to gambling and there are twice as many addicted gamblers as cancer patients (USA gambling addiction statistics, 2003). It might be the lottery, bingo, or poker and the Slots game (online). Cunningham-Williams et al. (2005) have found that the number of problem gamblers is growing as the availability of legal gambling increases in the US. It is estimated that the rate for problem gambling in the UK is either 0.7% or 0.9%. These rates are similar to those in other European countries (such as Germany and Norway) and are lower than countries such as the USA and Australia (www.gambleaware.co.uk, 2012).

Drug use in Muslim countries

Despite the fact that drugs and tobacco smoking are forbidden (*haram*) in Islam, alcohol and illicit drug use are widespread in many predominantly Islamic countries or countries with a significant Muslim population. Although data and information are limited, indirect indicators show that, in terms of treatment demand and social expression, related crime, HIV and hepatitis C, and abuse of all kinds of drugs are increasing in these countries (Toufiq, 2012).

In recent years, the Middle East has emerged as a major new market for amphetamines, with demand for pills called Captagon. This was a brand name for a discontinued product that contained fenethylline, but these pills today mostly consist of amphetamine and caffeine (UNODC, 2010). Use of cannabis, commonly known as marijuana, is widespread, while Libya and Bahrain in particular have large numbers of heroin users (Toufiq, 2012). In addition, Lebanon, with its clubbing scene, has a higher incidence of the use of designer-drugs such as ecstasy. Two-thirds of opium that is not converted to heroin is consumed in the Islamic Republic of Iran (42%), Afghanistan (7%) and Pakistan (7%) (UNODC, 2010). A survey conducted in Afghanistan suggests that the country has one of the highest opiate use prevalence rates in the world (UNODC, 2010). In Central Asia, Kazakhstan in particular has a high opiate use prevalence rate, followed by Uzbekistan and Kyrgyzstan but lower in Tajikistan and Turkmenistan. In Africa, Egypt is one the countries in the region with the highest prevalence of opiate use. However, the data available do not show a clear picture of the nature and extent of drug use in Muslim countries.

Many Muslim countries are protected from HIV/AIDS due to religious and cultural norms. However, they are now facing a rapidly rising threat due to changes of lifestyle and behaviours. 'Premarital sex, adultery, prostitution, homosexuality and intravenous drug use' are the major key factors for spreading HIV/AIDS in the Muslim countries (Eberstadt and Kelley, 2005). Various studies show that as many as four in ten injecting drug users in Algeria, five in ten in Egypt and Morocco, and six in ten in Lebanon have used non-sterile syringes (UNODC, 2010). However, the reliability of the available data on HIV/AIDS incidence, prevalence and mortality for Muslims is low because many Muslim countries either do not report their statistics or are under-reporting (Hasnain, 2005).

Islamic perspective on addiction

In Islam, there is a zero-tolerance policy toward addictive behaviours such as drug use and gambling. Any substance affecting the nervous system that can change consciousness, mood, thoughts and behaviours is prohibited. Muslim scholars are unanimous on the prohibition of more modern forms of street drugs such as nicotine, amphetamine, cocaine, opium, heroin and cannabis. The scholars have used principles of Islamic jurisprudence (*Fiqh*) to derive judgements regarding many of the illicit drugs available today that were unknown at the time of the revelation of the Qur'aan. Regarding the use of cannabis (hashish), it is argued that the application of the texts of the Qur'aan and Sunnah to hashish is similar to that of wine. Sheikh ibn Taymiyah stated that: 'This solid grass (hashish) is *haram*, whether or not it produces intoxication. Sinful people smoke it because they imagine it producing rapture and delight, an effect similar to drunkenness. While wine makes the one who drinks it active and quarrelsome, hashish produces dullness and lethargy; furthermore, smoking it disturbs the mind and temperament, excites sexual desire, and leads to shameless promiscuity, and these are greater evils than those caused by drinking. According to Sheikh Yusuf Al-Qaradawi (2007), drugs such as cannabis, heroin, cocaine, opium and the like 'are taken as a means of escape from the inner reality of one's feelings and the outer realities of life and religion into the realm of fantasy and imagination'.

Prior to the advent of Islam, gambling was not only customary but also taken to be a cause of pride, nobility and honour. For excessive show of pride, these people would distribute their share of the winnings amongst the poor

(Tafseer-ul-Kabeer Lir-Razi). Allah says in the Qur'aan (interpretation of the meaning):

> ☐ *O you who have believed, indeed, intoxicants, gambling, [sacrificing on] stone alters [to other than Allah], and divining arrows are but defilement from the work of Satan, so avoid it that you may be successful.* (Al-Mā'idah [The Table] 5:90)

In the above verse, Allah has described intoxicants and gambling amongst other things as being appalling, despicable and hateful acts of Satan and has commanded us to abstain from them because intoxicants, apart from sowing the seeds of enmity, also stop the remembrance of Allah (Islam and Drugs). The Almighty put intoxicating substances in the same category as gambling, where most people lose their savings, become addicted and destroy their lives. The harms of gambling include emotional problems and isolation; impact on family and children; financial problems; health problems including anxiety, depression and stress-related problems such as poor sleep, ulcers, bowel problems, headaches and muscle pains; gambling problems can lead to physical or emotional abuse of a partner, elder parent or child. Philips stated that 'By classifying drugs on a par with games of chance, idolatrous practices and the fortunetelling, all of which have been pronounced as absolutely forbidden, the prohibition of drugs is further emphasized.' He further suggested that 'Allah identified the origin of drugs for humans to realize that they are weapons of their most avowed enemy, Satan. In the battle for human souls, Satan uses a variety of tools which he beautifies and makes alluring in order to trap human beings' (Philips). The failure to abstain from intoxicants prevents us from the remembrance of Allah. The Messenger of Allah said: 'Whoever says to his companion: come let us place a game of haphazard, should give alms (as atonement)' (Bukhari). And he also stated that 'Whoever plays Chess is as if he dyes his hands with the flesh of swine and its blood' (Muslim). And 'He who plays backgammon disobeys Allah and His Messenger Muhammad' (Abu Dawud).

Prevention and public health

Islam has always been in the forefront in dealing with public health issues. The Qur'aan and the Hadith offer numerous directives about maintaining health, at the community, family and individual levels. Although care of the individual is important, safeguarding communities, including their weakest members, is of paramount importance (Stacey, 2010). However, to ignore Islam and its role in a community invites failure for any public health programme, whether it be polio eradication, HIV prevention or tobacco control (Simpson, 2005).

Harm reduction approaches have been advocated in dealing with both drug use and injecting behaviour, and the control of HIV. Harm reduction programmes include information about safer drug use and safer sex, needle exchanges schemes (pharmacy-based needle exchange or other forms of needle exchange), programmes to reduce the risks associated with HIV and hepatitis, and the supervision of the consumption of methadone or other opiate substitutes. In relation to the control of the HIV pandemic, there is evidence to suggest that harm reduction approaches had some success in the Islamic Republic of Iran, Malaysia and Indonesia where both needle exchange programmes and opioid substitution therapy have been implemented (Mesquita et al., 2007; Razzaghi et al., 2006; Reid et al., 2007). However, Iran remains the only country in the region where access to both needle exchange programmes and opioid substitution therapy has been dramatically scaled up (Cook, 2010).

Some Muslim countries such as Libya, Syria and Jordan have rejected the harm reduction approaches in dealing with injecting drug use-driven HIV epidemics (IHRA, 2010). Since 2008, Tunisia has introduced pilot needle and syringe programmes (NSPs). Morocco has increased its service provision and several needle and syringe programmes are now operating through both fixed and mobile units (IHRA, 2010). Some provision of opioid substitution therapy has been reported in Iran, Lebanon and Morocco. It has been reported that there are three opioid substitution therapy sites in the United Arab Emirates; no further details on service provision is available and the existence of sites has been disputed by civil society in the region (Toufiq, cited in Cook, 2010). Iran, Lebanon and Morocco currently include harm reduction as part of their national policies on HIV and drugs.

There are many Islamic countries that does not support the policy and practice of harm reduction despite the nature and extent of drug misuse and injecting drug use-driven HIV epidemics. The religious and political leaders have traditionally opposed harm reduction approaches on the basis that distribution of needles and condoms would encourage and imply acceptance of drug use and illegal sexual relations and that opioid substitution therapy would compromise the nation's goal to become drug free (Mandani et al., 2004; Reid et al., 2007; Todd et al., 2007). That means that harm reduction approaches contradict Islamic rules and values and, as such, cannot be used as valid and acceptable strategies to prevent the spread of this infection in Islamic countries (Mandani et al., 2004). It has been suggested that the preventive strategies to prevent HIV infection in Islamic countries should include strengthening of both Islamic and health education, encouraging people to follow and implement the Islamic rules and values that prohibit adultery, homosexuality, and intravenous drug use, and to practise safe sex only through legal marriage (Mandani et al., 2004).

The advocates of harm reduction approaches in Islamic countries to control the drug-driven HIV epidemics based their arguments on 'the Islamic principles of the preservation and protection of the faith, life, intellect, progeny and wealth' (Kamarulzaman and Saifuddeen, 2010). That is, the '*maqasid al-shari'ah*' framework. The authors argued that 'harm reduction programmes are permissible, and in fact, provide a practical solution to a problem that could result in far greater damage to the society at large if left unaddressed'. According to Kamarulzaman and Saifuddeen (2010), the principle of injury (*darar*) in Islam asserts that no one should be hurt or cause hurt to others. That is, the 'lesser of the Two Evils' principle, which is used to justify the permissibility of harm reduction approaches, as drug use and HIV pertain to matters of life and death. Another principle is the necessity to overrule prohibition in situations where there is great necessity: something that was originally prohibited may become permissible, quoting verse 173 of Surah Al-Baqara (Kamarulzaman and Saifuddeen, 2010). Other principles include: 'harm must be treated and benefits must be brought forth' and 'public interest should be given priority over personal interest'. The above principles have been used to implement harm reduction approaches in a few Islamic countries.

Islamic response to addictive behaviours

Addiction affects not only the individual drug user or gambler but the whole extended family. Family members who are affected by addiction face a form of chronic stress that impacts upon them at a number of different levels, including daily hassles of an unpleasant kind as well as relationships that deteriorate over what may be a very lengthy time span (Orford, 2012). There is much uncertainty for family members, and safety issues for the family, particularly for children. The focus of the family is on the addict rather than on their own specific needs and happiness. Some families become co-dependent, that is, they are part of the process of enabling the addict to continue using drugs or gambling activity. Providing for the needs of the addict or controlling the addict cause the family members to sacrifice their self-worth, personal growth and needs (Motivational Assessment Process for Families Members, 2002).

Most Muslim families are ashamed to ask for help when they think everyone will find out about their family problem. The result is that families often employ strategies that focus not on seeking professional help for the addict, but on denying the situation and hiding it from the extended family and the rest of their community (Fountain). Consequently, the family is always pretending, covering up for and bailing the addict out of trouble. This co-dependence is counterproductive for both the family and the individual addict. It has been stated that families can empower themselves by learning new patterns of thinking, feeling behaving and relating to others (Ajri and Sabran, 2011). For some families, participating in a self-help group or programme for families of an addict/alcoholic would be desirable. The findings of a study (Ajri and Sabran, 2011) indicate that a '12-step program' is an effective programme which enabled co-dependents to have a positive self-image and take care of themselves more than another group who did not participate in this programme. For others, it has been suggested that the family can learn to modify their own behaviour (*Sadaqah*) and become an important part of recovery programmes (Garrett et al., 1998). Some examples include:

- The addict must turn to Allah, making sincere repentance (*Tawbah*) for their own sins and shortcomings.
- Remember Allah's favours and mercy with gratitude and humbleness.
- Put their trust in and reliance on Allah, with sincerity, as He has the power to do anything.
- Have hope but remember to accept Allah's predestination (*Qadar*).
- Keep company with other Muslims who are practising their Islamic way of life correctly.
- The family should remind themselves that the addicts are responsible for their own choices and actions, and their own deviant behaviours.
- The family should not remind the addict of past mistakes or negative incidents.
- The family should focus on the positive aspects of the addict's behaviour.
- The family should avoid confrontation or being drawn into arguments with the addict.
- The family should have clear boundaries such as not tolerating the addict using drugs in the family home.
- Explain to the addicts that their addiction is their own problem and if they choose to disobey Allah by using drugs or gambling then they can do it without your help.
- Release the addict into the care of Allah, you have no power over his/her addiction.
- Let the addicts face the consequences of their own actions if they are in debt.
- But let them know that if and when they choose to take steps to get help to quit, then you will be there to help and support them.
- You can inform them that there are places they could go to for help; perhaps offer them some literature to read.
- The Muslim family can play a significant role in the care and treatment of the addict during the stage of detoxification, rehabilitation and after-care.

- Muslims should always have hope that Allah will help us out of our difficulties, and should not despair. Allah says in the Qur'aan (interpretation of the meaning):
- *'... and whoever fears Allah, He will make for him a way out'*
- *'... and whoever relies upon Allah, then indeed He is sufficient for him'* (Aṭ-Ṭalāq [The Divorce] 65:2–3).

One the biggest roadblocks to recovery and awareness is the denial, feelings of guilt, fear of being stigmatised, and cultural and social restrictions which may impede Muslim addicts from admitting to their addiction. They are also among the reasons why many Muslims fail to seek help, support and treatment from mainstream addiction agencies. In addition, the reality is that there are limited culturally congruent services offering help for Muslims struggling with addictive behaviours. Many Muslim addicts are reluctant to go to non-Muslim agencies for help and advice, because of fears about confidentiality and the lack of cultural competence of service providers. In addition, there is the perception that the service providers will not meet their cultural and religious needs or may provide advice or treatment that is un-Islamic. The findings of a study indicated that the majority of the drug users who had accessed mainstream drug treatment services rated them poorly, not only because their expectations were unmet, but also because of the perceived lack of cultural and religious competence in the service (Fountain). Even when external help is sought for a drug user by their family, mainstream drug services are rarely considered (Fountain). However, the family could receive help from a Muslim doctor, *Imam*, Islamic counsellor or Islamic organisations. If they fail to get access to the above, or if the above are unable to offer immediate help, the family should consider those service provisions that are culturally sensitive and understand the specific needs of the Muslim addict.

Nursing interventions

An assessment is a brief process that aims to determine whether an individual has a drug or gambling problem, or health-related problems and risk behaviours. The assessment should focus on the current pattern of drug use, the quantities, and associated problems. In order to ascertain the level of dependence, it is important to ask about experiences of withdrawal symptoms or any psychological complications. For a comprehensive account describing the taking of a drug history, see Rassool (2009, 2011). A mental state assessment should be undertaken when psychiatric symptoms are evident. A urine or saliva sample should be obtained for laboratory analysis. Nurses should provide health information about the prevention of blood-borne viruses (such as HIV and hepatitis B and C), including reducing risky injecting and sexual behaviours. Provision such as pre-test advice and post-test counselling should be made available for those requiring tests for HIV. When assessing the needs of the patient, the nurse should take account of any religious, ethnic or cultural factors. Other additional factors, such as physical or learning disabilities, sight or hearing problems, or difficulties with reading or speaking English, should be considered (NICE, 2007). An interpreter or an advocate (someone who supports you in putting across your views) should be made available if needed.

It is important at the initial assessment to assess for signs of withdrawal and monitor for life-threatening conditions. Nurses should provide information about the various treatment options, drug-withdrawal symptoms, and how to cope with them. Explanation should also be given about the 'loss of tolerance' and the risk of overdose if these drugs are consumed whilst in the abstinence stage. Some drug users such as those using opioids must undergo a detoxification process as part of the initial stage of the treatment plan. Detoxification is the process of allowing the body to rid itself of the substance, while managing the symptoms of withdrawal or 'cold turkey'. This involves the prescribing of medication to enable the individual to stop using drugs. The treatments for drug misuse include: detoxification; abstinence-based treatment; psychosocial interventions; harm reduction; maintenance treatment (for heroin users); taking an opioid substitute (such as methadone or buprenorphine); residential rehabilitation; and aftercare and self-help groups (NICE, 2007; Rassool, 2009). It is also important to prepare the patient during the rehabilitation/aftercare phase about stress management, coping skills, nutrition, relapse prevention, and healthy lifestyle choices. Information about self-help groups (such as 12-step groups, Alliance, or Narcotics Anonymous) should be provided.

There are many signs and symptoms of gambling behaviour. Behavioural, financial, psychological and health signs can all indicate problem gambling. For a more comprehensive account see Rassool (2011). The nurse's role already includes caring for patients with substance misuse, and this should extend to caring for patients with gambling problems. Nurses in the primary healthcare team are in a unique position to recognise patients who might be experiencing gambling problems, and to provide information, interventions (health education, harm reduction) and referral. It is important to include questions about gambling during the initial process and this should be as routine as asking about a patient's alcohol and tobacco use. The early identification of problem gambling improves patients' outcomes and reduces the harm to themselves and their families. If the patient is assessed as having a problem with gambling, it is best practice to refer them for treatment to a specialist practitioner. There are several tools available to assist in the screening process.

The treatment interventions for problem gamblers include both pharmacological and psychological therapies. Pharmacological interventions in the treatment for pathological gambling include opioid antagonists, serotonin re-uptake inhibitors (SRIs) and mood stabilisers. Mood stabilisers such as lithium carbonate have also been used as pharmacological interventions. Cognitive behavioural therapies and brief solution-focused therapy for the treatment of problem gambling are beginning to be examined. Gamblers Anonymous (GA) is the most widely available form of help accessible for individuals with gambling problems. Based on the 12-step philosophy originally used in Alcoholics Anonymous, GA can be accessed via the internet (www.gamblersanonymous.org). In addition to self-help groups for problem gamblers, similar options are available for friends, family members, or others affected by people with gambling problems.

Reflective Activity 13.2

Case Study

Farhana is a 20-year-old married woman who was brought by her family to the specialist drug centre established to meet the needs of her community. Both Farhana and her family were reluctant to attend the centre as they were mistrustful of the local drug services. However, they were persuaded to seek treatment and were referred to the specialist centre by the local *Imam*. Farhana had a normal childhood and did well at primary school, and attended the local Madrassa (Islamic school) after school hours. At 16 she got with the wrong crowd and was introduced to cannabis by her peers. She later started to smoke heroin. Things quickly spiralled out of control as she sought greater highs, and the social and psychological dynamic of shame, guilt and remorse led to the problem getting worse. She later got married, in the hope of changing her drug behaviour. She continues to use heroin during the marriage as her husband has a history of drug misuse. If she cannot obtain enough heroin, she uses diazepam which was prescribed by her doctor for a general anxiety disorder. She states that she has not had her menstrual period in the last 12 weeks and is certain that she is pregnant. However, she plans to make a new start in her life to have the baby.

- Why is the family reluctant to attend the local drug service?
- What are the main barriers in the utilisation of mainstream services by Muslim communities?
- What drug(s) does Farhana seem to be most addicted to?
- During the assessment process, you notice that Farhana avoids making eye contact. Why?

- What is your goal for Farhana?
- What interventions will you implement for the achievement of that goal?
- What would happen to Farhana if she stops her heroin use while she is pregnant?
- What are the cultural and religious issues regarding the care and treatment of Farhana?
- What should the counsellor or nurse do to maintain the privacy of Farhana?
- If Farhana speaks little English, which are the correct ways to communicate with the patient through an interpreter?

Comments on Activity 13.2

The family is reluctant to attend the local drug service for a variety of reasons. Findings from a study (Pe-Pua et al., 2010) indicate that a range of factors that influenced people's help-seeking behaviour include preference for seeking help from informal sources; different cultural perceptions of support; unfamiliarity with the 'system'; levels of language (or literacy) competency; concerns about immigration status; demographic factors (age, gender); limited social and family networks; and concerns about confidentiality. There are other cultural factors, such as attitudes to health and the causes of illness, and the appropriate treatment methods (Mohammadi, 2008), which deter families from seeking help from mainstream services. Some Muslims would turn to traditional healers or religious figures. Katz (1996), for example, found that UK Muslim families (Bangladeshi and Pakistani) did not access child and adolescent psychiatric services because they perceived their children's challenging behaviour as a religious problem, and believed the solution was to ensure that the child spent more time at the madrassa (religious school or college) supervised by an *Imam*.

During the process of assessment the least useful technique to use would be to explain to the patient that her beliefs about the drug problem are not correct. The patient may be reluctant to disclose personal information if the nurse or counsellor makes an attempt to correct the patient's different beliefs about the drug problem. This is a case where a non-judgemental approach is more effective. Questioning the validity of the patient's beliefs about her problems may also inhibit an effective nurse–patient therapeutic relationship. Privacy is important during the encounter between nurse and patient. The nurse should always begin a relationship by seeing an adult patient alone, and draw the family in as needed. In the case of Farhana's culture, as a Muslim, the individual's health problems are also considered the family's problems, and it is considered threatening to exclude family members from any nursing or medical interaction. However, the family should be reassured that they will be invited to join the meeting at a later stage.

If Farhana speaks little English, the correct way to communicate with the patient through an interpreter is to give her your full attention by looking directly at her rather than at the interpreter. Non-verbal communication, in the form of body language, facial expression, gestures, silences and signals, are also subject to cultural and individual differences and may be misinterpreted. For cultural or religious reason, the amount of eye contact that individuals make may differ between cultures. In some cultures, direct eye contact may be seen as impolite and disrespectful, whilst for others, avoidance of eye contact may be interpreted as a lack of interest or untrustworthiness (Black and Ethnic Minority Working Group, 2010). In order to maintain a therapeutic relationship with the patient, nurses are taught that making eye contact is essential. However, Muslim patients may see the avoidance of eye contact as a sign of respect.

When taking a drug history from a patient with a limited ability to speak English, the nurse should avoid asking closed questions involving a simple 'yes' or 'no' answer. Research indicates that when clients, regardless of cultural background, are asked, 'do you understand?' many will answer 'yes' even when they really do not understand (Black and Ethnic Minority Working Group, 2010). It has also been suggested that some patients will disclose more information about the state of their health problem through storytelling than by answering direct questions.

In relation to Farhana's multiple drug problem, she seemed to be dependent on heroin and diazepam. In fact, the diazepam withdrawal is more dangerous than heroin withdrawal. Diazepam withdrawal symptoms may include headache, muscle pain, extreme anxiety, tension, restlessness, confusion, irritability, tremor, abdominal and muscle cramps, vomiting and sweating. In more severe cases of diazepam withdrawal, symptoms may consist of depersonalisation, increased sensitivity to light or physical contact, hallucinations or epileptic seizures. Higher doses and prolonged use of diazepam would entail more severe withdrawal symptoms. In Farhana's case, if she suddenly stops her normal heroin intake it could cause severe withdrawal symptoms for her foetus and this could greatly increase the possibility of spontaneous abortion and foetal death. In some countries, methadone maintenance therapy is considered the standard care for pregnant women dependent on heroin. There is evidence to suggest that pregnant women enrolled in a substance-use disorders treatment programme are more likely to receive prenatal care, have infants of higher birth weight and be discharged home with their neonate (Burns et al., 2007). Methadone maintenance is only part of the overall package of pharmacological and psychosocial interventions. Farhana needs to go through several stages of interventions (maintenance, detoxification, rehabilitation, etc.) before she can remain drug free. She would need to have a 'road map' or care plan for her treatment journey, which is a key component of structured drug treatment interventions.

Conclusion

Drug use, HIV epidemics and gambling addiction are public health problems which constitute a grave and persistent threat to the political, economic, social, and cultural health of Islamic societies and communities. Service provision for Muslim drug users and problem-gamblers need to be considered in the context of cultural and religious perspectives. Muslims who take drugs or gamble are no different from the population sub-culture of those with addictive behaviours. Their needs are the same as others, with the exception of their spiritual needs. The issues related to working with Muslim patients include language, culture, patriarchy, gender issues, religious beliefs, family pride, health beliefs, stigma, confidentiality, oppression and racism. Another aspect of Islamic teachings which can be used in planning for the prevention of addictive behaviours rests on the activation of the role played by individuals and the community in providing mental, spiritual and social support to those having addictive problems. The Muslim family also is an important resource and asset in the social rehabilitation of the individual. In this respect, any programme addressing addictive behaviours should have a component of working with and through families and carers. Culturally appropriate health information and education in local languages on addiction and the danger of addictive substances (the relationship with HIV) and activities and should be addressed by the Muslim communities.

References

Abu Dawud, Sunan of Abu-Dawud, Hadith 4920. Narrated by AbuMusa al-Ash'ari, www.islam.com/questions/11752/playing-chess, date accessed 6 August 2013.

Ajri, Z. and Sabran, S. (2011) 'Changing of Self-Care Behavior by Practicing 12-Step Program among Codependents in Iran', *Journal of American Science* 7, 1, 170–3.

Black and Ethnic Minority Working Group (BEMWG) (2010) *Cultural Competency Toolkit: Health and Social Care* (London: BEMWG).

Bukhari and Muslim, cited in www.missionislam.com/family/gambling.htm, date accessed 6 August 2013.

Burns, L., Mattick, R.P., Lim, K. and Wallace, C. (2007) 'Methadone in Pregnancy: Treatment Retention and Neonatal Outcomes', *Addiction* 102, 2, 264.

Cook, C. (2010) *Global State of Harm Reduction: Key Issues for Broadening the Response* (London: International Harm Reduction Association).

Cunningham-Williams, R.M., Grucza, R.A., Cottler, L.B., Womack, S.B., Books, S.J., Przybeck, T.R., Spitznagel, E.L. and Cloninger, C.R. (2005) 'Prevalence and Predictors of Pathological Gambling: Results from the St Louis Personality, Health and Lifestyle (SLPHL) Study', *Journal of Psychiatric Research* 39, 4, 377–90.

Eberstadt, N. and Kelley, L.M. (2005) *Behind the Veil of a Public Health Crisis: HIV/AIDS in the Muslim World*. National Bureau of Asian Research, www.aei.org/home, date accessed 6 August 2013.

Fountain, J. *Issues Surrounding Drug Use and Drug Services among the South Asian Communities in England* (London: UCLAN/National Treatment Agency), www.nta.nhs.uk/uploads/1_south_asian_final.pdf, date accessed 6 August 2013.

Garrett, J., Landau, J., Shea, R., Stanton, M., Baciewicz, G. and Brinkman-Sull, D. (1998) 'The ARISE Intervention Using Families and Network Links to Engage Addicted Persons in Treatment', *Journal of Substance Abuse Treatment* 15, 4, 333–43.

Hasnain, M. (2005) 'Cultural Approach to HIV/AIDS Harm Reduction in Muslim Countries', *Harm Reduction Journal* 2, 1, 23. Doi: 10.1186/1477-7517-2-23.

IHRA (2010) *Middle East and North Africa*, Regional Update (London: International Harm Reduction Association).

Islam and Drugs. Student of Darul Uloom, Holcombe, UK, www.inter-islam.org/Prohibitions/drugs.htm, date accessed 6 August 2013.

Kamarulzaman, A. and Saifuddeen, S.M. (2010) 'Islam and Harm Reduction', *International Journal of Drug Policy* 21, 2, 115–18.

Katz, I. (1996) 'The Sociology of Children from Minority Ethnic Communities – Issues and Methods', in I. Butler and I. Shaw (eds), *A Case of Neglect? Children's Experience and the Sociology of Childhood* (London: Avebury).

Mandani, T.A., Al-Maazrou, Y.Y. and Al Jeffri, M.H. (2004) 'Epidemiology of the Human Immunodeficiency Virus in Saudi Arabia: 18-year Surveillance Results and Prevention from an Islamic Perspective', *BMC Infectious Diseases* 4, 25. Doi: 10.1186/1471-2334-4-25.

Mesquita, F., Winsarno, I., Atmosukarto, II., Eka, B., Nevendorff, l., Rahmah, A., Handoyo, P., Anastasia, P. and Angela, R. (2007) 'Public Health the Leading Force of the Indonesian Response to the HIV/AIDS Crisis among People who Inject Drugs', *Harm Reduction Journal* 17, 4, 9.

Mohammadi, N. (2008) *A Hermeneutic Phenomenological Inquiry into the Lived Experience of Muslim Patients in Australian Hospitals*. PhD Thesis, University of Adelaide.

Motivational Assessment Process for Families Members (2002) *Saskatchewan Alcohol and Drug Services: Motivational Assessment Process for Families Members*, www.saskatoonhealthregion.ca/your_health/calder_documents/ MAPforFamiliesMembers–Apr02rev1.pdf, date accessed 6 August 2013.

Muslim Hadith 5612. Narrated by Buraydah ibn al-Hasib, www.islam.com/ questions/11752/playing-chess, date accessed 6 August 2013.

National Institute for Clinical Excellence (NICE) (2007) *Treatments for Drug Misuse*. NICE clinical guidelines 51 and 52, www.nice.org.uk/nicemedia/ live/11813/36009/36009.pdf, date accessed 6 August 2013.

Orford, J. (2012) 'Re-Empowering Family Members' Disempowered by Addiction: Support for Individuals or Collective Action?' *Global Journal of Community Psychology Practice* 3, 1, www.gjcpp.org/en/resource.php?issue=10& resource=47, date accessed 6 August 2013.

Pe-Pua, R., Gendera, S., Katz, I. and O'Connor, A. (2010) *Meeting the Needs of Australian Muslim Families: Exploring Marginalisation, Family Issues and 'Best Practice' in Service Provision* (Sydney: University of New South Wales, Social Policy Research Centre), Report prepared for the Australian Government Department of Immigration and Citizenship.

Philips, A.B. *War on Drugs Began 14 Centuries Ago*, www.islamhouse.com/p/ 318545, date accessed 6 August 2013.

Rassool, G. Hussein (2009) *Alcohol and Drug Misuse – A Handbook for Students and Health Professionals* (London: Routledge).

Rassool, G. Hussein (2011) *Understanding Addiction Behaviours: Theoretical and Clinical Practice in Health and Social Care* (Basingstoke: Palgrave Macmillan).

Rassool, G. Hussein and Winnington, J. (2006) 'Framework for Multi-dimensional Assessment', in G. Hussein Rassool (ed.), *Dual Diagnosis Nursing* (Oxford: Blackwell Publications).

Razzaghi, E., Nassirimanesh, B., Afshar, P., Ohiri, K., Claeson, M. and Power, R. (2006) 'HIV/AIDS Harm Reduction in Iran', *The Lancet* 368, 9534, 434–5.

Reid, G.A., Kamarulzaman, A. and Sran, S.K. (2007) 'Malaysia and Harm Reduction: the Challenges and Responses', *International Journal of Drug Policy* 18, 2, 136–40.

Sheikh al-Islam Ibn Taymiyah, Fatwa Ibn Taymiyah, 4, 262, As Siyasah, AshShar'iyyah, www.islamonline.net/servlet/Satellite?pagename=Islam Online-English-Ask_Scholar/FatwaE/FatwaE&cid=1119503545310#ixzz1D XTWyIRX, date accessed 6 August 2013.

Sheikh Yusuf Al-Qaradawi (2007) *How Much Alcohol and Drugs does the Religion Allow?* (30 May), www.islamonline.net/servlet/Satellite?page

name=IslamOnline-English-Ask_Scholar/FatwaE/FatwaE&cid=111950
3545310#ixzz1DXTWyIRX, date accessed 6 August 2013.

Simpson, B.W. (2005) *The Muslim Mosaic – Islam and Public Health*, www.
jhsph.edu/publichealthnews/magazine/archive/mag_spring05/muslim_
mosaic/index.html, date accessed 6 August 2013.

Stacey, A. (2010) *How Islam Recommends Dealing with 21st Century Illnesses*,
IslamReligion.com, www.islamreligion.com/articles/2534, date accessed
6 August 2013.

Tafseer-ul-Kabeer Lir-Razi, 2, 231.

Todd, C.S., Nassiramanesh, B., Stanekzai, M.R. and Kamarulzaman, A. (2007)
'Emerging HIV Epidemics in Muslim Countries: Assessment of Different
Cultural Responses to Harm Reduction and Implications for HIV Control',
Current HIV/AIDS Reports (4 December) 4, 151–7.

Toufiq, J. (2010) 'National Center on Drug Abuse Prevention and Research,
Morocco. Global State of Harm Reduction Information Response', in
C. Cook, *Global State of Harm Reduction 2010: Key Issues for Broadening
the Response* (London: International Harm Reduction Association), www.
ihra.net.

Toufiq, J. (2012) Cited in Muslims WorldWide, *Saudi Arabia: Report shows
Islamic Countries have the Highest Drug-addiction Problem in the World*,
27 August, http://themuslimissue.wordpress.com/2012/08/27/report-
shows-islamic-countries-have-the-highest-drug-addiction-problem-in-the-
world/, date accessed 6 August 2013.

UNODC (2010) *World Drug Report 2010*, www.unodc.org/documents/wdr/
WDR_2010/Executive_summary.pdf, date accessed 6 August 2013.

UNODC (2012) *World Drug Report 2012*, www.unodc.org/documents/data-
and-analysis/WDR2012/Executive_summary_24may.pdf, date accessed
6 August 2013.

USA gambling addiction statistics, http://nogamblingaddiction.com/
addiction-statistics.htm, date accessed 6 August 2013.

WHO (2004) *Why Tobacco is a Public Health Priority*, www.who.int/tobacco/
health_priority/en/, date accessed 6 August 2013.

WHO (2008) *WHO wants Total Ban on Tobacco Advertising*, www.who.int/
tobacco/wntd/2008/en/index.html, date accessed 6 August 2013.

WHO (2009) *Report on the Global Tobacco Epidemic, 2009: Implementing
Smoke-free Environments*, www.who.int/tobacco/mpower/2009/en/index.
html, date accessed 6 August 2013.

www.gambleaware.co.uk/gambling-facts-and-figures/, date accessed 6 August
2013.

Alcohol: the Forbidden Nectar

14

G. Hussein Rassool

Learning Outcomes:

- Have an awareness of the extent of alcohol use in Muslim countries and countries where there is a significant Muslim population.
- Discuss the consumption and prohibition of alcohol use from an Islamic perspective.
- Examine the rationale for most observant Muslims avoiding alcohol in any form, even small amounts that are sometimes used in cooking.
- Discuss the nursing management of alcohol withdrawal.
- Describe the intervention strategies for a Muslim with alcohol problems.

Reflective Activity 14.1

State whether the following statements are true or false. Give reasons for your answers.

	True	False
1 Alcohol is part of the social and cultural fabric of Judeo-Christian societies.		
2 The word 'alcohol' comes from the Arabic language, and may be derived from the *al-kuḥl*.		
3 Alcohol is not regarded as a psychoactive substance.		
4 Only beer and wine are forbidden in Islam.		
5 The general rule in Islam is that any beverage that causes intoxication when taken is unlawful, in both small and large quantities.		

	True	False
6 In Muslim countries, the abstention rate is substantially higher among men than among women.		
7 Muslims are forbidden from praying while drunk, for one does not know the meaning of what one is saying in that state.		
8 Muslims who consume alcohol, no matter what the amount, are not breaking the rule and going against the decree set by God.		
9 For Muslims, the ultimate salvation from alcohol is to turn to Allah (God), read the Noble Qur'aan, and seek Allah's forgiveness and help.		
10 Participation in religious communities may reduce the likelihood of choosing friends who use alcohol.		
11 Muslim patients with alcohol-use disorders may tend to hide their alcohol dependence from hospital staff.		
12 It is more likely that the patient will not disclose their level of alcohol consumption if the healthcare professional is a non- Muslim.		

Introduction

Alcohol is part of the social, religious and cultural fabric of Judeo-Christian societies and is enjoyed by the majority of the world's adult population. It is also becoming an irreplaceable component of leisure, as being our 'favourite drug'. Groups from all walks of life and ages celebrate intoxication as a rite of passage applauded by their peers whilst at the same time the effects of intoxication are negatively moralised and marginalised (Room, 2005). Public health problems associated with alcohol consumption have reached alarming proportions, resulting in physical, psychological, social, economic and legal consequences. Alcohol consumption is one of the major avoidable risk factors (WHO, 2004), and actions to reduce the burden and costs associated with alcohol should be urgently increased (Rehm et al., 2009). This chapter examines alcohol from an Islamic perspective, focusing on the historical context of alcohol use, the global burden, the extent and nature of alcohol use, the detrimental effects of alcohol and the intervention strategies adopted.

Historical context

The word 'alcohol' comes from the Arabic language, and may be derived from *al-kuḥl*, the name of an early distilled substance, or perhaps from *al-gawl*, meaning 'spirit' or 'demon' and akin to liquors being called 'spirits' in English. It also means fermented grains, fruits, or sugars that form an intoxicating beverage. *Khamr* or *khamrah* is the word used in the Qur'aan to denote a fermented beverage that intoxicates a person when he/she drinks it (www. quranandscience.com). The first declaration made by Prophet Muhammad concerning this matter was that not only is *Khamr* (wine or alcohol) prohibited, but the definition of *Khamr* extends to any substance that intoxicates, in whatever form or under whatever name it may appear. Thus, beer and similar drinks are absolutely forbidden (*haram*) (Al-Qaradawi, 1982).

In ancient Egypt and Assyria, alcoholic beverages were used for pleasure, nutrition, medicine, ritual, remuneration and funerary purposes. At the height of the Roman Empire, the shift from ceremonial drinking, confined to banquets and special occasions, to casual, everyday drinking was accompanied by an increase in chronic drunkenness, which today would be labelled 'alcoholism' (Babor, 1986). It is argued that the early ritualisation of alcohol in Christian Europe, and the revulsion against mind-altering psychoactive substances by the church, added to alcohol achieving dominance in European nations (Gossop, 2007). By the first millennium, the most popular form of festivities in England was known as 'ales', and both ale and beer were at the top of lists of products to be given to lords for rent.

In pre-Islamic society, the Arabs had harsh lives and felt that alcohol was an indispensable way to cope with their problems. Among the predicaments that the Arab people had to face before Islam were: tribal warfare, excessive pride and competition, prostitution, insecurity, broken homes, and female infanticide. Women were treated as slaves, and children were deprived of affection, while men were expected to be tough and competitive. *Khamr* shops and bars were open 24 hours a day (www.quranandscience.com). In fact, one of the foremost qualities of pre-Islamic Arabs was their praise of wine-drinking, not because it was worth boasting about but because 'it was a means of displaying hospitality and pampering the soul' (Al-Mubarakpuri, 2002). It is stated that, for this reason, the 'grape vine was called *Karm*, the same word used for honour, and wine was called the daughter of *Karm*' (Al-Mubarakpuri, 2002).

The most important development regarding alcohol throughout the Middle Ages was probably that of distillation. The isolation of ethanol (alcohol) as a pure compound was first achieved by Muslim chemists who developed the art of distillation during the Abbasid caliphate, the most notable of whom were Jabir ibn Hayyan (Geber), Al-Kindi (Alkindus) and Al-Razi (Rhazes) (Al-Hassan,

2001; Al-Hassan and Hill, 1986). Pure distilled alcohol was first produced by Muslim chemists in the Islamic world during the 8th and 9th centuries. Geber (Jabir Ibn Hayyan) (721–815) invented the alembic still; he observed that heated wine from this still released a flammable vapour, which he described as 'of little use, but of great importance to science'. Not much later, al-Razi (864–930) described the distillation of alcohol and its use in medicine (Al-Hassan and Hill, 1986). The word 'alcohol' was introduced into Europe, together with the art of distillation and the resulting substance itself, around the 12th century by various European authors who translated and popularised the discoveries of Islamic and Persian alchemists (Al-Hassan, 2001).

In summary, alcohol throughout history has been valued by various cultures and societies. From the earliest times, alcohol has played an important role in religious worship, as a source of nutrients and calories, as a substitute for polluted water, for medicinal and therapeutic purposes and as a social lubricant. However, the general rule in Islam is that any beverage that makes people intoxicated when taken is unlawful, in both small and large quantities, whether it is alcohol, fermented raisin drink, or something else.

Alcohol and the Islamic perspective

The prohibition of consumption of alcohol and intoxicants is one of the 'distinctive' marks of the Islamic world. In Islam, the Noble Qur'aan forbids the use of intoxicants or psychoactive substances, that which makes one forgetful of God and prayer, whether it be wine, beer, gin, whisky, or other alcoholic beverages. Intoxicants were forbidden in the Qur'aan through several separate verses revealed at different times over a period of years. The first Qur'aanic verse (chronologically) to deal with alcohol was revealed in Makkah (interpretation of the meaning):

☐ *And from the fruits of date-palms and grapes, you derive strong drink (this was before the order of the prohibition of the alcoholic drinks) and a goodly provision. Verily, therein is indeed a sign for people who have wisdom. (An-Naĥl [The Bee] 16: 67)*

This verse is referring to the drinks that people make from the fruits of the date palm and grapevine, and what they used to do with intoxicating *Nabidh* (a drink made from dates) before it was forbidden (Ibn Kathir). This also alludes to the fact that there are both evil and good possibilities in certain drinks. After hearing this verse, some Muslims started to wonder about the correctness of taking *khamr* (www.quranandscience.com). That is why all the verses relating to the use of intoxicating drinks should be considered in the context of the whole Qur'aan. A later verse was revealed which said that alcohol contains some good and some evil, but that the evil is greater than the good. This was the next step in turning people away from its consumption. The verse is as follows (interpretation of the meaning):

☐ *They ask you (O Muhammad) concerning alcoholic drink and gambling: 'In them is a great sin, and (some) benefit for men, but the sin of them is greater than their benefit.' And they ask you what they ought to spend. Say: 'That which is beyond your needs.' Thus Allah makes clear to you His Laws in order that you may give thought.* (Al Baqara [The Cow] 2: 219)

After this verse was revealed, most of the early reverters to Islam continued to drink but some began to abstain or reduce their intake. However, it is said that particular Muslims had been abstinent even in the pre-Islamic days, most notably, Uthman Ibn Affan, who later was the third Caliph (ruler) (www.quranandscience.com). Uthman said, 'Al-khamr "robs" the mind totally; and I have not yet seen anything which when entirely "robbed" or curtailed will come back in its original intact form!' (www.quranandscience.com).

The third mention of alcohol in the Qur'aan appeared as follows (interpretation of the meaning):

☐ *O you who believe! Approach not As-Salaat (the prayer) when you are in a drunken state until you know (the meaning) of what you utter.* (An-Nisā' [The Women] 4:43)

According to Ibn Kathir, in this Qur'aanic verse, Allah forbade the Muslims from praying while drunk, for one does not know the meaning of what one is saying in that state. This was one of the stages in turning people away from the consumption of alcoholic beverages. Finally, the focus of the rulings was on total abstinence as alcohol tended to turn people away from God and make them forget about prayer, and Muslims were ordered to abstain. The following verse was revealed (interpretation of the meaning):

☐ *O you who believe! Intoxicants (all kinds of alcoholic drinks), gambling, Al-Ansab, and Al-Azlam (arrows for seeking luck or decision) are an abomination of Shaitan's (Satan's) handiwork. So avoid (strictly all) that (abomination) in order that you may be successful.* (Al-Mā'idah [The Table Spread] 5:90–1)

The Prophet Muhammad said that 'Alcohol is the mother of all evils and it is the most shameful of evils' (Ibn-Majah [a]). The Prophet Muhammad also instructed the people to avoid any intoxicating substance whether it intoxicates in a large amount or even when taken in a small amount. 'Anything which intoxicates in a large quantity, is prohibited even in a small quantity' (Ibn-Majah [b]). For this reason, most observant Muslims avoid alcohol in any form, even small amounts that are sometimes used in cooking. Not only those who drink alcohol are cursed but also those who deal with them directly or indirectly are cursed by Allah. In another hadith, the Prophet said: 'God's curse falls on ten groups of people who deal with alcohol. The one who distills it, the one for whom it has been distilled, the one who drinks it, the one who transports it, the one to whom it has been brought, the one whom serves it, the one who sells it, the one who utilizes money from it, the one who buys it and the one who buys it for someone else' (Ibn-Majah [c]).

Muslims who consume alcohol, no matter what the amount, are breaking the rule and are going against the decree set by God (Allah), and what the individual is doing is unlawful (*haram*). The Prophet Muhammad issued a warning of the punishment in Islam for alcohol drinkers: 'Whoever drinks *khamr* and becomes intoxicated, his prayers will not be accepted for 40 days, and if he dies he will enter Hell, and if he repents Allah will accept his repentance. If he drinks again and becomes intoxicated again, his prayers will not be accepted for 40 days, and if he dies he will enter Hell, and if he repents Allah will accept his repentance. If he drinks again and becomes intoxicated again, his prayers will not be accepted for 40 days, and if he dies he will enter Hell, and if he repents Allah will accept his repentance. If he drinks a fourth time, Allah promises that He will make him drink from the mud of *khibaal* on the Day of Resurrection. The people asked, "O Messenger of Allah, what is the mud of *khibaal*?" He said, "The juice of the people of Hell"' (Ibn Majah [d]). Another hadith of the Prophet Muhammad stated that: 'Whoever dies and has the habit of drinking *khamr*, he will meet Allah as one who worships idols' (Al-Tabaraani and Al-Albani). However, there are no prohibitions on using alcohol for scientific, medical, industrial or automotive use (as a biofuel, solvent or a coolant, for instance) (Attar).

Alcohol consumption in non-Muslim and Muslim countries

From a public health perspective, the global burden related to alcohol consumption, in terms of both morbidity and mortality, is considerable in most parts of the world. The World Health Organization (WHO, 2004) estimates that there are about 2 billion people worldwide who consume alcoholic beverages and 76.3 million with diagnosable alcohol-use disorders. One in 25 deaths around the world is caused by alcohol consumption, and it is now as damaging to global health as tobacco was a decade ago (Rehm et al., 2009). In Europe, alcohol is public health enemy number 3, behind only tobacco and high blood pressure, and ahead of obesity, lack of exercise, or illicit drugs (Anderson and Baumberg, 2007). In the UK, alcohol consumption and related problems appear to be comparatively lower in Muslim communities than in the population at large. For example, findings from reports and surveys indicate relatively high levels of non-drinkers amongst most Pakistani and Bengali men and women (Alcohol Concern, 2003; Information Centre, 2004; National Centre for Social Research, 2001). It is reported that in France, one-third of Muslims (originally from Algeria, Morocco, Tunisia and sub-Saharan Africa) drink alcohol (IFOP, 2011). The findings of a study with a sample of the population of Albania (Burazeri and Kark, 2010), one of the few predominantly Muslim countries in Europe, showed that alcohol consumption appeared to be more frequent among Albanian men and was extremely low in women. In a study of immigrants with backgrounds from Iran, Turkey and Pakistan (Amundsen, 2012), it was found that Muslim immigrants reported a significantly lower drinking frequency than non-Muslims, although this did not apply to Iranians. In the United States, there is a low rate of alcohol misuse for adherent Muslim populations (Hanolt, 2006). However, Muslims born in the US are more likely to drink than immigrant Muslims (Haddad and Lummis, 1987). Although American Muslim students had a low rate of drinking in the previous year (46.6%) compared with their non-Muslim US college counterparts, they had a higher rate of alcohol consumption compared with their counterparts in predominately Muslim countries (Abu-Ras et al., 2010).

The World Health Organisation's annual reports place Muslim countries at the bottom of the list in per capita alcohol consumption. All but four of the 43 Muslim countries surveyed are below the median in alcohol consumption. Of the four above the median, two (Azerbaijan and Kyrgyzstan) are former republics of the USSR with large non-Muslim Russian populations, and the other two (Burkina Faso and Lebanon) are nearly half non-Muslim (WHO, 2004, pp. 11–12). These figures are 'reported' and may not be representative of the total consumption, as alcohol is smuggled in or produced as traditional beverages in the home. It is difficult to know how much of the alcohol is consumed by natives and how much by tourists and other expatriates in the Muslim countries (Michalak and Trocki, 2006). 'Alcohol and Islam: an Overview' (WHO, 2004) gives estimates of unrecorded drinking for a number of countries, 15 of which are Muslim. These estimates range from 0.3 litres of alcohol per adult in Algeria to 4.0 litres in Tajikistan. The estimate of unrecorded drinking in Saudi Arabia is 0.6 litres per person. Although the norm for alcohol use in Muslim countries is abstention, in Albania, Azerbaijan, and Turkmenistan more than half the population drink alcohol (WHO, 2004). In Muslim countries, as in all countries, the abstention rate is substantially higher among women than among men.

There is a constant increase in the use of alcohol in several countries where Islam is the major religion. In North-west Africa, in the countries of the Maghreb, problem-drinking certainly exists, despite the delicate silence that surrounds this (Chaib, 2000, p. 98). It is reported that 'alcoholism is now common in the Sudan' (Suliman, 1983). Severe or heavy episodic drinking are reported in five Muslim countries, with rates from 0.2% in the Comoros to 12.3% in Chad, meaning that in Chad 12.3% of the population consumes five or more drinks per sitting at least once a week, more than double the rate in the US (WHO, 2004, pp. 28–9). Another survey of alcohol dependence ranges from very low in Egypt (0.2%), Syria (0.2%), and Indonesia (1.0%); to fairly low in Turkey (1.3%); to high in Iran (7.3%) (WHO, 2004, p. 30). However, one should take these figures with caution as the definitions used for 'heavy episodic drinking' and 'alcohol dependence' vary from country to country. However, it is worth nothing that in countries such as Egypt, Tunisia, Morocco, and the United Arab Emirates, the consumption rate is directly linked to tourist flows. There are variations between Muslim countries in their patterns of beverage preference. For example, Algerians consume 56% of their net alcohol intake as beer, while Tunisians prefer wine (52%), and Syrians prefer spirits (67%) (WHO, 2004). No data are available on the use of alcohol amongst women in Muslim countries.

The methodological problems associated with the survey in Muslim countries include the use of different terminology associated with alcohol problems; the sample size being inadequate or not representative of the population; and the problems of denial by the respondents. It has been stated that Muslims tend to respond in absolute negatives more than Western respondents, due to 'culturally determined tendencies to respond in the negative to guilt-provoking issues', and give 'culturally desired responses' (Bilal et al., 1990; Neumark et al., 2001).

Assessment and intervention strategies: nursing implications

For a summary of the harms associated with alcohol use and the screening tools that are available to identify current or potential alcohol problems, see Rassool (2009). Where alcohol causes physical withdrawal syndromes, detoxification is a treatment intervention. The principles of nursing care in alcohol detoxification include: monitoring of dehydration, blood pressure, dietary intake; orientation to time, place and person; sleep; poor physical health; fear of withdrawal symptoms; risky behaviours; anxiety; guilt; and spiritual needs (Rassool, 2009, 2010). The standard treatment for alcohol misuse may include pharmacotherapy to alleviate withdrawal symptoms and the prevention and management of more serious complications, and preparation for more structured psychosocial and educational interventions (Rassool, 2009). Psychological interventions include brief interventions, motivational interviewing and other cognitive–behavioural approaches.

Spiritual interventions

For Muslims, the ultimate salvation from alcohol is to turn to Allah (God), read the Noble Qur'aan, and seek Allah's forgiveness and help (Rassool, 2013). In addition, the problem drinker needs to seek professional help for their drinking behaviour. Muslims are required to seek such treatment and the method of treatment is clearly prescribed. The Prophet Muhammad stated that 'There is a cure for every disease. Whenever an illness is treated with its right remedy, it will, by Allah's permission, be cured' (Muslim [a]). Islam does not 'shame' its believers when they come for treatment and this is based on the understanding that Allah forgives and that we, as humans, have the responsibility to support and assist in recovery whenever possible (Muhammad, 2000). It is stated that religion may inhibit alcohol use through at least three possible mechanisms: positive peer groups, moral values, and increased coping skills. More specifically, participation in religious communities may reduce the likelihood of choosing friends who use alcohol (Koenig et al., 2001). It is the process of acculturation into peer groups characterised by non-alcohol-using norms that serves to instil moral values that discourage alcohol use (Hodge, 2011).

The treatments for alcohol disorders have been subjected to criticism by Muslim Scholars (Badri, 1976; Suliman, 1983). Badri (1976) criticises Western alcoholism treatments such as chemically induced aversion, defends Islamic remedies, which he says have been mischaracterised, and concludes that Muslim therapists should use 'the potential power of Islam as a force of persuasion and aversion' (pp. 1, 50, 55). Suliman (1983) advocates that a remedy for alcoholism is to return to 'the therapeutic village and the mosque' (p. 65). It is argued that the deeper integration of Muslims into their communities can be both prevention and cure for alcoholism; at the same time, there may be non-religious therapies for alcoholism which could be combined with Islamic therapies (Michalak and Trocki, 2006). However, in order for any modern psychological treatments to be effective, it has been suggested that education is needed about the correct interpretation of belief (*Aqeedah*), devotion

(*Ibadah*) and practice of virtue, morality and manners (*Akhlaq*) (Alias and Majid, 2005).

Ito and Donovan (1986) suggested that a well-planned programme for continued assistance will increase the problem drinker's chances of a successful long-term outcome. The aftercare programme may include residential rehabilitation and further psychological interventions such as counselling or marital therapy, in combination with attending self-help groups such as Alcoholics Anonymous. A twelve-step recovery programme for persons who experience problems associated with addiction, based upon Islamic principles, has been established at the *Millati Islami* (www.millatiislami.org). *Millati Islami* is a 'fellowship of men and women [who] look to Allah (God) to guide us on Millati Islami (the Path of Peace). While recovering, we strive to become rightly guided Muslims, [who have] submitted our will and services to Allah.' These recovery support groups have adapted the 12 Steps to incorporate Islamic principles in their treatment programmes. However, the prime treatment will be spiritual growth and development based on Islamic principles.

Reflective Activity 14.2

Case Study

A 28-year-old Muslim executive, married with two children, presented at the local Accident and Emergency unit with severe hand tremors, headache, and nausea, including heightened autonomic activity such as agitation, sweating, and tachycardia. He was also found to be confused and disoriented. His blood urea, electrolytes, liver function test, and complete blood count were all within normal limits. His complaints strongly indicated the presence of alcohol withdrawal – delirium tremens triggered by abstinence from alcohol consumption. He refused to disclose his pattern of alcohol consumption because of shame and guilt. Approximately 12 months ago, he had been hospitalised for alcohol withdrawal syndrome during the month of Ramadan (fasting).

- What would be the immediate intervention required?
- What other withdrawal symptoms or behavioural problems may be observed?
- What are the short-term goals for this patient?
- What are the long-term goals for this patient?
- Outline a care plan for this patient for the management of withdrawal?
- What are his special needs as a Muslim during hospitalisation?

General comments in relation to Reflective Activity 14.2

Although it is forbidden for Muslims to drink alcohol, some Muslims do not follow this strict abstinence especially when they live in a non-Muslim society. Many Muslim patients who engage in behaviours prohibited by Islam during other months, such as consuming alcohol, abstain throughout the month of Ramadan. This sudden abstinence from alcohol consumption would be expected to cause distress and anguish especially during the initial days of fasting, depending on the level of alcohol consumption. The present case illustrates the impact of Ramadan fasting on the pattern and timing of severe alcohol withdrawal delirium. It is often difficult for the nurse or healthcare professional to determine the pattern of alcohol use and the level of consumption from the patient as Muslim drinkers often hide their consumption.

There is evidence to suggest that Muslim patients with alcohol-use disorders may tend to hide their alcohol dependence from hospital staff (Dotinga et al., 2004). Concealing use may stem from their religious obligation and the shame and guilt experienced by the individual. In addition, there is also the perception of a fear of punishment or disapproval from partners, family, and the Muslim community. The essence here is not to reject the alcohol drinker from the mainstream community but to be there to provide help and support, and opportunities for education, discussion and guidance. Rejection, fear of criticism, or marginalisation of the problem drinker by the community or family, would be counterproductive. In this context, it is important to invite the individual within the fold of Islam 'in a kind and gentle manner with beautiful exhortation from time to time, whilst praying for him in his absence that he be guided, seeking out times when supplications are answered, especially the last third of the night' (islamqa., 145587). In fact, behaviours and actions that are teeming with love and compassion are more effective and more likely to be accepted. The Messenger of Allah enjoined us to be kind, and he said: 'There is no kindness in a thing but it adorns it, and it is not taken away from a thing but it makes it defective' (Muslim [b]).

Good practice guidelines

- It is more likely that the patient will disclose their level of alcohol consumption or pattern of drinking if the healthcare professional is a non-Muslim.
- Promote client safety.

- Patients need a non-stimulating and non-threatening environment, and low lighting at night will help reduce perceptual disturbances.
- Maintain physiological stability during the withdrawal phase.
- Psychological elements require observation and management, including auditory and visual hallucinations, delirium, altered mental states, hyper-vigilance, anxiety, paranoia, depression, tactile hallucinations, and the levels of risk.
- Monitoring of the withdrawal syndrome.
- Screening for drug and alcohol problems (assessment, urine/saliva testing).
- Meeting physical and psychological needs.
- A contact point for further help (self-help groups).
- Harm-reduction advice.
- Provision of appropriate referral and follow-up.

A framework for the nursing management of alcohol withdrawal is presented in Table 14.1.

Table 14.1 A nursing practice framework for alcohol withdrawal

Physical needs	Interventions
General	Assess level of consciousness.
Environmental stimuli	Nursing in quiet area with only one member of staff in contact.
Body temperature	Control body temperature: apply or remove bed clothing when necessary.
Blood pressure	Monitor blood pressure.
Foods and fluids	Offer fluids every 60 minutes and record fluid intake.
Rest and sleep	Allow rest or sleep between monitoring of vital signs.
Elimination	Assist to bathroom and record output.
Seizure	Monitor for epileptic seizure.
Physical comfort/Sleep	Change position if necessary. Institute measures to help patients to sleep.
Withdrawal	Monitor vital signs and amount of withdrawal.
Psychological needs	
Reality orientation	Time, place and person. Assess presence of hallucinations or delusions.
Risk behaviour	Assess for suicidal ideation.
Providing positive reinforcement	Reinforce positive elements of the intervention.

Conclusion

Despite the prohibition of alcohol in Islam, some Muslims consume intoxicating substances, whether it be wine, beer, gin, or whisky. The main reason why alcohol is forbidden in Islam is because of its ability to lead to many negative issues, such as health, social and economic problems, and damage to their relationships with God. However, the use of alcohol remains an under-identified problem. Many Muslims go to great lengths to hide the fact that they drink, from society, family and friends. This is because there are some extremely negative social consequences to drinking, including arrest, and being shunned or socially excluded. Many Muslims who reside in Europe and the United States may consume alcohol publicly, simply because alcohol is the norm in those societies, as compared with those Muslims who live in countries where Islamic laws are staunchly adhered to. Many Muslims consuming alcohol tend to abstain throughout the month of Ramadan. This sudden abstinence from alcohol consumption would be expected to lead to withdrawal syndrome. However, owing to the difficulty of identifying and treating alcohol-use disorders in Muslim patients, services need to develop an outreach approach through the local *Imam* (priest) and the Mosque. Multi-dimensional pharmacological and psychosocial interventions and a multi-professional approach coupled with culturally sensitive care are required, to provide better and more effective outcomes for those with alcohol-related problems.

References

Abu Dawud and at-Tirmidhî, cited in 'The Lawful and the Prohibited in Islam', http://islamdrugfree.blogspot.com/2011_08_01_archive.html, date accessed 7 August 2013.

Abu-Ras, W., Ahmed, S. and Arfken, C.L. (2010) 'Alcohol Use among US Muslim College Students: Risk and Protective Factors', *Journal of Ethnicity in Substance Abuse* 9, 3, 206–322.

Alcohol and Islam: An Overview (2006), http://goliath.ecnext.com/coms2/gi_0199-6796414/Alcohol-and-Islam-an-overview.html, date accessed 7 August 2013.

Alcohol Concern (2003) *Alcohol Drinking among Black and Minority Ethnic Communities (BME) in the United Kingdom* (London: Acquire).

Al-Hassan, A.Y. (2001) *The Different Aspects of Islamic Culture, Science and Technology in Islam*, Vol. 4, Part II, UNESCO (Cambridge: Cambridge University Press).

Al-Hassan, A.Y. and Hill, D. (1986) *Islamic Technology: An Illustrated History*, UNESCO (Cambridge: Cambridge University Press).

Ali, O., Abu-Ras, W. and Hamid, H. (2009) *Muslim Americans*, Statistics and Services Research Division (New York: Nathan Kline Institute for Psychiatric Research), http://ssrdqst.rfmh.org/cecc/index.php?q=node/25, date accessed 26 February 2013.

Alias, A. and Majid, A.H.S. (2005) 'Psychology of Learning from an Islamic Perspective'. Paper presented at the 3rd International Seminar on Learning and Motivation, 12 September 2005, Kedah, Malaysia.

Al-Mubarakpuri, Safi-Ur R. (2002) *The Sealed Nectar: Ar Raheeq Al- Makhtum, Biography of the Noble Prophet (PBUH)* (Riyadh, Saudi Arabia: Darussalam).

Al-Qaradawi, Y. (1982) *The Lawful and the Prohibited in Islam (Al-Halal wal Haram fil Islam)* (New York/India: Islamic Book Service).

Al-Tabaraani, 12/45, and Al-Albani, in Saheeh al-Jaami', 6525.

Amundsen, E.J. (2012) 'Low Level of Alcohol Drinking among Two Generations of Non-Western Immigrants in Oslo: a Multi-ethnic Comparison', *BMC Public Health* 12, 535. Doi: 10.1186/1471-2458-12-535

Anderson, P. and Baumberg, B. (2007) *Alcohol and Public Health in Europe* (London: Institute of Alcohol Studies).

Attar, S. *The Alcohol and Drug Abuse: The American Scene and the Islamic Perspective*, www.islamcan.com/youth/the-alcohol–drug-abuse-the-american-scene-and-the-islamic-perspective.shtml, date accessed 7 August 2013.

Babor, T. (1989) *Alcohol – Customs and Rituals* (London: Burke Publishing).

Badri, M.B. (1976) *Islam and Alcoholism* (Tacoma Park, MD: Muslim Students Association of the US and Canada).

Bilal, A.M., Makhawi, B., Al-Fayez, G. and Shaltout, A.F. (1990) 'Attitudes of a Sector of the Arab-Muslim Population in Kuwait towards Alcohol and Drug Misuse: an Objective Appraisal', *Drug and Alcohol Dependence* 26, 55–62.

Burazeri, G. and Kark, J.D. (2010) 'Alcohol Intake and its Correlates in a Transitional Predominantly Muslim Population in Southeastern Europe', *Addictive Behaviours* 35, 7, 706–13.

Chaib, Y. (2000) *L'émigré et la mort: La mort musulmane en France* (Aix-en-Provence, France: Edisud), p. 98.

Dotinga, A., van den Eijnden, R.J., Bosveld, W. and Garretsen, H.F. (2004) 'Methodological Problems Related to Alcohol Research among Turks and Moroccans Living in the Netherlands: Findings from Semi-structured Interviews', *Ethnicity and Health* 9, 139–51.

Gossop, M. (2007) *Living with Drugs* (Aldershot: Ashgate).

Haddad, Y. and Lummis, A. (1987) *Islamic Values in the United States: A Comparative Study* (New York: Oxford University Press).

Hanolt (2006) cited in Ali, O., Abu-Ras, W. and Hamid, H. (2009) *Muslim Americans*, Statistics and Services Research Division (New York: Nathan Kline Institute for Psychiatric Research), http://ssrdqst.rfmh.org/cecc/index.php?q=node/25, date accessed 7 August 2013.

Hodge, D.R. (2011) 'Alcohol Treatment and Cognitive-Behavioral Therapy: Enhancing Effectiveness by Incorporating Spirituality and Religion', *Social Work*, http://findarticles.com/p/articles/mi_hb6467/is_1_56/ai_n56639867/, date accessed 7 August 2013.

Ibn Kathir. *Tafsir of Ibn Kathir*, www.tafsir.com/default.asp?sid=16&tid=27841, date accessed 7 August 2013.

Ibn Majah [a], Sunan Ibn-I-Majah, Volume 3, Book of Intoxicants, Chapter 30, Hadith No. 3371.

Ibn Majah [b], Sunan Ibn-I-Majah, Volume 3, Book of Intoxicants, Chapter 30, Hadith No. 3392.

Ibn Majah [c].,Sunan Ibn-I-Majah, Volume 3, Book of Intoxicants, Chapter 30, Hadith No. 3380.

Ibn Majah [d], Chapter 6, no. 3377; see also *Saheeh al-Jaami'*, 6313.

IFOP (2011) *Enquête auprès de la population d'origine musulmane*, www.ifop.fr/media/poll/1499-1-study_file.pdf, date accessed 7 August 2013.

Information Centre (2004) *Health Survey for England 2004: The Health of Minority Ethnic Groups* (Leeds: The Information Centre).

Ito, J.R. and Donovan, D.M. (1986) 'Aftercare in Alcoholism Treatment: a Review', in W.R. Miller and N. Heather (eds), *Treating Addictive Behaviours: Processes of Change* (New York: Plenum Press).

Koenig, H.G., McCullough, M.E. and Larson, D.B. (2001) *Handbook of Religion and Health* (New York: Oxford University Press).

Michalak, L. and Trocki, K. (2006) 'Alcohol and Islam: an Overview', *Contemporary Drug Problems* 33 (Winter), http://ipac.kacst.edu.sa/eDoc/eBook/2476.pdf, date accessed 7 August 2013.

Muhammmad, J. (2000) *Islam and Addiction*, www.islamonline.net/servlet/Satellite?c=Article_C&pagename=Zone-English-Family/FYELayout&cid=1157365822643, date accessed 7 August 2013.

Muslim [a], Fiqh-us Sunnah, Section 59,44 Sickness, Expiation of Sins, Section: Seeking Medical Treatment.

Muslim [b], 2594, www.islam-qa.com/en/consult/93775, date accessed 7 August 2013.

National Centre for Social Research and Department of Epidemiology and Public Health at the Royal Free and University College Medical School (2001) *The Health of Minority Ethnic Groups '99 (Health Survey for England)* (London: Office for National Statistics).

Neumark, Y., Tahav, G., Teichman, M. and Hasin, D. (2001) 'Alcohol Drinking Patterns among Jewish and Arab Men and Women in Israel', *Journal of Studies on Alcohol* 62, 4, 443–7.

Rassool, G. Hussein (2009) *Alcohol and Drug Misuse: A Handbook for Student and Health Professionals* (London: Routledge).

Rassool, G. Hussein (2010) *Addiction for Nurses* (Oxford: Wiley-Blackwell).

Rassool, G. Hussein (2014) *Health Psychology from an Islamic Perspective: A Guide for Health Professionals* (Riyadh, Saudi Arabia: IIPH) (Forthcoming).

Rehm, J., Mathers, C., Popova, S., Thavorncharoensap, M., Teerawattananon, Y. and Patra, J. (2009) 'Global Burden of Disease and Injury and Economic Cost Attributable to Alcohol Use and Alcohol-use Disorders', *Lancet* 373, 9682, 2223–33.

Room, R. (2005) 'Stigma, Social Inequality and Alcohol and Drug Use', *Drug and Alcohol Review* 124, 143–55.

Suliman, H. (1983) 'Alcohol and Islamic Faith', *Drug and Alcohol Dependence* 7, 63–5.

World Health Organization (WHO) (2004) *Global Status Report on Alcohol* (Geneva: WHO).

www.millatiislami.org, date accessed 7 August 2013.

www.quranandscience.com, date accessed 7 August 2013.

Rites de Passage: Birth, Death and Bereavement

15

S. Majali

Learning Outcomes:

- Have an awareness of the influence of religious and cultural beliefs of a Muslim woman post-natally.
- Discuss the Islamic perspectives on (a) breastfeeding; (b) circumcision; (c) illness; and (d) dying.
- Examine the approaches in the provision of support to individuals and key people during end-of-life care.
- Describe the procedures and protocols involved following the death of a Muslim in hospital.
- Examine the ways in which the spiritual dimension can be incorporated into the nursing care of the dying.

Reflective Activity 15.1

State whether the following statements are true or false. Give reasons for your answers.

	True	False
1 Rubbing a softened date upon the child's palate (*Tahneek*) is recommended for new-born Muslims.		
2 It is Islamic practice to put on the baby charms or amulets or blue beads to shield the baby from the evil eye.		
3 Circumcision is not obligatory for men.		

	True	False
4 For Muslims, it is a recommended to shave off the hair of the new-born a week after birth.		
5 Breastfeeding is encouraged in Islam for a period of two years.		
6 Breastfeeding benefits the child both physically and psychologically, but not the mother.		
7 Like Christians, Muslims believe in life after death, and the death of a loved one is seen as a temporary separation.		
8 Muslims are always buried, never cremated.		
9 All Muslims wear black during the period of mourning.		
10 A Muslim burial should take place as soon as possible, preferably within 24 hours.		
11 It is permissible for family members to mourn for three days.		

Introduction

As nurses we come into contact with people from a variety of cultures and faiths and we feel at a loss when we are unable to meet their needs because of cultural and religious differences. This problem is intensified when a Muslim woman is having a baby or a patient is terminally ill. The purpose of this chapter is to describe Islamic teachings and practices concerning birth, death, dying and bereavement. It is hoped that this will enable nurses and other health professionals to provide culturally appropriate care to Muslim patients.

Birth: passage into life

There are some rituals that accompany the new-born in a Muslim family. First we need to ask God to bless the new baby and to make him/her among the righteous. There is a tradition amongst Muslims that the prayer call (*Adhan*) and *iqaamah* should be recited into the baby's ear. On this issue, Sheikh Al-Munajjid stated that 'Among the Sunnah for welcoming the new-born, the scholars mentioned that the *Adhan* should be recited into the baby's right ear so that the first thing he hears in this world will be the words of *Tawheed* which will have a blessed effect on the child. With regard to reciting the *iqaamah* in the child's left ear, there is nothing to prove that this is required' (Sheik Al-Albani [a]). One should restrict oneself to the authentic Sunnah, beginning with rubbing a softened date upon the child's palate (*Tahneek*). Nurses or obstetricians attending the mother during the delivery can facilitate the father's carrying out this rite, and it does not harm the baby in any way. Family, friends and any person handling the baby are expected to say '*MashaAllah*' (What God wills) as a way to ward off evil (Wehbe-Alamah, 2008). Babies may be given gifts with some verses of the Qur'aan, or other charms or amulets, or blue beads to shield the baby from the evil eye – a cultural belief which is very common among Arabs and Muslims (Wehbe-Alamah, 2008). However, this is not Islamic practice.

Tahneek

Tahneek means putting something sweet, such as dates or honey, in the child's mouth when first born. It is a 'preferred' or recommended action to do *tahneek* for the baby and to pray for the child on the day of the birth (Sheikh Muhammed Salih Al-Munajjid). Dates have played an important part in the history of the Muslim world and in the Arab countries, where they are part of the daily food of many people. It is believed that babies need glucose after birth, which helps provide the new-born with the energy it needs and strengthens the muscles of the mouth (Al-Baar, 2005). Soon after the birth a respected elder can place a small amount of date paste on his clean finger and insert it in the baby's mouth and rub it on the upper palate, thereby the soft date becomes the first food that enters the baby's mouth, even before breast milk (Sheikh and Gatrad, 2008).

Al Aqiqah

Another practice, which families carry out on the seventh day after the birth of a baby, is the slaughtering of a sheep or two and distributing the meat to the family and the needy as a way of showing thanks to Allah (Wehbe-Alamah, 2008). It is traditional (*sunnah*) to slaughter one sheep for a baby girl and two sheep for a baby boy.

Shaving the hair

The Messenger of Allah said: 'A boy is ransomed by his *aqeeqah*. Sacrifice should be made for him on the seventh day, he should be given a name and his head should be shaved' (Tirmidhî et al.). It is a tradition to shave off the hair of the new-born a week after birth. Then it is prescribed that there should be given in charity gold or silver equal in weight to the hair. This does not have to be done by actually weighing the hair; if it is too difficult to do that, it is sufficient to estimate the weight and give paper currency equivalent to the price of that amount of gold or silver (Sheikh Al-Munajjid, Fatwa 7889).

Circumcision

Male babies are circumcised as it is considered to help maintain a man's hygiene (Wehbe-Alamah, 2008). It is feared that without circumcision some urine remains under the foreskin and will soil the clothes and break the ablution (Gulam, 2003; Sheikh and Gatrad, 2008). Frequent nappy changes and the use of barrier creams are recommended after circumcision (Sheikh and Gatrad, 2008). There is no fixed time for circumcision as it depends on family, region and country. Some Muslims are circumcised as early as on the seventh day after birth. Researchers have noted that the wives of circumcised men have less risk of getting cervical cancer than the wives of uncircumcised men (Al-Baar, 2005, p. 76) and that male circumcision reduces the incidence of cancer of the penis (Larke et al., 2011). Female circumcision (removing the prepuce of the clitoris) is only recommended, for females, and not mandatory as it is for the male (Ibn Qudamah). According to Dhami and Sheikh (2008), this is the least invasive procedure involved and the only form that can be accurately termed circumcision. Female genital mutilation (FGM), different from male circumcision, is a procedure that has been made illegal in many countries in Europe, North America and the Southern hemisphere including Australia and New Zealand.

Breastfeeding

Breastfeeding is encouraged in Islam for a period of two years. The World Health Organisation (www.who.int) strongly recommends exclusive breast-feeding for the first six months of life. From six months, other foods should complement breastfeeding for up to two years or more. In addition, breastfeeding should begin within an hour of birth, and should be given 'on demand', as often as the child wants, day and night; bottles or pacifiers should be avoided. Breastfeeding benefits mother and child both physically and psychologically. Breast milk provides the nutrients new-borns and infants need for healthy development and contains antibodies. Breastfeeding also benefits mothers. The practice, when done exclusively, often induces a lack of menstruation, which is a natural (though not fail-safe) method of birth control. It reduces risks of breast and ovarian cancer later in life, helps women return to their pre-pregnancy weight faster, and lowers rates of obesity.

The Qur'aan states that (interpretation of the meaning):

☐ *The mothers shall give suck to their children for two whole years, (that is) for those (parents) who desire to complete the term of suckling, but the father of the child shall bear the cost of the mother's food and clothing on a reasonable basis. No person shall have a burden laid on him greater than he can bear. No mother shall be treated unfairly on account of her child, or father on account of his child. And on the (father's) heir is incumbent the like of that (which was on the father). If they both decide on weaning, by mutual consent, and after due consultation, there is no sin on them. And if you decide on a foster suckling-mother for your children, there is no sin on you, provided you pay (the mother) what you agreed (to give her) on a reasonable basis. And fear Allah and know that Allah is All-Seer of what you do.* (Al-Baqara [The Cow] 2:233)

This is a command, in the Qur'aan, to mothers to breastfeed their children naturally. The scholars mentioned that one part of breastfeeding is obligatory, which is the yellow substance (colostrum) that is produced at the beginning of breastfeeding and which is known medically to be of great benefit in building the immune system of the child. Undoubtedly, in carrying out the commands of Allah there is great blessing (Sheikh Muhammed Salih Al-Munajjid, Fatwa 13750). Mothers whose own milk is lacking, who are sick or who are too busy working sometimes buy milk from a milk bank. According to Sheikh Muhammad ibn Salih al-'Uthaymin (islamqa, Fatwa No. 4049), for Muslims it is not permissible to establish this kind of bank, because this is human milk, and the milk from different mothers will be mixed, so that no one will know who is the mother. In Islam, drinking the milk of a woman creates the same relationship as does a close tie by blood (for example, it has an effect on whom one may and may not marry). Babies who have shared breast milk from the same mother are considered to be siblings and cannot marry each other in the future. If the milk is of any kind other than human, then there is nothing wrong with milk banks. In order to preserve a woman's modesty, it is important to provide access to women's changing rooms or a room where women can breastfeed their children in private.

Health and sickness

Those who care for the sick, whether they are doctors, nurses or other healthcare professionals, or even relatives, are urged to be gentle, humble, modest, kind, tolerant, patient, and show compassion. Islam preaches kindness and generosity on the part of Muslims at all times. The Noble Qur'aan says (interpretation of the meaning):

☐ *And by the Mercy of Allah, you dealt with them gently.* (Āli 'Imrān [Family of Imran] 3:159)

Muslim patients expect their family or caregivers to take care of them as they would for their own relatives, with love, compassion and understanding. In a Muslim family, the authority of the family overrules the individual's autonomy (Al-Shahri, 2002) and the husband or the eldest son is usually the decision-maker. Nurses need to identify who is the decision-maker in the family so that they can follow up with them on issues regarding the patient's care. Even a patient's diagnosis or bad news is shared first with the family rather than the patient, which causes an ethical dilemma for nurses and others.

Muslims are encouraged to visit the sick, with the purpose of taking their mind off their illness and generating hope in their hearts, and to pray for them to be cured by Allah (Ott et al., 2003; Sheikh and Gatrad, 2008). There are several accounts of the Prophet visiting the sick, laying his hands on them, praying for them and encouraging others to do the same. The Prophet said, 'He who visits a sick person who is not on the point of death and supplicates seven times: *As'alullahal-'Azima Rabbal-'Arshil-'Azimi, an yashfiyaka* (I beseech Allah the Great, the Rabb of the Great Throne, to heal you), Allah will certainly heal him from that sickness' (Abu Dawud and Tirmidhî). The Messenger of Allah said: 'When a Muslim visits a sick Muslim at dawn, seventy thousand angels keep on praying for him till dusk. If he visits him in the evening, seventy thousand angels keep on praying for him till the morning; and he will have (his share of) reaped fruits in *Jannah* (paradise)' (Tirmidhî). Muslim nurses and doctors are obligated to make every effort to relieve the suffering of their patients, be it physical or mental. Doctors have no right to terminate any human life under their care. Whilst Islam gives importance to saving life, it also makes clear that dying is a part of the covenant, and the final decision about the term of life is up to Allah. Islam does not believe in prolonging life, as everyone has been created for a particular life journey (Rassool, 2004). Muslim physicians are not encouraged to prolong artificially the suffering of someone in a vegetative state: they are ordained to help alleviate suffering (Athar, 1988).

Muslims are encouraged to have their wills prepared at all times because no one knows when death might occur (Al Shafii, 2002, p. 575). Patients who have little chance of recovery should make an effort to give people their rights whether these are debts, or deposits given to the patient for safe keeping. The sick are supported in making arrangements for someone to care for their children during their sickness and after their death. Muslims believe that death is a departure from the life of this world, but not the end of a person's existence. Like Christians, Muslims believe in life after death and that the death of a loved one is a temporary separation. Death is seen as the beginning of eternal life (Ott et al., 2003). Thus, nurses will find Muslim patients and their families at peace with illness, calamity and death, affirming their faith, and saying (interpretation of the meaning),

☐ *Truly! To Allah we belong and truly, to Him we shall return.* (Al-Baqara [The Cow] 2:156)

In order to understand the Islamic attitude towards death and dying it is necessary to begin with the Qur'aan's portrayal of creation (interpretation of the meaning):

☐ *Then We made the Nutfah into a clot (a piece of thick coagulated blood), then We made the clot into a little lump of flesh, then We made out of that little lump of flesh bones, then We clothed the bones with flesh, and then We brought it forth as another creation. So blessed be Allah, the Best of creators. After that, surely, you will die. Then (again), surely, you will be resurrected on the Day of Resurrection.* (Al-Mu'minūn [The Believers] 23:14–16)

The Qur'aan announces not only the inevitability of death, but also the Day of Resurrection. Creation, death and resurrecting are, therefore, sacred and inexorably linked from the beginning (Kramer, 1988). Another version describing creation elaborates this (interpretation of the meaning):

☐ *O mankind! If you are in doubt about the Resurrection, then verily! We have created you (i.e. Adam) from dust, then from a Nutfah (mixed drops of male and female sexual discharge i.e. offspring of Adam), then from a clot (a piece of thick coagulated blood) then from a little lump of flesh, some formed and some unformed (miscarriage), that We may make (it) clear to you (i.e. to show you Our Power and Ability to do what We will). And We cause whom We will to remain in the wombs for an appointed term, then We bring you out as infants, then (give you growth) that you may reach your age of full strength. And among you there is he who dies (young), and among you there is he who is brought back to the miserable old age, so that he knows nothing after having known.* (Al-Ĥaj [The Pilgrimage] 22:5)

Addressed to those who may have doubts about resurrection, these verses indicate that Allah's creations are too wonderful to end with death. Death is perceived not as a negative phenomenon but as a positive state. Just as life is creation, so death is also an act of creation. In the Noble Qur'aan, Allah says (interpretation of the meaning):

☐ *Who has created death and life, that He may test you which of you is best in deed.* (Al-Mulk [The Sovereignty] 67:2)

It is also stated:

☐ *And it is He Who gives life and causes death.* (Al-Mu'minūn [The Believers] 23:80)

Furthermore, these stages have no meaning until one completes the full cycle – through them the soul develops. Life, then, is a preparation for the soul to pass through the stage of death, and to be fit to progress into the life of death (Wehbe-Alamah, 2008).

Suicide and euthanasia (*Qatl al-rahma*)

Islam has made human life sacred and has safeguarded its preservation. No one knows where, how and when he or she will die (interpretation of the meaning),

☐ *Verily, Allah! With Him (Alone) is the knowledge of the Hour.* (Luqmān [Luqman] 31:34)

Muslims believe that the time of death is predetermined by God, and may feel that it is wrong to struggle once God's will is clear (Ott et al., 2003). Therefore, suicide, euthanasia and denial of nutrition or hydration are forbidden in Islam, but discontinuation of life support can be authorised by the elder son or senior male member of the family (Hedayat and Pirzadeh, 2001). Since God is the creator of life, a person does not 'own' his or her life and therefore, cannot terminate it (interpretation of the meaning):

☐ *And do not throw yourselves into destruction (by not spending your wealth in the Cause of Allah), and do good.* (Al-Baqara [The Cow] 2:195)

☐ *And do not kill yourselves (nor kill one another). Surely, Allah is Most Merciful to you.* (An-Nisā' [Women] 4:29)

Wishing for death is discouraged, and so is praying for it, if this is done because a person is going through difficulties such as sickness, poverty, or other worldly afflictions. The Prophet said: 'None of you should hope for death because of some harm that has come to him. If he has wish such, he should say, "O Allah, give me life if You know that life is better for me. And give me death if You [know] that death is better... for me' (Bukhari and Muslim). This indicates that Islam is against euthanasia, because it is seen as interfering with a person's destiny and in what God has decided for each person, and with the purpose of the person's life or death (interpretation of the meaning):

☐ *And no person can ever die except by Allah's Leave and at an appointed term.*
   (Āli `Imrān [The Family of Imran] 3:145)

Muslim practices during a person's last hours

Generally, the Muslim tradition dictates that a person who shows signs of dying should be positioned on his or her back, facing the *Qibla* (in the direction of the Holy Kaa'ba in Makkah), although there is no foundation in the practice of the Prophet (Abu Aisha, 2010). At the same time, verses from the Qur'aan are recited by the dying person or, if he/she is unable, by a relative in order to comfort the dying person. Sheikh 'Abd al-'Azeez ibn Baaz stated that 'reciting Qur'aan in the presence of one who is sick is a good thing, and Allah may benefit him through that. But with regard to singling out *Surah Yaa Seen*, the basic principle is that the hadith is weak (*da'eef*) so there are no grounds for singling out this surah' (Fatawa Ibn Baaz, 13/93). Sheikh Al-Albani said: 'With regard to reciting *Surah Yaa Seen* in the presence of the dying person, and turning him to face the *Qiblah*, there is no authentic (*Saḥīḥ*) report concerning that.' And Allah knows best. It is helpful if a copy of the Qur'aan is made available for family members if they did not bring their own. Then the basic creed of Islam (*Shahadatain*) is recited:

☐ *There is no God but Allah and Mohammed is his Prophet.*

The dying person is expected to repent of all his earthly sins, but sins are not confessed to another person before death. If no family members are present, any practising Muslim may be asked to give help and religious comfort. It is probably best in such cases for hospital staff to contact the local mosque or *Imam*, provided it is the patient's wish, and to ask someone to come to attend the patient. When the patient seems to be approaching death, those of his family and relatives who are present must stay with him. If they notice signs of panic and terror they must remind him of his good works, the immensity of Allah's mercy, His forgiveness of the sinful and His pardon of peoples' 'misdeeds'.

Body disposition

For Muslims there are certain practices related to body disposition after death. Once the person is dead, the mouth and eyes are closed and the face is bandaged around the chin. The head is turned towards the right shoulder; this is so that the body can be buried facing towards Makkah. The feet are tied together and the body is straightened. This is done by flexing the elbows, shoulders, knees and hips before straightening them. This is thought to ensure that the body does not stiffen, thus facilitating its washing and shrouding (Siala, 1996). The body is usually taken home or to the mosque. It is the responsibility of the family to wash the person according to the Islamic rites for washing the deceased (*ghusul*) (Siala, 1996). Two or three persons may perform the washing. Those who take on the responsibility of washing the dead should be the most knowledgeable concerning the procedures. Women relatives wash a female corpse and men wash a male corpse; for a married person, a spouse may perform the washing. The persons should be trustworthy and honest adult Muslims. The washing should be carried out in a clean and private place and where water is available. The washer should start the washing by saying '*Bismillah*', 'In the name of Allah'. The body should be washed a minimum of three times and the water should have in it some cleaning agent like soap or disinfectant. It is stated that the Prophet came among us while we were bathing his daughter and he said, 'Begin with her right side and the places of *Wudu*' (Bukhari [a]). The final washing should have in it some perfume such as camphor or lotus leaves (if available). During the washing, the private parts (*aura*) of the deceased should be covered with a piece of cloth. The body should then be dried and the hair combed out. In the case of women, the hair should be plaited into three braids, one from the front and two from the sides, and placed behind her head (Bukhari [b]). After the washing, the body should be dried and covered totally with a white sheet (Siala, 1996). Once the body is cleaned and wrapped, no one should view it. Those who wash the dead are recommended to take an Islamic bath (*ghusl*) afterwards.

Funerals and burials

Muslims do not cremate the deceased but always bury them. Only the males attend funerals (*janaza*). The ceremony is simple but solemn and can be performed at any time, but this depends on the local authorities or services. Prayers for the dead are performed in a disciplined manner by the company present at the funeral, usually an *Imam* and his followers, who say customary prayers for the deceased, some silently and some out loud. Prayers for the dead are recited in a standing position only, for in Islam no bowing or prostrations are allowed, except before Allah (Kramer, 1988). Prayers remind the mourners that through death we return to await our fate, and that we will be raised at the Last day of Judgement (Kramer, 1988).

A Muslim burial should take place as soon as possible, preferably within 24 hours. Delay can cause distress to the relatives and, if unavoidable, the reasons should be explained carefully to the relatives. The deceased is placed in a plain wooden coffin, which is narrow at the feet and wider at the shoulders. It is carried to the place of burial. There is no specific prayer to say, as it is better to remain silent and think of our own death. The body is taken from the coffin before it is buried in order to speed decomposition and is lowered into a grave six feet deep (equal to the height of an average man). It is preferable to place a body in the grave with its feet first; also to place the body on its right side facing the *Qiblah*. It is desirable that those who attend the burial throw three handfuls of soil over the grave (Siala, 1996). After the burial, it is desirable to pray individually, with sincerity, for forgiveness of the deceased and acceptance (of his conduct by Allah), because after a short while the deceased will be questioned about his life.

Mourning

The question of mourning for the deceased is an interesting one in Islam, and it is clear from the tradition that the Prophet forbade it. However, grief at the death of a friend or relative is normal and weeping is allowed. In Arab and Muslim cultures grieving normally does take the form of clear outward lamenting, sometimes loud and prolonged wailing (Abu Aisha, 2010). It is permissible for the family members to mourn for three days. For the widow, the period of mourning is 4 months and 10 days if she is not pregnant. If she is pregnant, the mourning ends as soon as the baby is delivered. Condolences may be offered in any words so long as they lighten the distress, induce patience, and bring solace to the bereaved. Muslims are encouraged to show empathy towards the bereaved, but it should be done without exaggeration: comforting and supporting the bereaved as long as it remains necessary. Thus the bereaved should be visited from time to time.

The family does not normally cook on the day of the funeral, it is *sunnah* that friends and relatives bring food to the house for them (Siala, 1996). Endurance should be shown by the bereaved, who are recommended to praise God and say, 'We belong to him, and to him we return.' In some countries it is customary to wear black during mourning but this is not a religious requirement (Siala, 1996) and is prohibited. If the person died in debt, it is the responsibility of the relatives to discharge the debt and any bequests as

Table 15.1 A summary of considerations after death

- Once death is pronounced, the eyes of the deceased should be closed.
- Cover the deceased with a piece of cloth. A woman's hijab should be kept on as if she was alive. This is to safeguard the respect and dignity of the deceased in death.
- Any connected tubes, false teeth, contact lenses, artificial limbs, and jewellery should be removed.
- Wounds or weeping incisions should be packed with bandage to prevent leakage.
- The mouth should be held in a closed position. This is achieved by tying the lower jaw to the top of the head with a bandage to prevent sagging of the jaw.
- Arms should be positioned straight at the sides.
- The ankles should be tied together to avoid dropping during transferring of the body.
- Autopsy or post-mortem examinations are not permitted except for legal reasons, and if permitted, should be done with the utmost respect for the dead.
- The body should be released to the family as soon as possible.
- Nurses should not try to hug or physically touch family members but may show sympathy and support.

---

soon as possible, provided that this is within their capacity (Al Shafii, 2002, pp. 943–4). There is a concern that a Muslim who dies in a non-Islamic institution may not be treated in accordance with the Islamic tradition (Salman and Zoucha, 2010). It is extremely important to follow the Islamic rituals when death becomes inevitable and treatment measures fail. A summary of considerations after death is presented in Table 15.1

Reflective Activity 15.2

Case Study 1

Zahra has just delivered a healthy baby boy. She overhears Ali, Zahra's husband, talking about the circumcision of the baby. Being Zahra's nurse, you believe that circumcision is painful for the baby and is not beneficial.

- How would you respond to this situation, as this is not part of your religious/cultural practice?

- What are some of the main points that you need to include in your discussion with Zahra and Ali?
- How would you enable Zahra and Ali to fulfil their religious requirement?
- What services are provided by your local health authorities or Islamic organisations regarding circumcision?

Comments on Reflective Activity 15.2

Circumcision is a common practice in Muslim communities. It is considered a hygienic practice since some urine might remain under the foreskin during ablution. There is scientific evidence that demonstrates the potential medical benefits of circumcision for the new-born male (American Academy of Pediatrics, 1999). Circumcision prevents urinary tract infections, sexually transmitted infections and cancer of the penis. At present, this procedure is usually carried out in the hospital during the first few days after birth. You can assist the family by providing them with information about the specialist unit or the surgeons who are willing to perform the circumcision, or the local Mosque/Islamic organisation who can help. The parents will need instructions on how to keep the penis clean, watch out for complications and relieve the baby's discomfort during and after the procedure. The most common complications include infection, bleeding, and not removing enough of the foreskin. Parents should be prepared for how the freshly circumcised penis will appear. Typically, there may be swelling and bruising noted after the circumcision as a secondary effect of the injection of anaesthesia. The swelling should subside over the next week. Frequent changing of the infant's diaper is required in order to prevent irritation from soiling.

Reflective Activity 15.3

Case Study 2

Lamia has been on your unit for the past three weeks; she has uterine cancer and has received several chemotherapy treatments without much success. During the past week she has deteriorated and is in her final stages. You notice that the family are confused and do not know what to do. They appear to be devout Muslims.

- How would you approach the family and help them through this stressful time?
- How would you meet the spiritual needs of Lamia?

- What are some of the practices that are carried out by Muslim families in caring for their dying relative?
- What arrangement should be made after death has been confirmed?

Comments on Reflective Activity 15.3

This is a highly sensitive time for the family, who need support and understanding from the healthcare team. If there is a nearby Muslim cultural centre or Mosque then you can ask the Sheikh or *Imam* to talk to the family. If there is no religious person available you need to provide some information to the family and help them implement some of the practices, such as positioning the patient in the direction of Makkah, and preparation of the body for the ritual washing. Allowing the family to be near the patient so that they can recite the Qur'aan is also helpful.

Conclusion

There are some rituals that accompany the new-born, and also death in a Muslim family. For Muslims there are ways of welcoming a new-born child into the community (*Ummah*). Among the Sunnah for welcoming the new-born, the scholars mentioned that the *Adhan* should be recited into the baby's right ear so that the first thing he or she hears in this world will be the words of *Tawheed*. Unlike birth, which is the start of a temporary existence on earth, Muslims believe that death is a departure from the life of this world to the hereafter, which is eternal. Nurses should be fully cognisant of the 'rites of passage' of a Muslim from birth to death so that they can adopt culturally congruent and sensitive care in meeting the needs of the Muslim patient.

References

Abu Aisha, B. (2010) *Funeral Rites and Regulations in Islam*, www.missionislam. com/knowledge/funeral.htm, date accessed 7 August 2013.

Abu Dawud and Tirmidhî, Arabic/English book reference: Book 7, Hadith 906, http://sunnah.com/riyadussaliheen/7, date accessed 7 August 2013.

Al-Baar, M. (2005) *al-Khitaan*, p. 76, www.islam-qa.com/en/ref/7073, date accessed 7 August 2013.

Al Shafii, Y. (2002) *Riyad Al-Saleheen* (Beirut, Lebanon: Dar Al Kitab Al Arabi).

Al-Shahri, M. (2002) 'Culturally Sensitive Caring for Saudi Patients', *Journal of Transcultural Nursing* 13, 2, 133–8.

American Academy of Pediatrics (1999) 'Task Force on Circumcision', *Pediatrics* 103, 686–93.

Athar, S. (1988) *Guidelines for Health Care Providers when Dealing with Muslim Patients*, Medical Ethics Committee, Islamic Medical Association North America, www.imana.org, date accessed 7 August 2013.

Bukhari [a], Sahih Al-Bukhari, vol. 2, p. 195, no. 346.

Bukhari [b], Sahih Al-Bukhari, vol. 2, p. 197, no. 350.

Bukhari and Muslim, cited in www.fatwaislam.com/fis/index.cfm?scn=fd&ID= 505, date accessed 7 August 2013.

Dhami, S. and Sheikh, A. (2008) 'The Family: Predicament and Promise', in A. Sheikh and A.R. Gatrad (eds), *Caring for Muslim Patients*, 2nd edn (Oxford: Radcliffe Medical Publishing).

Gulam, H. (2003) 'Care of the Muslim Patient', *Australian Nursing Journal* (August) 63, 1–3.

Hedayat, K. and Pirzadeh, R. (2001) 'Issues in Islamic Biomedical Ethics: a Primer for Pediatricians', *Pediatrics* 108, 4, 965–71.

Ibn Qudamah, al-Mughni 1/70, cited in http://answers.yahoo.com/question/index?qid=20121104162352AA914YV, date accessed 7 August 2013.

Kramer, K. (1988) *The Sacred Art of Dying: How World Religions Understand Death* (New York: Paulis Press).

Larke, N.L., Thomas, S.L., dos Santos Silva, I. and Weiss, H.A. (2011) 'Male Circumcision and Penile Cancer: a Systematic Review and Meta-analysis', *Cancer Causes Control* 22, 8, 1097–110.

Ott, B., Al-Junaibi, S. and Al-Khadhuri, J. (2003) 'Preventing Ethical Dilemmas: Understanding Islamic Health Care Practices', *Pediatric Nursing* 29, 3, 227–30.

Rassool, G. Hussein (2004) 'Commentary: an Islamic Perspective', *Journal of Advanced Nursing* 46, 3, 281–3.

Salman, K. and Zoucha, R. (2010) 'Considering Faith Within Culture When Caring for the Terminally Ill Muslim Patient and Family', *Journal of Hospice and Palliative Nursing* 12, 3, 156–63.

Sheikh, A. and Gatrad, A. (2008) 'Birth Customs: Meaning and Significance', in A. Sheikh and A. Gatrad (eds), *Caring for Muslim Patients*, 2nd edn (Oxford: Radcliffe Medical Publishing).

Sheikh 'Abd al-'Azeez ibn Baaz. Fatawa Ibn Baaz, 13/93, http://islamqa.info/en/ref/72201/DEATH%20AND%20DYING, date accessed 7 August 2013.

Sheik Al-Albani [a], Silsilat al-Ahaadeeth al-Da'eefah wa'l-Mawdoo'ah, http://islamqa.com/en/ref/7889/when%20a%20baby%20is%20born, date accessed 7 August 2013.

Sheikh Al-Albani, in Ahkaam al-Janaa'iz: 'Reciting Soorat Yaa-seen for the Dying Person', http://islamqa.info/en/ref/72201/DEATH%20AND %20DYING, date accessed 7 August 2013.

Sheikh Muhammad ibn Salih al-'Uthaymeen. Fatwa No 4049, Q & A, http://islamqa.info/en/ref/4049, date accessed 7 August 2013.

Sheikh Muhammed Salih Al-Munajjid. Fatwa 7889, Islamic actions for welcoming a new baby, from http://islamqa.com/en/ref/7889/when%20a%20baby%20is%20born, date accessed 7 August 2013.

Sheikh Muhammed Salih Al-Munajjid. Fatwa 13750, Islam Q & A, http://msapubli.com/islam-qa/Volume_26/Chapter_3.htm, date accessed 7 August 2013.

Siala, M. (1996) *Authentic Step by Step Illustrated Janazah Guide*, Salman Al-Farisi Islamic Center, cited in www.missionislam.com/knowledge/janazahstepbystep.htm, date accessed 7 August 2013.

Tirmidhî, 1522; al-Nasa'i, 4220; Abu Dawud, 2838; cited in http://islamqa.info/en/ref/7889, date accessed 7 August 2013.

Tirmidhî, Sunnah.com reference: Book 7, Hadith 6, Arabic/English book reference: Book 7, Hadith 899, http://sunnah.com/riyadussaliheen/7, date accessed 7 August 2013.

Wehbe-Alamah, H. (2008) 'Bridging Generic and Professional Care Practices for Muslim Patients through Use of Leininger's Culture Care Modes', *Contemporary Nurse* 28, 1–2, 83–97.

Organ and Blood Donation and End-of-Life Decisions

16

G. Hussein Rassool and C. Sange

Learning Outcomes:

- Identify the reasons why Muslims are more reluctant to refuse to donate organs for transplantation than other religious groups.
- Examine the Islamic ethical approach to: (a) organ donation; and (b) blood donation.
- Examine the Islamic ethical approach to: (a) post-mortem examination; and (b) end-of-life decisions.
- Discuss the criteria to be met before organ transplantation for Muslim patients.
- Discuss the arguments against euthanasia from an Islamic perspective.

Reflective Activity 16.1

State whether the following statements are true or false. Give reasons for your answers.

	True	False
1 Organ donation is against the Muslim religion.		
2 Even if I am healthy, I cannot be a living donor.		
3 Hundreds of people's lives are saved each year by organ transplants.		
4 If I agree to donate my organs, the hospital staff won't work as hard to save my life.		

	True	False
5 Organs that can be donated by people who have died include the heart, lungs, kidneys, liver, pancreas and small bowel.		
6 Violating the human body, whether living or dead, is not forbidden in Islam.		
7 Because of my medical conditions, nobody would want my organs or tissues.		
8 Muslims may carry donor cards.		
9 In the absence of a card or an expressed wish to donate organs, the family may not give permission to obtain organs from the body to save other people's lives.		
10 I'm aged under 18. I'm too young to make this decision.		
11 I'm too old to donate. Nobody would want my organs.		
12 Organ donation results in blemish of the body.		

Introduction

The technological advances in medicine and health care in such diverse areas as organ transplantation, blood donation and end-of-life decisions, including the development of kidney dialysis and respirators, posed novel questions to Muslim scholars and jurists regarding when and how care might be withdrawn. Approaches to organ and blood donation, post-mortem examinations and end-of-life decisions are all governed according to religious and cultural views. Lovering (2008) stated that Muslim and non-Muslim nurses approach ethical dilemmas, such as assisting with organ donation, end-of-life practices with a critically ill patient, and assisting with procedures such as abortion and sterilisation, from different ethical perspectives. In this chapter we aim to examine the Islamic ethical approach to organ transplantation, blood transfusion, post-mortem and end-of-life decisions, with reference to the Qur'aan and Hadith. For a more comprehensive examination of the ethical dimensions in caring from an Islamic perspective, see Chapter 4.

Understanding organ and blood donation

Organ donation means taking healthy organs and tissues from one individual for transplantation into another. Organs that can be donated include:

- Internal organs: kidneys, heart, liver, pancreas, intestines, lungs
- Skin
- Bone and bone marrow
- Cornea.

In England, the Human Tissue Act states that:

> if a person has, while alive and competent, given consent for some or all of their organs or tissue to be donated following his or her death (by joining the NHS Organ Donor Register or by other means, such as discussing their wishes with those closest to them), then that consent is sufficient for the donation to go ahead. Once consent is established, relatives or other relevant people should be advised of the fact and encouraged to respect the deceased's wishes. [The relatives] have no legal right to veto or overrule them . . . .
>
> If there is no record of the deceased's wishes, the medical staff will approach the relatives or other relevant people to establish any known wishes of the deceased. If these are not known, and the deceased has nominated a person to deal with the use of their body after death, then consent can be given by that person.
>
> If neither of the above apply, consent to donate can be given by someone in a 'qualifying relationship' immediately before the death of the deceased person. (NHS Blood and Transplant [a])

Most organ and tissue donations occur after the donor has died. But some organs and tissues can be donated while the donor is alive. Organ transplantation in Islam is seen as a means of alleviating pain or saving life on the basis of the rules of the Shari'ah (Islam and Organ Donation). Everyone, irrespective of age or health and who is considered legally competent, can join the Donor Register in the UK. This is a way to give legal consent or authorisation for donation to take place. Children can register but their parents, guardians or those with parental responsibility will be asked to provide their consent should the child's death lead to donation being considered (NHS Blood and Transplant [a]). Having a medical condition does not necessarily prevent a person from becoming an organ or tissue donor except for those diagnosed with HIV or who have, or are suspected of having, Creutzfeldt-Jakob disease (CJD). In the US, the United Network for Organ Sharing (UNOS) manages the national transplant waiting list, matching donors to recipients; monitors every organ match; ensures that organ allocation policies are followed; maintains the database; and educates professional groups about their important role in the donation process.

Islamic perspectives on organ donation

Since there are no specific codes on transplant and organ donation in Islamic law (*Shar'iah*), there are different approaches to treatment. Some scholars and jurists believe that organ donation is not permissible and hold the view that this does not fall under the criteria of the Islamic principle of *al-darurat tubih al-mahzurat* (necessities overrule prohibition) due to other overriding Islamic principles (Islam and Organ Donation). However, there are also a significant number of Muslim scholars who suggest Islamic law permits such practices. The resolutions of the Islamic Fiqh Council of the Organisation of the Islamic Conference, stated that it is permissible to donate organs. This is most likely to be the correct view, so long as the donation will not lead to the death of the donor (islamqa.info/en/ref/107690). In 1995, the Muslim Law (Shar'iah) Council UK issued a fatwa (religious opinion) on organ donation. The Council resolved that:

- The council supports organ transplantation as a means of alleviating pain or saving life on the basis of the rules of the Shar'iah.
- Muslims may carry donor cards.
- The next of kin of a dead person, in the absence of a card or an expressed wish to donate their organs, may give permission to obtain organs from the body to save other people's lives.

Muslim scholars of the most prestigious academies are unanimous in declaring that organ donation is an act of merit and in certain circumstances can be an obligation. Generally, the violation of the human body, whether living or dead, is forbidden in Islam, but the consensus of the most eminent Islamic scholars is that this can be overruled when saving another person's life. Preserving life is a fundamental function of the Shari'ah, hence organ donation and transplantation within this view becomes permissible in the Islamic world.

The Shar'iah Academy of the Organisation of the Islamic Conference (representing all Muslim countries), the Grand Ulema Council of Saudi Arabia, the Iranian Religious Authority and the Al-Azhar Academy of Egypt call upon Muslims to donate organs for transplantation. Both viewpoints, of permissibility and non-permissibility, take their evidence from the Qur'aan and the Hadith and therefore individual Muslims should make a decision according to their understanding of the Shar'iah, or seek advice from their local *Imam* or scholar (Islam and Organ Donation). However, there are certain limits and conditions in place to protect donors and those who are in need of donation. The following requirements should be met before transplantation (Sarhill et al., 2001):

- A transplant is the only form of treatment available.
- The likelihood of success is high.
- The consent of the donor or next of kin is obtained.
- The death of the donor has been established by a Muslim doctor.
- There is no imminent danger to the life of a living donor.
- The recipient has been informed of the operation, and of its arrangement for ritual body wash.

In addition, organ donation is permissible so long as it does not exploit donors, and if recipients are granted fair access to donated organs regardless of race/ethnicity, religious identity, class, or financial situation (Budiani and Shibly, 2006). According to Budiani and Shibly (2006), these conditions aim to prevent exploitation of the poor, who might sell their organs to wealthier but ailing patients, and to ensure equitable access to donated organs and tissues. The Islamic Medical Association of North America (IMANA) supports transplantation in general – both the giving and receiving of organs are allowed for the purpose of saving life – and has issued guidelines for giving and receiving organs (see Table 16.1).

Table 16.1   Guidelines for giving and receiving organs

This has to be done under the following guidelines:

- The medical need has to be defined.
- The possible benefit to the patient has to be defined.
- Consent from the donor as well as the recipient must be obtained.
- There must be no financial incentive to the donor or his/her relatives for giving the organs (a voluntary gift may be permitted).
- Any permanent harm to the donor must be avoided.
- One may not transplant sex organs (testicles, ovaries), which would violate the sanctity of marriage.
- There should be no sale of organs by any party.
- There should be no cost to the family of the donor for removing the organ.
- Cadaver donation is permitted but only if specifically mentioned in that person's will or driving licence.
- Blood transfusion is permissible. Giving or receiving blood from people of other faiths is permissible.

Source: Adapted from IMANA Ethics Committee, 'Islamic Medical Ethics: the IMANA Perspective', www.imana.org/?page=%20IslamicMedicalEthic, date accessed 8 August 2013. Reproduced with kind permission from IMANA.

Muslims and organ donation

In the UK the prevalence of established renal failure (ERF) is at least three times greater amongst people of South Asian background than in the Caucasian population (Raleigh, 1997). Muslims are more likely to need a kidney transplant because they are more susceptible to developing diabetes and high blood pressure, which can lead to kidney failure. As a result of higher demand and a shortage of organ donors, Black and Asian people have to wait on average five years or more for a kidney transplant, twice as long as the rest of the population (NHS Blood and Transplant [b]). According to Hayward and Madill (2003), Muslims are more likely to refuse to donate than other religious groups, and also are the least likely to have been approached for such requests. Research findings have shown that reasons why certain religious groups do not participate in organ donation include knowledge and understanding of organ donation, rather than cultural and religious practices (Randhawa, 1998; Sheikh and Dhami, 2000). The findings of a study by Clarke-Swaby (2010) showed that Black Africans, Caribbeans and Asians were concerned by the waiting times for transplants. The study also identified that age, beliefs, culture and lack of knowledge were some of the factors associated with not wanting to donate organs. A qualitative study of the attitudes of 141 UK Muslim Indo-Asians to organ donation showed that the participants' 'culture-specific issues arguing against donation included a sense of the sacredness of the body, a fatalistic approach to illness, a belief that organs took on an independent role as "witnesses" to an individual's life on Judgement Day and an anxiety that the donor would have no control of the probity of the recipient of an organ' (Alkhawari et al., 2006). The Muslim Health Network is supporting UK Transplant's organ donation campaign, which has targeted the Asian community, especially the Muslim community.

Reflective Activity 16.2

State whether the following statements are true or false. Give reasons for your answers.

		True	False
1	Blood donation is not acceptable in Islam.		
2	There is a distinction to be made between Muslims and non-Muslims in donating and receiving blood.		
3	It is permissible for Muslims to donate blood to non-Muslims.		

	True	False
4 Buying and selling of the blood is permitted in Islam.		
5 It is acceptable for a Muslim to think and talk about death.		
6 When a Muslim dies, there are very specific rituals in caring for the dead body.		
7 When a Muslim dies, the body should ideally be positioned facing the direction of Makkah.		
8 Islam supports euthanasia and the right to die voluntarily.		
9 Islamic law forbids mutilation of the corpse, as in the case of a post-mortem.		

Blood donation

Islamic views on blood donation are similar to those on organ donation and transplantation. Blood donation is considered an extremely meritorious and rewarding act of charity in Islam; since Islam exhorts us to be charitable to all of God's creation, we cannot think of any charity greater than the gift of life (Sheikh Ahmad Kutty). Blood donation is considered a rewarding act of charity in Islam, and a way of pleasing Allah (interpretation of the meaning):

☐ *And if anyone saved a life, it would be as if he saved the life of all mankind.* (Al-Māʾidah [The Table Spread] 5:32)

There is no distinction to be made between Muslims and non-Muslims in donating and receiving blood. So, it is permissible to receive blood from the Blood Bank even if the donor was a non-Muslim. Likewise, it is also permissible to donate blood to non-Muslims. Blood donation and transfusion under Islamic law must consider the following:

- The donor is mature and sane.
- The donor is willing to donate.
- There is no risk to the life of the donor.
- There is a definite risk to the receiver's life.
- There is no alternative.
- Buying and selling of blood is not permitted in Islam.

Blood donation, without doubt, tops the list of charitable deeds; it is a duty for every Muslim not only to participate in it but also to take initiatives in their communities to organise blood banks. From a Shar'iah perspective, it will not be permissible for anyone to sell his/her blood to the bank; rather, it must be donated freely.

Euthanasia, dying and the believing Muslim

Practices, beliefs and customs surrounding death and end-of-life decisions are common to all religions and cultures. There is no doubt that the only thing guaranteed in life and promised to all by God is *death*. Death for a Muslim marks the transition from one state of existence to the next as part of the divine plan. Islam places great emphasis on the sanctity of life and the reality of death (interpretation of the meaning):

☐ *Every soul shall taste death.* (Āli'Imrān [The Family of Imran] 3:185)

For a Muslim, life on earth is viewed as a test of resistance from all forbidden things, and of the maintenance and duration of one's belief in Allah and the teachings of Islam. Life after death is then seen as eternal, where one repays for one's deeds, either in heaven or in hell. Islam teaches the continued existence of the soul and a transformed physical existence after death. Muslims believe there will be a day of judgement when all human beings will be divided between the eternal destinations of Paradise and Hell. Death is not considered as taboo in Islam because for Muslims death should always be present in their thoughts, and they should reflect upon it constantly, and on a daily basis. When a Muslim dies, there are very specific rituals in caring for the dead body. See Chapter 15 for a comprehensive account of the Islamic traditions and customs following death.

Islam does not believe in prolonging life, as everyone has been created for a certain life span. Prolongation of life by artificial means (such as a life support machine) is strongly disapproved of unless there is evidence that a reasonable quality of life will result (Rahman, 1987). At the Islamic Juridical Council (IJC) meetings, Muslim jurists of different schools ruled that once invasive treatment has been intensified to save the life of a patient, life-saving equipment cannot be turned off unless the physicians are certain about the inevitability of death (Sachedina, 2005). According to the Islamic point of view, spiritual health, moral elevation and purity are very important in determining the quality of life, in addition to physical health and comfort. Thus, a patient's suffering might be the divine will for her/his purification and spiritual maturity (Zahedi et al., 2007).

However, in a case of the occurrence of brain death caused by irreversible damage to the brain, including loss of spontaneous respiration, the jurists ruled that if three attending physicians attest to a totally damaged brain that results in an unresponsive coma, apnoea, and absent cephalic reflexes, and if the patient can be kept alive only by a respirator, then the person is biologically dead, although legal death can be attested only when the breathing stops completely after the turning off of life-saving equipment (Al-Qarar, 1990). Islamic law permits withdrawal of futile and disproportionate treatment on the basis of the consent of immediate family members, who act on the professional advice of the physician in charge of the case (Sachedina, 2005).

In the US and Europe, organisations exist which promote euthanasia as an ethical action, a 'rational' alternative to life, especially if the individual is overwhelmed by severe infirmity or serious suffering. According to Al-Qaradawi (2005), 'Euthanasia or Mercy Killing is the act or practice of ending the life of an individual suffering from a terminal illness or an incurable condition, through lethal injection or the suspension of extraordinary medical treatment.' With the advent of patients' advocacy and healthcare rights, patients are increasingly asking nurses and other healthcare professionals to 'intervene' to achieve a 'good death' (Rassool, 2004). Islam, and the other two main monotheistic faiths (Christianity and Judaism), agree that 'life cannot be taken save by an express mandate'. This covenant is in the hands of God. With regard to human life and suffering, three 'commands' may be envisaged: (1) the duty to preserve life, (2) the obligation to alleviate suffering, and (3) the duty to recognise that life has an end (Rassool, 2004). This covenant is stated in the Qur'aan (interpretation of the meaning):

□ *We ordained for the Children of Israel that if anyone killed a person not in retaliation of murder, or (and) to spread mischief in the land – it would be as if he killed all mankind, and if anyone saved a life, it would be as if he saved the life of all mankind.* (Al-Mā'idah [The Table Spread] 5:32)

Islamic jurisprudence does not recognise a person's right to die voluntarily. The Islamic arguments against euthanasia can be summarised in two main reasons: (1) life is sacred and euthanasia and suicide are not included among the reasons allowed for killing in Islam; and (2) Allah decides how long each of us will live, and two verses support this reason (Aramesh and Shadi, 2007). Islam places great emphasis on the sanctity of life and the reality of death, and decrees that life cannot be terminated by any form of euthanasia (mercy killing) or rational suicide. Similarly, the killing of a terminally ill person, whether it be doctor assisted or family member assisted, is regarded as disobedience against God's will. However, there is a clear distinction between active and passive euthanasia. The Islamic ethical rule 'No harm shall be inflicted or reciprocated in Islam' could be understood as allowing for important distinctions and rules about life-sustaining treatments in terminally ill patients; the distinctions on which ethical decisions are made include the difference between killing (active euthanasia) and letting die (passive euthanasia) (Sachedina, 2005). For instance, withholding or withdrawing treatment in a brain-dead patient would not be considered a form of euthanasia, and thus is permissible (Hedayat and Pirzadeh, 2001). The decision to end the life of a loved one is difficult regardless of one's religious or ethnic background.

The European Council for Fatwa and Research (ECFR) (2008) stated that having considered the different legal stances Western countries take concerning Euthanasia, both in approval and in rejection, the Council decided the following:

> The prohibition of the direct active euthanasia and the prohibition of suicide and assisting in bringing it about, for according to Shar'iah, killing a patient suffering from a terminal illness is not permissible for the physician, the patient's family or the patient himself. The patient whatever his illness and however sick he (or she) is shall not be killed because of desperation and loss of hope in recovery or to prevent the transfer of the patient's disease to others, and whoever commits the act of killing will be a deliberate killer. The Qur'aanic text confirms without a shadow of a doubt that homicide is forbidden absolutely, as Allah Almighty says (interpretation of the meaning): 'And take not life, which Allah has made sacred, except by way of justice and law' (Al-'An'ām 6:51), and as Allah Almighty also says (interpretation of the meaning): 'Because of that We ordained for the Children of Israel that if anyone killed a person not in retaliation of murder or for spreading mischief in the land – it would be as if he killed all mankind' (Al-Mā'idah [The Table Spread] 5:32).

It is unlawful for the patient to kill himself (or herself) and it is unlawful for somebody else to kill him (or her) even if given leave to kill him. The former case will be suicide and the latter will be aggression against the other by killing him, for the patient's permission does not render the unlawful act lawful. The patient does not possess his own soul to permit somebody else to take it.

Post-mortem examinations

Islam requires that a Muslim be buried straight away following death, and post-mortem is not allowed by the religion. Islamic law forbids mutilation of the corpse. Post-mortem is permissible when it is deemed necessary to establish the cause of death because of significant public health interest or when required by law. It is not acceptable to undertake a post-mortem examination for routine documentation. Whilst Islamic jurists have long argued that this prohibition does not apply to respectful legal and medical procedures necessary to determine a cause of death, Qur'aanic statements about the resurrection of the physical body influence cultural resistance to the procedure (Lawrence, 2001). The prohibition of post-mortem is also based on a statement by the Prophet Muhammad: 'To break the bone of a dead person is like breaking the bone of a living person' (Abu Dawud).

This indicates that a dead person is not to be treated with disrespect, just as a living person is not to be treated with disrespect (Al-Teebi). This also means that an individual has the same level of sanctity when dead as when alive, and that breaking his bone when he is dead is forbidden just as it is forbidden to break it when he is alive (Al-Baaji). In addition, the loss of a loved one is extremely difficult for any family to deal with and the thought of an invasive post-mortem can compound the grief and distress. Using the Muslim's body as material for dissection, training and teaching is contrary to the honour that Allah has bestowed upon him. A statement to that effect was issued by the Council of Senior Scholars, in which it says: 'And since dissecting involves a loss of dignity, and since there is no necessity for dissecting them because it is possible to obtain dead bodies that are not protected by Shari'ah, the Council believes that dissections should be restricted to such bodies and not bodies of people who are protected by Shari'ah' (Abhaath Hay'at Kibaar al-'Ulama' (2/84).

Since post-mortem can take time, it poses a problem for Muslims as the Shari'ah encourages burial as soon as possible. It is not permissible to delay burial except within the limits of what is needed to prepare the body or to wait for the relatives or neighbours to come, if that will not take too long according to local custom, because the Prophet has said: 'Hasten to bury your dead' (Malik et al.).

Reflective Activity 16.3

Case Study

A 35-year-old Muslim man was admitted to the intensive care unit of the hospital via emergency medical services after suffering a severe closed-head injury resulting from a car accident. A computed tomography (CT) scan of the head revealed a subdural haematoma with right-to-left shift and effacement of the right ventricle. After evaluating the patient and the CT scan, the neurosurgeon determined that the patient would not benefit from surgery and that the injury may have been fatal. The trauma surgeon and neurosurgeon recommended that medical care, including hyperventilation to reduce cerebral oedema, be continued until a period of observation could allow determination of the extent and irreversibility of the injury. Next of kin were notified of the patient's injuries, condition, and grim prognosis, which were discussed at length with the family. Further physical examination and brain blood flow study results were consistent with brain death. During this conversation with the family, the doctor suggested that organ donation might be an option for this patient. The patient's family was very upset upon hearing that the patient had died and immediately expressed negative feelings about organ donation. The family claim that organ donation is against their religion.

- How would you respond to the relatives' immediate grief and loss?
- The family is not clear about 'brain death'. How would you explain this to the family?
- How would you approach the family about organ donation?
- What further information could be provided to the family about organ donation?
- What impact might the organ donation process have on the family?

Comments on Reflective Activity 16.3

For Muslims, death is divinely willed and when it arrives it should be readily accepted as there should be no reasoning by the bereaved as to why they have lost their loved one (Sajid, 2003). At the death of this individual, the family would invoke Allah and say 'Verily we belong to Allah, and truly to Him shall we return' (*Inna lillahi wa inna ilayhi raji'un*). Once the death has been confirmed and the family has been told about the bad news, the nurse would be the first line of support for the family. The family present should also be left alone to enable them to work through their intense emotions. When Muslims feel sorrow over a loss, or grief overwhelms them, they should draw comfort from their faith and find solace in spiritual practices. Religious practices encourage sharing of grief and provide the means for absolving it. For some, it may be valuable to talk to the *Imam* to gain spiritual comfort. The extended family network can also provide a great deal of support for the bereaved. When offering condolences, words should be chosen carefully and said gently to convey empathy. For Muslims, it is a duty for them to offer condolences, comfort, and sympathy to the family and to encourage the family to accept Allah's will.

How individuals would react to this situation will depend on the context and on personality factors. As this event was unexpected, there would be many questions the family would need to ask. It would be ideal at this stage to leave the family alone with the assurance that any help or information they require will be provided. The best possible approach through which any condition can be explained to the family is via a doctor, with nurses being present at the time. It is important not to use language that would be too technical for the family members to understand. Nurses can play a significant role in clarifying this state. The relatives would need to understand that once a patient has been classed as being 'brain dead', or having suffered 'brain death', that means there is no activity of the brain. One could give the following explanation: brain death is a legal definition of death. It is the complete and irreversible cessation (stopping) of all brain function. It means that, as a result of severe trauma or injury to the brain, the body's blood supply to the brain is blocked, the brain dies and it cannot be revived. A doctor conducts the required medical tests to make the diagnosis of brain death. These tests are based on sound and legally accepted medical guidelines that comply with legal requirements (www.kidney.org).

The family have already been approached regarding organ donation but have rejected this on the basis that it was against their religion. However, this cannot be imposed on the family. A more effective approach is to provide them with information, for example, 'Islam and Organ Donation' in the appropriate language, and let them make the decision based on an informed choice. In this context, leaflets should be readily available for potential donors, but having an *Imam* available who could provide advice on the religious rulings on organ transplants would be helpful as well. The nurse may also be able to clarify the issue of the acceptability of organ donation in Islam. If the family agrees to organ and/or tissue donation, the patient will remain on the ventilator and is supported with fluids and medications to keep blood flowing to the organs and tissue. Tests are performed to determine the medical suitability of the organs and tissues for transplantation. In the meantime, other medical personnel identify potential recipients for the different organs and tissues that can be transplanted. These procedures may take up to 12 hours to arrange. The deceased person is then taken into surgery to remove the donated organs or tissue, or both. After they are removed, the ventilator is disconnected (www. kidney.org).

Literature on the psychological impact that the organ donation process can have on the family has been limited. The findings of a study (Merchant et al., 2008) indicated that the vast majority of respondents feel something good and useful has come out of their loss, and that donation has a beneficial effect on bereavement. However, the respondents also reported that they experienced some negative or upsetting things, such as feeling confused about brain death and feeling rushed into making decisions. Providing clear, consistent, and timely information to the family about the patient is essential to establish trust. In this case the doctor has just disclosed the death of the patient, and subsequently also discusses organ donation. The process of organ donation or discussion around this issue cannot begin until the family knows of and accepts their relative's death. The timing of information is vital. The more time and attention the healthcare team give to the family members, the more likely these relatives are to give consent. Health professionals can feel encouraged about addressing families during this tragic period.

Conclusion

Organ and blood donation and end-of-life decisions are not only a matter of professional and Western medicine, but rather must include aspects of personal choice, and a recognition of cultural, social and religious values. Although the availability of organ transplants has spread across the globe, there still remains a scarcity of organ donors. The situation is similar to that of people donating blood. It appears to be generally related to the vagueness amongst people of all religions regarding religious tenets and organ/blood donation. This uncertainty does impact on the number of donors available, and on those who are waiting for donations. It is important that Islamic cultural and religious organisations work in partnership with healthcare services or other organisations to enable the promotion and delivery of an educational campaign on organ donation and transplants, to Muslim communities.

For Muslims, it is permissible to allow transplants of organs and blood donations as long as certain conditions are satisfied. According to Gatrad (1994), discussions concerning organ transplantation should be initiated by the transplant team: other professionals have in the past relayed conflicting advice to parents and this has resulted in the patient in need of a transplant not being treated. This team should include a liaison officer who works in the Muslim communities providing advice and support to families of patients needing organ transplantation and also to those families whose children have undergone a transplant operation. In relation to post-mortems, the Government in England is to allow Muslims (and Jews) to opt for alternative examinations of their loved ones by pathologists, which will not delay burial or involve invasive procedures. Those who object to post-mortem on religious grounds, will be allowed to ask for a Magnetic Resonance Imaging (MRI) scan of the bodies to be carried out instead (*Telegraph*, December 2009). A trial has seen pathologists using MRI scanners instead of post-mortem. Under the new system, coroners will be able to consider faith issues and the wishes of bereaved families when deciding what type of post-mortem should take place.

From an Islamic perspective, there are sharply delineated rules that inform nurses or healthcare professionals on what to do in the case of euthanasia, rational suicide or assisted suicide. Muslim healthcare professionals must maintain life, alleviate suffering, and have no right to assist in the termination of any human life under their care (Rassool, 2004).

References

Abhaath Hay'at Kibaar al-'Ulama' (2/84), http://islamqa.info/en/ref/140779, date accessed 8 August 2013.

Abu Dawud, 3207, cited in Fatawa Islamiyah, Vol. 7, pp. 191–3, Darussalam, www.fatwaislam.com/fis/index.cfm?scn=fd&ID=522, date accessed 8 August 2013.

Al-Baaji. al-Muntaqa Sharh al-Muwatta' (2/63), http://islamqa.info/en/ref/140779, date accessed 8 August 2013.

Alkhawari, F.S., Stimson, G.V. and Warrens, A.N. (2006) 'Attitudes toward Transplantation in UK Muslim Indo-Asians in West London', *American Journal of Transplantation* 6, 6, 1493.

Al-Qaradawi, Y. (2005) *Fatwa on Euthanasia*, www.IslamOnline.net, Living Shar'iah: Fatwa Bank, date accessed 8 August 2013.

Al-Qarar (1990) 'al-Thani bi-sha'n mawdu' taqrir husul al-wafat wa raf'ajhizat al-in'ash min jism al-insan', *Majalla al-buhuth al-fiqhiyya almu'asira* 4, 159–60.

Al-Teebi. *Is it Permissible for a Muslim to Donate his Body for Medical Research after HeDdies?* http://islamqa.info/en/ref/140779, date accessed 8 August 2013.

Aramesh, K. and Shadi, H. (2007) 'Euthanasia: an Islamic Ethical Perspective', *Iranian Journal of Allergy, Asthma and Immunology* 6, 5, 35–8.

Budiani, D. and Shibly, O. (2006) *Islam, Organ Transplants, and Organs Trafficking in the Muslim World: Paving a Path for Solutions*, submitted as a paper for the volume entitled, *Muslim Medical Ethics: Theory and Practice* (October 2006), cofs.googlecode.com/svn/trunk/ . . . /Budiani_and_Shibley.doc, date accessed 8 August 2013.

Clarke-Swaby, S. (2010) *Exploring the Understanding and Cultural Beliefs Surrounding Organ Donation amongst Black Africans, Caribbean and Asian Population Affected with Kidney Diseases in Lambeth, Southwark and Lewisham*, Mary Seacole Development Award winner 2009. Department of Health, Comms. No. 0193.

European Council for Fatwa and Research (ECFR) (2008) *Final Statement: Eleventh Ordinary Session of the European Council for Fatwa and Research*, www.e-cfr.org/ar/, date accessed 8 August 2013.

Gatrad, A.R. (1994) 'Muslim Customs Surrounding Death, Bereavement, Post-mortem Examinations, and Organ Transplants', *British Medical Journal* 30, 521. Doi, http://dx.doi.org/10.1136/bmj.309.6953.521, date accessed 8 August 2013.

Hayward, C. and Madill, A. (2003) 'The Meaning of Organ Donation: Muslims of Pakistani Origin and White English Nationals Living in North England', *Social Science and Medicine* 57, 3, 389–401.

Hedayat, K.M. and Pirzadeh, R. (2001) 'Issues in Islamic Biomedical Ethics: a Primer for the Pediatrician', *Pediatrics* 108, 4, 965–71.

IMANA Ethics Committee. 'IMANA Islamic Medical Ethics: the Position of Islamic Medical Association of North America', *On Issues of Medical Ethics*, www.imana.org/Ethics/ethics.html, date accessed 8 August 2013.

Islam and Organ Donation: A Guide to Organ Donation and Muslim Beliefs, www.organdonation.nhs.uk/newsroom/fact_sheets/religious_leaflets/islam_and_organ_donation/islam_and_organ_donation.pdf, date accessed 8 August 2013.

islamqa.info/en/ref/107690, Islamic Fiqh Council of the Organisation of the Islamic Conference, Ruling on Organ Donation, http://islamqa.info/en/ref/107690, date accessed 8 August 2013

Lawrence, S. (2001) 'Autopsy', in C. Blakemore and S. Jennett (eds), The Oxford Companion to the Body (Oxford: Oxford University Press).

Lovering, S. (2008) *Arab Muslim Nurses' Experiences of the Meaning of Caring* [Professional Doctorate] (Sydney, Australia: University of Sydney), http://hdl.handle.net/2123/3764, date accessed 10 August 2013.

Malik and Ahmad, 2/240; and by al-Bukhari, 2/87–88, http://islamiliveforit.blogspot.com/2012/09/hurry-up-with-dead-ahadith-1099-1101.html#sthash.lXGMfvZc.dpuf, date accessed 8 August 2013.

Merchant, S.J., Yoshida, E.M., Lee, T.K., Richardson, P., Karlsbjerg, K.M. and Cheung, E. (2008) 'Exploring the Psychological Effects of Deceased Organ Donation on the Families of the Organ Donors', *Clinical Transplantation* 22, 341–7.

NHS Blood and Transplant [a], www.uktransplant.org.uk/ukt/newsroom/statements_and_stances/statements/opt_in_or_out.jsp, date accessed 8 August 2013.

NHS Blood and Transplant [b]. News Release 10 March 2011, www.nhsbt.nhs.uk/news/2011/newsrelease100311.html, date accessed 8 August 2013.

Rahman, F. (1987) *Health and Medicine in the Islamic Tradition* (New York: Crossroad).

Raleigh, V.S. (1997) 'Diabetes and Hypertension in Britain's Ethnic Minority Communities: Implications for the Future of Renal Services', *British Medical Journal* 314, 7078, 209–12.

Randhawa, G. (1998) 'An Exploratory Study Examining the Influence of Religion on Attitudes towards Organ Donation among the Asian Population in Luton – UK', *Nephrology: Dialysis Transplantation* 13, 8, 1949–54.

Rassool, G. Hussein (2004) 'Commentary: an Islamic Perspective', *Journal of Advanced Nursing* 46, 3, 281–3.

Sachedina, A. (2005) 'End-of-Life: the Islamic View', *Lancet* 366, 9487, 774–9.

Sajid, A. (2003) *Death and Bereavement in Islam*, The Muslim Council for Religious and Racial Harmony (Hove: Brighton Islamic Mission), www.mcb.org.uk/downloads/Death-Bereavement.pdf, date accessed 8 August 2013.

Sarhill, N., LeGrand, S., Islambouli, R., Davis, M.P. and Walsh, D. (2001). 'The Terminally Ill Muslim: Death and Dying from the Muslim Perspective', *The American Journal of Hospice and Palliative Care* 18, 4, 251–5.

Sheikh, A. and Dhami, S. (2000) 'Attitudes to Organ Donation among South Asians in the UK', *Royal Society of Medicine* 93, 3, 161–2.

Sheikh Ahmad Kutty. *Can Muslims Donate Blood?* http://islamnewsroom.com/news-we-need/479-organdonors1, date accessed 8 August 2013.

Telegraph (2009) 'Muslims and Jews to be Allowed to have Different Post-mortem', 21 April.

www.kidney.org. *Brain Death: A Simple Explanation for Donor Families*, www.kidney.org/transplantation/donorFamilies/infoBooksBrain.cfm, date accessed 8 August 2013.

Zahedi, F., Larijani, B. and Bazzaz, J.T. (2007) 'End of Life Ethical Issues and Islamic Views', *Iran Journal of Allergy, Asthma and Immunology* 6 (Suppl. 5), 5–15.

17 Putting Cultural Competence All Together: Some Considerations in Caring for Muslim Patients

G. Hussein Rassool

Learning Outcomes:

- Discuss how Islam focuses on human behaviours and forbids practices that are a risk to health.
- Discuss the importance of valuing the patients' religious beliefs and practices.
- Critically analyse the need for cultural competence in caring for Muslim patients.
- Examine the effects of health literacy in caring for Muslim patients.
- Discuss culturally appropriate approaches in dealing with sensitive issues.
- Identify resources available in culturally competent care.
- Discuss the major challenges for nurses in developing and implementing culturally competent care for Muslim patients in a multi-ethnic and multi-cultural society.

Reflective Activity 17.1

State whether the following statements are true or false. Give reasons for your answers.

	True	False
1 Cultural diversity exists amongst the Muslim population.		

	True	False

2 Islamic injunctions do not focus on every single aspect of human lives through the maintenance of healthy behaviours and lifestyle.

3 Purification is not obligatory in Islam prior to worship.

4 The Qur'aan and the Hadith offer numerous directives about maintaining health at the community, family and individual levels.

5 The focus of a public health approach is its emphasis on religious and ethical values and on encouraging healthy behaviours.

6 The nurse does not need to understand the patients and their worldview with regard to their illness.

7 The development of a therapeutic relationship between the patient and nurse is the hallmark of the engagement stage of nursing care and treatment.

8 'Acculturation' means a merging of cultures as a result of prolonged contact.

9 Research has shown that family involvement in care has not been a major factor in both providing nursing care as well as the overall emotional, social, and psychological well-being of the patient.

10 In the Islamic culture, although patients reserve the right to make their own decisions, doctors or nurses should communicate with the family before they communicate with the patient.

11 Understanding the degree of acculturation is an important place to start in assessing the impact of a patient's personal culture and faith on health practices.

12 The nurse should protect information and treat it as confidential, and is not allowed to share information which is required for the purposes of safeguarding and/or public protection.

13 The delivery of culturally sensitive care is not possible without adequate educational preparation of nurses and other healthcare professionals.

Introduction

Due to the increase in globalisation and immigration of the Muslim population in many parts of the world, the delivery of health care to Muslim patients has become more challenging for policy makers, and for health and social care professionals. Thus, it is reasonable to assume that nurses and allied healthcare professionals will come into contact with Muslim patients as part of their caseload. Muslim patients are not a homogeneous group of people as cultural and linguistic diversity exists amongst the Muslim population. Muslims are from different sub-cultures and it would be thoughtless to perceive all Muslims as having the same normative behavioural patterns and acculturation. However, the similarities or homogeneity that are found within the Muslim communities are related to health beliefs and practices, access and utilisation of health care, health risks, family dynamics, and decision-making processes. The acknowledgement that most countries in the Northern Hemisphere are now multi-ethnic and multi-racial, and the compelling evidence of racial and ethnic health disparities, are the driving forces for incorporating cultural and religious perspectives into nursing practice. Thus, the need for educational preparation of nurses is beyond dispute. It should be possible for nurses to develop levels of awareness, skills, and religio-cultural sensitivity that can be applied to interactions with Muslim patients, their family, and their significant others. This chapter aims to synthesise the contents of previous chapters and provide a framework that is applicable in caring for Muslim patients from a nursing perspective.

Public health and promoting health behaviours

Islam, through the Qur'aan and Hadith, provides teachings that can be used to promote behaviours that might lead to a healthy lifestyle. Religion and spirituality directly affect mental and physical health, for they influence coping strategies, health behaviours, and health care-seeking attitudes (Koenig, 2009). For a Muslim, taking good care of one's health is a religious duty as Islam attaches great importance to health. As Al-Khayat (2004) pointed out,

> since its advent, Islam has prioritised health, placing it as second in importance to faith. In fact, embedded in the very essence of the divine law is the protection of the five essential needs: faith, life, progeny, property, and mind. And, with only a little reflection, it becomes apparent that 60% of these essentials (three out of the five), namely life, progeny and mind, cannot be adequately safeguarded without the protection and preservation of health". Thus, we as Muslims and humanity as a whole, need to preserve and safeguard our health

to utilise it to our optimum potential to further our journey as servants of Allah. (Rassool, 2013)

From the Islamic perspective, our body has rights over us and God has entrusted the human body to the individual, who has the responsibility to maintain healthy behaviours. Islamic injunctions focus on every single aspect of human lives. This is reflected in the prevention of risk behaviours, and the set rules for nutrition, exercise and physical activity, personal and public hygiene and other health-related practices. When it comes to personal hygiene, there are the traditions of Prophet Muhammad, which include advice about actions that are part of a natural way to maintain personal hygiene. The Prophet emphasised oral hygiene and recommended using the *miswak* to clean the teeth and refresh the breath. The *miswak* is a small branch of the *Salvador perscia* plant, which was shown later to be a good source of fluoride, silica, chloride, and Vitamin C (Yosef). Purification is obligatory in Islam prior to worship. Muslims are required to wash the exposed body parts five times a day before each prayer and before touching the Qur'aan.

In relation to dietary regulations, pork and related products, animals found dead, carnivorous animals, or wild animals that use their claws or teeth to kill their prey, are foods that are prohibited by Islamic law as they are considered unhealthy or harmful to the body. Muslims consume foods that are permissible or prepared according to Islamic law, a *halal* diet. Eating healthy food, such as honey, olives, figs, dates, milk, and related products, is encouraged. Muslims vary in their adherence to the Islamic rules, due to cultural influences on these dietary prescriptions. However, Islamic law provides for exceptions in order to save a person's life.

Islam also focuses on human behaviours and forbids practices that risk human health. These include smoking tobacco, drinking alcohol and using other psychoactive substances, gambling, and sexual relationships outside marriage. In view of this, the Prophet stated that 'There is not to be any causing of harm nor is there to be any reciprocation of harm' (Ibn Majah). This is the rule that defines the boundary of a person's behaviour so as not to cause harm to others (Gezairy). The prohibition of alcohol, drugs, gambling, and inappropriate sexual behaviours is in consequence of the physical, psychological, social, and economic harms they cause to individual, family, and community. In the past, some Muslim countries have been slow to confront public health issues such as alcohol, substance misuse, injecting drugs and HIV/AIDS because these health topics are not easily introduced in the conservative Islamic cultures. However, this is gradually changing as a result of the recognition of the need to challenge and overcome, by preventive health measures and psychosocial interventions, this new kind of threat to the Muslim communities. The focus of the public health approach is its emphasis on religious and ethical values and its encouragement of healthy behaviours as a preventive method to be used against the widespread affliction of alcohol, drugs, and HIV/AIDS. There are other health behaviours that Muslims are encouraged to perform including physical activities and exercise.

Cultural competence: major challenges for nurses

There are major challenges facing nurses in the provision of culturally competent care to Muslim patients with different cultural and ethnic backgrounds. The diversity of ethnicity and linguistic groups, with each having its own cultural characteristics and worldview of health and illness among Muslims, presents constant challenges to nurses and health service providers. Understanding these perspectives by nurses should inform efforts designed to achieve cultural competence and the delivery of culturally sensitive care.

There has not yet been a universally accepted definition of cultural competence, as the literature has yielded various definitions. 'Cultural competence' is defined as the ability of providers and organisations to effectively deliver healthcare services that meet the social, cultural, and linguistic needs of patients (Betancourt et al., 2002). A much simpler definition is that 'Culturally competent care includes knowledge, attitudes, and skills that support caring for people across different languages and cultures' (Seeleman et al., 2009). In nursing, cultural competence practice involves the use of cross-cultural knowledge and culturally sensitive skills in implementing culturally congruent nursing care (Douglas et al., 2011). However, culturally sensitive health care needs to be delivered clearly and effectively. This is achieved by creating awareness of the different cultural backgrounds in order to plan individualised courses of care. Both the nurse and the patient bring their own learned cultures and languages into their healthcare experiences. These experiences are more likely to succeed and to yield patient satisfaction, treatment adherence, and positive health outcomes when good communication between providers and patients is established. In addition to the patient's cultural beliefs, nurses must be aware of their own beliefs, practices, and perceptions as these may have an impact on the care they provide to clients from diverse cultural backgrounds (Rassool, 2006).

A limited amount of empirical evidence supports the assertion that cultural competence will lead to a reduction in racial and ethnic disparities in health care, and will improve rehabilitation outcomes, including the well-being of the diverse client populations (Geron, 2002; Goode et al., 2006). Furthermore, particular cultural competence interventions seem to have an effect on health services' utilisation, satisfaction, and increase in knowledge

(AHRQ, 2004). The findings of a study indicate that Muslim consumers of healthcare services suggested that cultural competence efforts would lead to (1) a greater understanding of Islam and Islamic culture, thereby improving the patient–provider relationship, and (2) improve Muslim experiences within the healthcare system, resulting in reduced challenges and increased accommodations (Padela et al., 2011). Meyer (1996) describes four major challenges for nurses in achieving cultural competence in health care. The challenges include recognising clinical differences among people of different ethnic and racial groups; communication (this deals with everything from the need for interpreters to understanding the nuances of words in various languages); ethics; and trust (the relationship between nurse and patient).

Value the patient's religious belief and practices related to health care

It is worth noting that the Nursing Code of Ethics in Islam is derived from this verse in the Qur'aan, in which Allah says (interpretation of the meaning):

☐ *And whoever saves one – it is as if he had saved mankind entirely.* (Al-Māʾidah [The Table Spread] 5:32)

One of the most important reasons to address Muslims' spiritual and religious beliefs in the healthcare setting is their impact on health-related behaviours. Muslim beliefs and practices have implications for a variety of healthcare issues, such as those related to sexual norms and to obstetrical and gynaecological care, including maternal and child health issues, and the stigma associated with mental health issues and HIV/AIDS (Hasnain, 2005). Nurses should value the patient's beliefs and practices and show continuous respect regardless of their age, gender, religion, social status, sexual orientation, ethnic background, and healthcare decisions. In addition, nurses should have self-awareness concerning their own personal beliefs while not being judgemental about patients' beliefs. They should have the competence to integrate a patient's beliefs and practices into the care plan.

Respect for the belief systems of others and the effects of those beliefs on health behaviours are critically important to culturally competent care. Religious beliefs and values also influence patients' notions of healing. The findings of a study (Padela et al., 2011) examining the healthcare needs of American Muslims showed that, in addition to prayer and supplication to God, human agents (for example, *Imams*, family members, healthcare providers, friends, and community members) played important roles in the healing process. Table 17.1 presents a summary of the religious beliefs and practices related to health care.

Table 17.1 A summary of religious beliefs and practices related to health care

Health & illness	Health practices
Autopsy	Not permitted unless required by law.
Assisted suicide and euthanasia	Not permitted.
Artificial reproductive technology	Is permitted between husband and wife only during the span of intact marriage.
Abortion	Not permitted except to save the mother's life. If it is reliably established that the continuation of a pregnancy will result in the death of the mother then an abortion is allowable. The mother's life takes precedence over that of the unborn baby because the mother is already established in life, with duties and responsibilities.
Blood donation	Is permitted
Blood transfusions	Are allowed after proper screening.
Breastfeeding	Recommended for a period of 2 years.
Birth control	Reversible methods of birth control are acceptable, as sexual intercourse is for pleasure, not merely for procreation. Irreversible methods, such as vasectomy, tubal ligation, or hysterectomy, are prohibited unless absolutely necessary for the health of the patient.
Circumcision	Circumcision of male infants is recommended. Circumcision occurs early in life, but at no particular age. The practice varies from culture to culture
Genetic engineering	Genetic engineering to cure disease is acceptable, but not cloning. Applications such as diagnosis, amelioration, cure or prevention of genetic disease are acceptable and commendable.
Gestational surrogacy	Where the surrogate mother is biologically unrelated to the child, gestational surrogacy is prohibited.
Homosexuality	While Islam opposes homosexuality, it does not prohibit Muslim physicians from caring for homosexual patients.

(Continued)

Table 17.1   Continued

Health & illness	Health practices
Life	Regard for the sanctity of life is an injunction.
Miscarriages	Miscarriages due to biomedical factors are not considered abortions as these occur without human interference.
Somatisation	Mental or emotional distress may be expressed somatically, as the locus of emotion, rationality and the soul is located in the physical heart in traditional Islamic psychology.
Organ donation	Acceptable.
Organ transplantation	Organ transplantation, both donating and receiving, is allowed with some restrictions (donor material of porcine origin).
Terminal patient	Maintaining a terminal patient on artificial life support for a prolonged period of time in a vegetative state is not encouraged.

Source: Adapted from S. Attar, 'Information for Health Care Providers when Dealing with a Muslim Patient', www.islam-usa.com/index.php?option=com_content&view=article&id=115:information-for-health-care-providers-when-dealing-with-a-muslim-patient&catid=60:articles&Itemid=145, date accessed 8 August 2013. (With Kind Permission.)

Culturally appropriate care: development of a therapeutic relationship

The development of a therapeutic relationship between the patient and nurse is the hallmark of the engagement stage of nursing care and treatment. The aims of this phase are to understand the patient and their worldview regarding their illness, to respond to their behaviour and language, to recognise their often unspoken needs, and thereby to develop some trust and genuineness. The sensitive understanding of the patient needs and acceptance of the patient as an individual, based on creating rapport in culturally appropriate ways, would enable the establishment of a trusting relationship. Trust, respect, honesty, and effective communication are key principles in establishing the therapeutic relationship.

The main source of problems in caring for Muslim patients or patients from diverse cultural backgrounds is a lack of understanding and tolerance and the inability to ask questions sensitively (Rassool, 2006). Accepting the patient, consistency, and listening are considered by clients to be critical at the beginning of the relationship (Forchuk et al., 2000; McKlindon and Barnsteiner, 1999). That is, good communication and open dialogue are the key to providing culturally sensitive care (Gulam, 2003). For a patient with limited spoken English and who is unfamiliar with the healthcare system, this phase in the nurse–patient interaction is vital in reducing anxiety or tension and providing support. Having empathy is crucial in the development of a therapeutic relationship. Empathy is defined as 'the ability of the nurse to enter into the client's relational world, to see and feel the world as the client sees and feels it, and to explore the meaning it has for the client. Empathy involves the nurse being able to attend to the subjective experience of the client and validate that his/her understanding is an accurate reflection of the client's experience' (Registered Nurses Association of Ontario, 2002). This means that the nurse must be able to view the patient's illness and situation from their position and not look down upon them from a paternalistic stance. Table 17.2 presents some

Table 17.2 Nurse–patient encounter

When	Statements	Rationale
Prior to nursing assessment	Development of therapeutic relationship	Generally, acknowledge and greet the patient first. Ask the patient for their preferred name and make note. Ask informed individuals what is culturally appropriate. Consider use of informal conversation prior to formal assessment.
	When possible: Would you prefer one of my female/male colleagues to assess you? Would you like the use of a professional interpreter?	Muslims may prefer a same-gender nurse provider. Patients may prefer to have an interpreter present during an examination, even if they can speak English.

(Continued)

Table 17.2   Continued

When	Statements	Rationale
	Communication: Eye contact Touch	Muslims will avoid direct eye contact during a conversation, as a sign of respect for the speaker. Keep the interactions going. For Muslims, it is inappropriate for women and men to shake hands, or to hug, or pat the shoulder. Take your cue from the patient.
	Would you like to include/ involve anyone else in this process?	Decision-making – In Islamic tradition, the male is head of the household, and the official decision-maker.
During the assessment	Tell me about how you are feeling? Do you have treatment preferences you would like me to include in your care plan? May I take your temperature, pulse, respiration and blood pressure?	Listen respectfully. When you speak, try to use plain language. Some may want to incorporate traditional healing and health practices with conventional medicine. Understand cultural norms about modesty. Explain what will be done and why.
	Do you have a special diet right now that is different from what you would normally eat?	Some patients may prefer certain foods and or drinks when they are ill. In addition, during fasting and religious seasons diets may be different and need to be considered during the process of determining the appropriate course of treatment.

(*Continued*)

Table 17.2 Continued

When	Statements	Rationale
	Would you like me to explain or go over anything again?	This gives the patient an opportunity to relate their understanding of the information about the condition and/or instructions that you have provided.
During and/or after the assessment	Would you like for me to explain the next steps/process?	Explain tests, procedures and treatments to the patient and appropriate family members. Use other health information (leaflets, booklets) professionally translated into the patient's preferred language to help you explain the situation.

examples of the nurse's encounter with the patient prior, during and after the nursing assessment.

There are many different strategies to building a trusting nurse–patient relationship, of which one of the most important and recognised is familiarity with different cultural backgrounds. This factor needs to be critically handled so as not to yield an offending response, which will later hold back the process of information gathering. Together, sensitivity, listening skills, and cultural awareness can help to form the trusting relationship that would help and encourage patients to share their thoughts, feelings, and information at times when their minds are cluttered with many concerns and fears.

Assessing the degree of acculturation

There are many important cultural issues that a nurse needs to consider during the assessment process. Knowledge of the range of culturally based beliefs and values in health practice provides a broad background for assessing and understanding an individual's explanatory models regarding an illness, and adherence to recommended health intervention strategies. Acculturation is defined as a 'cultural modification of an individual, group, or people by adapting to or borrowing traits from another culture; *also*: a merging of cultures as a result of prolonged contact' (Merriam-Webster). Acculturation or familiarity with Western health practices can bring ethnic minority patients to gradually subscribe to Western values and practices, along with their own traditional methods of health care (Woollett et al., 1995).

An understanding of the degree of acculturation is an important place to start in assessing the impact of a patient's personal culture and faith on the health practice (Salman and Zoucha, 2010). In the US and elsewhere, it is routine to assess the degree of acculturation. During the initial assessment, questions include the patient's length of residence in the host country, educational status, degree of exposure to the larger community versus the patient's ethnic community, religious and cultural practices, values, proficiency in the English language, and gender role (Luna, 1989). Giger and Davidhizar (2008) proposed six cultural phenomena that the nurse must understand in order to provide effective care for all patients: communication, space, social organisations, time, environmental control, and biological variation. A Transcultural Nursing Assessment Tool can be accessed at www. culturediversity.org/assmtform.htm.

Recognise health literacy

Health literacy is a worldwide concern. The World Health Organisation (2001) stated that 'Improved health literacy is necessary for people to increase control over their health and for better management of disease and risk. Communications strategies that increase access to information and build the capacity to use it can improve health literacy, decision-making, risk perception and assessment, and lead to informed action of individuals, communities, and organizations.' According to Healthy People (2010), an individual is considered to be 'health literate' when he or she possesses the skills to understand information and services and use them to make appropriate decisions about health. It is suggested that the areas commonly associated with health literacy include: patient–physician communication; drug labelling; medical instructions and medical compliance; health information publications and other resources; informed consent; responding to medical and insurance forms; giving patient history; public health training; and assessments for allied professional programmes, such as social work and speech–language pathology (National Institutes of Health).

Patients must possess the skills to understand health information and services and use them to make appropriate decisions about health, based on informed choices. The concept of health literacy extends to the materials, environments, and challenges specifically associated with disease prevention and health promotion (National Institutes of Health). Nurses need to identify and recognise patients who are at risk due to their low level of health literacy. Some of the warning signs of a lack of health literacy include: patients forgetting their reading glasses, bringing along a family member to hospital visits, and facing difficulties in filling in hospital forms. The nurses should ensure that they communicate effectively in ways the patients understand. This may be by explaining, talking supported by drawing pictures, and writing the essential health information. Repetition or reinforcement of the message should be an integral part of the process. This is relevant in caring for Muslim patients. Health education materials should be developed in the patients' own language and written appropriately for those with limited literacy.

Providing culturally competent care for Muslims

Caring for Muslim patients involves meeting their physical, social, psychological and spiritual needs. Although nurses have been moving away from the bio-medical model there is inherent conflict in meeting the spiritual needs of Muslim patients. This may be due to ethnocentrism. Nurses demonstrating ethnocentrism could be a potential danger to their patients as they can impose their own beliefs on their patients, and causing the patients' cultural needs to be unmet (Okrentowich, 2007). For example, an ethnocentric nurse will apply the same approaches or strategies in all patients' care, ignoring the patients' cultural or religious background.

There is a dearth of literature on addressing the matching and mismatching of nurses' cultural values and patient values, and the experiences of caring for a Muslim patient in a non-Muslim country. This is a brief review of the literature addressing critical issues when providing culturally competent care for Muslims patients. Few studies have addressed the emotion and frustration of nurses addressing the conflicts between their own cultural values and patients' values. The findings of a descriptive study of six critical-care (non-Muslim) nurses' experience with caring for Muslim patients in Saudi Arabia (Halligan, 2006) showed that family involvement in care was found to be a major factor in both providing nursing care as well as the overall emotional, social, and psychological well-being of the patient. The family unit often 'dictated the care' of the patient, even to the extent that the physician would discuss treatment options and decision-making solely with the family, without the patient's involvement. It was found that patients were eager to communicate with nurses in Arabic, even though they knew the nurses did not understand. Nurses admitted to often simply smiling and trying to listen. However, many nurses found it difficult to form patient bonds and develop the family's trust when communication was limited, and attempts to do so often resulted in frustration. The findings also showed that nurses often felt powerless in helping sad or depressed patients since comforting was not seen as part of the nurse's role. Attempts to be emotionally sensitive, especially through caring touch, were not welcomed or appreciated by most patients. Halligan (2006) also found that the cause of the stress and frustration experienced by nurses was conflicts experienced in balancing patients' care and dealing with their own emotions.

A study of expatriate non-Muslim nurses' experiences of working in a cardiac intensive care unit in Saudi Arabia (Van Bommel, 2011) found that the nurses had a culture shock, in relation to caring for Muslim patients. They also found it difficult to understand the Muslim patient's refusal to take treatment or undergo interventional procedures before prayer, and regarded the non-adherence to limited visiting hours as being unacceptable. This state of affairs in caring for Muslim patients is not only related to Middle Eastern countries, but a universal phenomenon. This lack of congruence is reflected in a statement from an American nurse who said: 'I have found caring for Muslim patients to be a very demanding and frustrating assignment. They ask for many things that we nurses are unfamiliar with and that can create problems in a hospital setting. For example, asking for lots of water to wash themselves before and after using the bathroom, this can make a mess, especially if bed rest was ordered. Can't they delay all these special requests until after they are discharged?' (El Gindy, 2004).

Worth et al. (2009) examined the care experiences of South Asian Sikh and Muslim patients in Scotland with life limiting illness, and their families, and attempt to understand the reasons for any difficulties with access to services and how these might be overcome. The findings showed that most healthcare and social care professionals expressed good intentions in striving to provide equitable care but were concerned by their lack of cultural understanding and were uncertain about how to adapt their usual care. In addition, the professionals were anxious about making a cultural blunder, particularly in fraught end-of-life situations. Some of the barriers among professionals include: cultural assumptions, particularly about family; lack of effective cultural awareness or training in diversity; institutional discrimination and direct racism; and language barriers and inability to access interpretation services at short notice.

Finally, other studies have shown how to promote culturally competent care. Wehbe-Alamah (2008) has demonstrated the promotion of culturally competent care by using Leininger's culture care preservation and/or maintenance, culture care accommodation and/or negotiation, and culture care re-patterning and/or restructuring action modes to bridge the gap between generic (folk) and professional care practices. Nooredin's study (2008), in Australia, showed how Muslim patients could be cared for in a culturally sensitive manner and led the reader to reflect on aspects of Muslim religious beliefs and practices and on how this may impact on individuals' experience when in hospital. Salman and Zoucha (2010) maintained that to deliver effective culturally competent care to a terminally ill Muslim patient, the Islamic rituals must be carried out in a way that recognises and respects the cultural differences of this particular population.

Nurses need to keep in mind when caring for Muslim patients that there are religiously based attitudes and dietary regulations that may influence a Muslim patient's adherence to a medication regimen. They may be related to one or a combination of beliefs such as that the medication is too strong, or the patient may not be familiar with the prescribed medication. In addition, a Muslim patient who is fasting (voluntarily) outside of the month of Ramadan and is not taking the prescribed dose. Muslim dietary regulations can affect patients' use of medications, especially drugs incorporating gelatine or alcohol. (If gelatine is made from a forbidden substance, such as pig meat, bones, skin, or the like, it is regarded as unlawful.) Religious scholars unanimously agree that lard (pig fat) falls under this prohibition. However, if the gelatine is free from any substance seen as unlawful, there is no harm in using it (Fatwas of the Permanent Committee – Fatwa no. 8039). Medications may be administered by injection, preferably from a same sex care provider. The acceptability of a type of medication may also be influenced by cultural values. Muslim patients tend to take suffering with emotional reserve and may hesitate to express the need for pain management. Some may even refuse pain medication if they understand the experience of their pain to be spiritually enriching. It is also important to check with the patient about the use of alternative or herbal medicines. Some culturally based herbal medications may be contraindicated when used in combination with other pharmaceuticals. Muslim patients need to feel reassured that these medications or herbal products would not be taken away from them. When feasible, consider incorporating them into the current treatment and management plan.

The implementation of culturally competent care involves the assessment of physical, psychological, social and spiritual needs. A care plan can then be developed based on the identified needs, with subsequent strategies for nursing interventions. The principles used by the ethicists include preservation of the patient's faith; the sanctity of life; alleviation of suffering; respect for the patient's autonomy, while achieving best medical treatment without harm; and always being honest and truthful in giving information (ISPI, 2006). Significant aspects in caring for Muslim patients are presented in Table 17.3.

Table 17.3 Significant aspects of caring for Muslim patients

Significant aspects	Nursing interventions
Identification	Identify Muslim patients with the word 'Muslim' in the chart or case note, and on the name tag or bracelet.
Physical examination	Always examine a female patient in the presence of another female.
Nutrition	Discuss their dietary choices with them, particularly if a *halal* menu is unavailable in the hospital. Allow the family to bring food if there are no restrictions.
Medication Pain management	Inform patients if their drug prescriptions contain animal products or compounds such as shortening, lard, pork, gelatine (e.g., gel capsules, insulin), or alcohol (e.g., cough medications). Narcotic pain medications may be resisted by some Muslim patients because of the belief that the experience of pain is a trial to be endured. Inform patients about the source and management of pain.
Fasting If the patient insists on fasting and refuses treatment	Nurses should explore ways for their Muslim patients to observe the fast safely. Discuss dietary alterations. Discuss potential health effects: caffeine withdrawal; nicotine withdrawal; and adapt the medication regime. Consult the *Imam*. Help the patient to understand the consequences of fasting if he/she is physically unable.
Sexual health	Muslims often express embarrassment or offence when questioned about their sexual relationships and when asked other personal questions. Explaining the reasons behind the questions may help allay some discomfort.
Use of the left hand	The left hand is considered unclean in many Muslim cultures. To avoid offence, use the right hand for feeding, administering medications, or handing something to a patient.

(*Continued*)

Table 17.3 Continued

Significant aspects	Nursing interventions
Modesty and respect	Allow Muslims patients – men and women – to wear long hospital gowns. A Muslim woman may wear a hijab during an examination or while in the hospital, removing it only when necessary. Announce your presence before entering, to allow the patient to cover the head or body.
Same-gender preference	Where possible, arrange for patients to be admitted to same-sex hospital wards or provide a same-sex healthcare person if possible.
Prayer	Allow them to pray if they can, and read the Qur'aan.
Rights	Inform them of their rights as patients, and encourage a living will.
Child birth	Preferably there should be no male in the delivery room except the husband.
Death	Allow the family and *Imam* to follow Islamic guidelines for preparing the dead body for an Islamic funeral. The female body should be given the same respect and privacy as if she was living.
Visitors	It is an Islamic cultural and religious practice to visit the sick. Be open and understanding of visits by family members and well-wishers when practical.

Dealing with culturally sensitive issues

Nurses should be adequately prepared by developing skills in dealing with sensitive issues and protecting the respect and dignity of the individual. These sensitive issues may include: grief, critical illness, emotional and physical abuse, sexual abuse and harassment, date rape, domestic violence, self-harm, unwanted pregnancy, sexually transmitted disease, and abortion. These issues may be distressing and confronting for Muslim patients. Always maintain privacy and confidentiality when dealing with sensitive or difficult information with the patients' families. Respect for a patient's right to confidentiality and rules concerning the disclosure of information are based on a nursing code of professional conduct, and in some cases on the law of the country in which you are practising.

For Muslims, the stigma of psychiatric disorders, sexually transmitted disease, unwanted pregnancy, or HIV may hinder Muslim patients from seeking care or disclosing information to a nurse or other healthcare professional. Transgression of these norms is not only regarded as sinful, but disclosure of such deviant practices may bring shame upon the family or the community (Boston Healing Landscape Project). Muslims often express embarrassment or are offended when questioned about their sexual relationships and other personal matters. Culturally competent care targets the whole patient, not just his or her physical ailment. The nurse needs to explain the reasons behind the questions, which may help allay some discomfort and should be non-judgemental. It is also valuable to reassure the patient regarding the confidentiality of the information. Use a positive and objective approach and discuss multiple sides of the issue. Refer patients to their families (if appropriate), religious leader, or counsellor for problems and concerns that go beyond the role of the nurse.

The extended Muslim family may also play an important role in receiving information about the medical status of the patient and in the medical decision-making process. In the Islamic culture, although patients reserve the right to make their own decisions, doctors or nurses should communicate with the family before they communicate with the patient, especially if there is bad news, for example, a fatal diagnosis (Salman and Zoucha, 2010). This decision-making involves the immediate family, for example, the husband, wife, children, and parents or elders. Some Muslim patients may prefer to be informed only of 'good news' about an illness or when receiving test or laboratory results. In the event of a medical emergency or a poor prognosis, the nurse or other healthcare professional would report the situation to the family, and they in turn would be responsible for informing the patient (Boston Healing Landscape Project). In many cases, patients are admitted to the hospital with a terminal illness, but they are not aware of the diagnosis because the family has kept it secret to protect their loved ones from bad news (Salman and Zoucha, 2010). It is also common for family members to become concerned with the care of an individual patient, and the elder or male family head may be involved in negotiating and approving a treatment plan, or determining the disclosure of medical information, such as a sensitive diagnosis or poor prognosis, for a female patient or a child (Boston Healing Landscape Project). Although this may be a more culturally based practice than a religious one, nurses should understand how much information they could disclose to the patient and family.

Educational model of cultural competence

There are several nursing models for culturally competent care, including the Campinha-Bacote Model (2008), Giger and Davidhizar's Model of Transcultural Nursing (2008), Leininger's Cultural Care Diversity and Universality Theory/Model (Leininger and McFarland, 2006), and the Papadopoulos et al. Model (1998). The Papadopoulos et al. Model (1998) consists of four stages. The first stage in the model is cultural awareness and is the basis for a critical examination of our personal values and beliefs. The nature of the construction of cultural identity as well as its influence on people's health beliefs and practices is viewed as a learning foundation. Cultural knowledge (the second stage) can be gained in a number of ways. Meaningful contact with people from different Muslim communities can enhance knowledge around their health beliefs and behaviours as well as raising understanding around the problems they face. An important element in achieving cultural sensitivity (the third stage), is how professionals view people in their care, and clients should be seen as equal partners. This includes trust, acceptance and respect as well as facilitation and negotiation. The achievement of the fourth stage (cultural competence) requires the synthesis and application of previously gained awareness, knowledge and sensitivity.

Cultural competence activities include the development of skills in the assessment of need, clinical diagnosis, and clinical skills. The practices are responsive to the culture and diversity within the populations served. A most important component of this stage of development is the ability to recognise and challenge racism and other forms of discrimination and oppressive practice. It is argued that this model combines both the multi-culturalist and the anti-racist perspectives and facilitates the development of a broader understanding around inequalities, and human and citizenship rights, whilst promoting the development of skills needed to bring about change at the patient/client level (Papadopoulos et al., 1998). Nurses should have some cultural knowledge about the traditions of the population they serve; the goal of the nursing care and interventions is the provision of culturally competent care that diminishes barriers and improves health outcomes. There is evidence to suggest that educational programmes and training in the area can improve the knowledge, attitudes and skills of nurses and providers working with diverse patient populations (Beach et al., 2005; Black et al., 2008).

Community resources for Muslims

The role of the *Imam* and the Mosque in the modern Western world is of huge significance and importance to Muslim communities as a resource. At the time of the Prophet, Mosques were used for a number of purposes including the following: as a centre of learning and training; a political platform; a charity distribution centre; a centre for the homeless; a place for social gatherings; for inter-faith activities; and for civic engagement (MINAB, 2011). The traditional role of an *Imam* is to lead prayers, deliver sermons, and conduct religious ceremonies, as well as to provide counsel to individuals and their families (Ali and Milstein, 2012). In the US, *Imams* actively counsel members of their congregation across a wide range of problems (Ali et al., 2005). With rapid change in national and international circles, the place of *Imams* and Mosques is becoming increasingly critical in relation to issues and problems faced by Muslim communities, especially in the area of health.

The *Imam* is a central figure in this process, for he delivers healthcare messages framed within an Islamic worldview, counsels the distressed, provides spiritual support, and facilitates healing through communal supplications or prescribing Qur'aanic litanies. Within the hospital, his role somewhat overlaps those of healthcare chaplains: he visits Muslim patients, is involved in patient–provider–family healthcare discussions, and serves as a religious 'translator' and cultural broker (Padela et al., 2011). Therefore, in times of duress, Muslim communities call on their *Imam* for help and support. *Imams* are de facto mental health care providers (Ali and Milstein, 2012). Hence, the nurse can use the *Imam* as a resource person in caring for Muslim patients in the provision of emotional and spiritual support.

Reflective Activity 17.2

Case Study

Jamal is 14 years old, and lives with his Muslim parents and three siblings in a terraced house in a deprived suburban area. Jamal and his siblings were born in England but his parents emigrated from Pakistan over 20 years ago. The area where Jamal's family lives consists mostly of Muslims communities. Much of his life revolves around the neighbourhood, at the cultural and Islamic centre, with his extended family, and the Muslim community. The children of the family speak English fluently, but the parents and grandparents converse in English only when they must. Jamal's mother stays home full time to care for Jamal and his three siblings, aged 3, 7 and 9. Mr Ahmad, Jamal's father, works for a family business, and when not working he is usually at the local Mosque and the cultural centre. Mr Ahmad and his family are devout Muslims.

Jamal was diagnosed with Duchenne muscular dystrophy when he was 7. It is the most common type of muscular dystrophy and is a sex-linked recessive trait. It affects young boys, in whom pseudo-hypertrophy of the calves and weakness of the hip and shoulder girdles progress from early childhood. A child who is diagnosed with muscular dystrophy gradually loses the ability to do things like walking, sitting upright, breathing easily, and moving the arms and hands. Jamal was confined to a wheelchair by the age of 10. His language and communication skills are impaired due to his learning disability. Frustration, depression, and other signs of emotional immaturity may be present in such children because of the intellectual limitation.

At the time of confirmation of Jamal's diagnosis, the multidisciplinary healthcare team recommended that his younger siblings have a physical examination and blood test to measure the levels of serum creatine kinase, an enzyme that is released into the bloodstream when muscle fibres are deteriorating. Elevated levels indicate that something is causing muscle damage. In addition, a DNA test for gene abnormalities can be performed to look for patterns of deterioration and abnormal levels of protein. However, the Ahmad family declined to undergo such tests and felt that their children's health was in Allah's (God's) hands. During childhood, Jamal came to the hospital because of his struggle to get up from a sitting position, and to swing-walk back and forth, and his difficulty going up stairs, and toe-walking.

Recently Jamal was admitted to hospital with respiratory problems and the healthcare team recommended that he should be hospitalised. Jamal's parents initially declined but agreed a week later. Once Jamal appeared to be responding to IV antibiotics, his parents pressured the healthcare team to allow him to complete his course of antibiotics at home. However, Jamal's conditions worsened and he was readmitted to hospital, as he needed to be intubated so that he could be placed on a ventilator to assist with his breathing. He also needed physical therapy and bracing to improve flexibility of his muscles. The parents appeared very concerned and distressed.

- What are the various ways in which religious beliefs can affect the understanding of illness?
- How would you assess the psychological, spiritual, and cultural needs of Jamal?
- What factors would you consider prior to providing care to Jamal?
- How would you ensure that Jamal's needs are met in a culturally sensitive manner?
- How will you communicate with Jamal?
- How do you ensure that Jamal understands your communication?
- What factors may cause nurses or other healthcare professionals to relate to patients in a prejudiced manner?
- What challenges do nurses face when trying to become more culturally competent?

Comments on Reflective Activity 17.2

The responses for some of the questions above are presented here. The world-view of Muslim patients towards health and illness incorporates the notion of receiving illness and death with patience, meditation, and prayers. Athar (1993, 1998) stated that Muslim patients consider an illness as atonement for their sins, and death as part of a journey to meet their God. The individuals' experiences of having a disability will depend on the severity and type of disability but also depend on the strengths of their faith or *Imaan*. The following statement (Example constructed by Miles, 2007, cited in Hasnain et al., 2008) is from an individual with a disability.

> This is my personal test with Allah, and it is my belief that Allah gives strength to meet every test. I laugh at the problems, because they are nothing compared with the mercy of Allah. I smile at the doctors, because they seem so burdened with all their medical knowledge and gadgets and rushing about. I laugh with the porter who pushes me on a trolley around the hospital, because he talks to me like a human, not just a sad case.

Muslims also believe that being disabled is a test from Allah in this life, and therefore can be a blessing in disguise. This belief may be quite surprising for a non-Muslim trying to make some sense of how being ill or having an illness could be a trial and tribulation from God. For Muslims even if they are pricked by a thorn, Allah washes away their sins, hence, with every pain that Muslims go through, be it mental, physical or spiritual, sins are being expiated. In contrast, some Muslims believe that having an illness is a curse or punishment from Allah. However, 'Islam views disability as morally neutral, neither a blessing nor a curse: It is considered an inevitable part of the human condition, one that Muslim society and individuals must address' (Hasnain et al., 2008, p. 31). Despite the concept of moral neutrality, disabilities, whether congenital, physical, or developmental, have sometimes been seen as punishment from God for poor character, in both rural and urban areas, depending on the multiple social factors linked to a family (Armstrong and Ager, 2005).

In order to provide interventions and meet Jamal's complex needs, the nurse needs to assess the physical, psychological, cultural, and spiritual needs of the patient and develop a care plan based on meeting those needs. A complete family and developmental history provides important diagnostic data for the patient with muscular dystrophy. Due to the complex needs of patients with muscular dystrophy, the patient should be managed by a multidisciplinary team. The nursing interventions and therapeutic management are focused on managing the symptoms, facilitating ambulation, managing respiratory and cardiac difficulties, and maintaining the highest level of functional independence possible. Because of the nature of muscular dystrophy, nursing interventions are primarily preventive and supportive. The nurse needs to explore the religious aspects of hygiene, washing and dressing in the Muslim traditional way. As the patient is a devout Muslim, assistance should be accorded for Jamal to make ablution before the regular five daily prayers. The nurse is also required to consider issues of privacy, dignity and modesty. Communication with Jamal may be a problem due to his language and communication deficit. The nurse will need to explore ways to communicate (verbal and non-verbal) with Jamal and to ensure that the communication is effective. For patients who are in a wheelchair, obesity frequently becomes a problem. A low-calorie, high-protein diet is recommended to avoid this complication because the additional weight places a strain on already compromised muscles. Constipation may also be a problem, which can be managed with added dietary fibres and extra fluids.

Nursing care involves psychological support of the patient and family, as serious disabilities may challenge a patient's beliefs or religious values, resulting in high levels of spiritual or psychological distress. The family needs opportunities to express feelings about the genetic transmission, progressive nature, and effect of the disease on the family. The status of the younger male children in this family may not be certain as Mr Ahmad was reluctant to have a physical examination and blood test performed for his younger children. This uncertainty also creates more anxieties and distress for the family. The nurse has an important role in providing both health information and support to the family in a culturally sensitive way to relieve their distress. Information should also be given to the Ahmad family about the local Muscular Dystrophy Association.

There are many factors that would cause nurses or other healthcare professionals to relate to patients in a prejudiced or culturally insensitive manner. First, comes the cultural conflict – this is to be expected in any healthcare setting with individuals from different cultural backgrounds. It is very challenging for some nurses to make patients and their families agree to something that is good for them, but that goes against their worldview or perception of illness. In this scenario, at the time of confirmation of Jamal's diagnosis, the multidisciplinary healthcare team recommended that his younger siblings have a physical examination and blood test to ensure their status in relation to muscular dystrophy. Secondly, poor cross-cultural communication between nurse and patient, and language barriers, may inhibit the provision of high quality care. Evidence clearly links clinician–patient communication to patient satisfaction, adherence, and health outcomes (Stewart et al., 1999). Our own attitudes and belief systems affect the way we interact and communicate with patients. Lopes (2001) stated that the most likely results of poor cultural competence are caused by a combination of factors including:

- Lack of knowledge, resulting in an inability to recognise and appreciate the factors that influence one's well-being.
- Self-protection/denial, leading to an attitude that differences are not significant, or that our common humanity transcends our differences.
- Fear – trying to understand something that is new, that does not fit into one's belief system, can be intimidating and challenging.
- Time constraints – feeling rushed and unable to look in depth at an individual patient's needs in a climate of managed care and cutbacks in health services.

Moreover, when health providers fail to consider socio-cultural factors, they may resort to stereotyping, which can affect their behaviour and clinical decision-making (van Ryn and Burke, 2000).

Conclusion: the way forward

Nursing is facing a daunting challenge in caring for patients of different cultures. In relation to the ICN Code for Nurses (ICN, 2006) it is anticipated that nurses will have the right attitudes, knowledge, and skills to work effectively within the cultural and religious context of the Muslim patient. The question that arises is: how does one become culturally competent? Does having more knowledge about Islam make nurses more competent? No, having knowledge about Islamic beliefs and practices does not make nurses more competent. What is fundamental in culturally competent care is being responsive to the health beliefs and practices of the Muslim patients, and to their cultural and linguistic needs. According to Pedersen (1997), the main features of cultural competence are self-awareness, knowledge about culture, and skills. That is, our cultural competence begins with self-awareness of our own values and biases, and is fortified by seeking cultural knowledge about Muslim patients. The nurses need to make genuine efforts to integrate their knowledge with the cultural knowledge of the Muslim patients. The ability to have this acceptance and understanding of Muslim patients' worldview means the nurse is able to demonstrate empathy towards the Muslims patients. According to Okrentowich (2007), 'Learning and experiencing different cultural backgrounds will result in ethno-relativism; the nurse will then appreciate the needs of patients of different cultures. This self-awareness will allow the nurse to adjust his or her practices to the needs of the patient.' That is, nurses should avoid judging patients by their own values or their own core cultural beliefs, and should not engage in negative stereotyping. Having the cultural skills would enable nurses to provide nursing interventions that are patient-centred. Being culturally competent is an ongoing process. It has been suggested that 'it is having the awareness that none of us ever knows everything there is to know, so we are always engaged in becoming more competent; according to the participants, it is about being a true advocate for our patient (Ahmed et al., 2011). Above all, we need to have respect and tolerance for culturally diverse patients.

The delivery of culturally competent care cannot be achieved without adequate educational preparation of nurses. Academic institutions providing education and training of nurses and other healthcare professionals and healthcare systems should consider re-examining their curriculum programme so that future nurse practitioners can become more aware in meeting the holistic needs of Muslim patients. Professional development will always be most effective when it is part of a strategic plan to create an organisational learning culture in the integration of cultural competence. If education and training in cultural competence for nurses and all healthcare professionals are to become a reality, policy-makers, professional associations, Mosques and *Imams*, Islamic cultural centres, educationalists and clinicians need to capitalise on the current political climate to focus on an effective strategy in order to meet the needs of the Muslim patients in a multicultural society. This is a major challenge. Allah knows best.

References

Ahmed, S., Wilson, K.B., Henriksen Jr., R.C. and WindWalker Jones, J. (2011) 'What Does It Mean to Be a Culturally-Competent Counselor?' *Journal for Social Action in Counseling and Psychology* 3, 1, 17–28.

AHRQ (2004) *Setting the Agenda for Research on Cultural Competence in Health Care: Introduction and Key Findings* (Rockville, MD: Agency for Healthcare Research and Quality).

Ali, O.M. and Milstein, G. (2012) 'Mental Illness Recognition and Referral Practices among *Imams* in the United States', *Journal of Muslim Mental Health* 6, 2, http://hdl.handle.net/2027/spo.10381607.0006.202, date accessed 9 August 2013.

Ali, O.M., Milstein, G. and Marzuk, P.M. (2005) 'The *Imam*'s Role in Meeting the Counseling Needs of Muslim Communities in the United States', *Psychiatric Services* 56, 202–5.

Al-Khayat, M.M. (2004) *Health as a Human Right in Islam. Health Education through Religion* (Cairo, Egypt: World Health Organisation, Regional Office for the Eastern Mediterranean).

Armstrong, J. and Ager, A. (2005) 'Perspectives on Disability in Afghanistan and their Implications for Rehabilitation Services', International Journal of Rehabilitation Research 28, 1, 87–92.

Athar, S. (1993) *Islamic Perspectives in Medicine. A Survey of Islamic Medicine: Achievements and Contemporary Issues* (Indianapolis, IN: American Trust Publications).

Athar, S. (1998) *Ethical Decision-Making in Patient Care: An Islamic Perspective* (Lombard, IL: Islamic Medical Association of North America).

Beach, M.C., Price, E.G., Gary, T.L. et al. (2005) 'Cultural Competence: a Systematic Review of Health Care Provider Educational Interventions', *Medical Care* 43, 4, 356–73.

Betancourt, J.R., Green, A.R. and Carrillo, J.E. (2002) *Cultural Competence in Health Care: Emerging Frameworks and Practical Approaches* (New York: The Commonwealth Fund).

Black, M., Soelberg, T. and Springer, P. (2008) 'Cultural Competency in Nursing Education', *Academic Exchange Quarterly* 12, 2, 245–9.

Boston Healing Landscape Project. *Islam and Health*, www.bu.edu/bhlp/Resources/Islam/health/guidelines.html#General, date accessed 8 August 2013.

Campinha-Bacote, J. (2008) *The Process of Cultural Competence in the Delivery of Healthcare Services*, www.transculturalcare.net/Publications.htm, date accessed 8 August 2013.

Douglas, M.K., Pierce, J.U., Rosenkoetter, M., Pacquiao, D., Callister, L.C, Hattar-Pollara, M., Lauderdale, J., Milstead, J., Nardi, D. and Purnell, L. (2011) 'Standards of Practice for Culturally Competent Nursing Care: 2011 Update', *Journal of Transcultural Nursing* 22, 4, 317–33.

El Gindy, G. (2004) 'Treating Muslims with Cultural Sensitivity in a Post-9/11 World', *Minority Nurse*, www.minoritynurse.com/cultural-competency/treating-muslims-cultural-sensitivity-post-911-world, date accessed 9 August 2013.

Fatwas of the Permanent Committee – Group 1 – Volume 22: Hudud – Slaughtering and Hunting – Foods – Ruling on Gelatine (Fatwa no: 8039, Part 22, page 261), www.alifta.com/Fatawa/FatawaChapters.aspx?View=Page&PageNo=1&FromMoeasrID=22084&PageID=8508&BookID=7, date accessed 8 August 2013.

Forchuk, C., Westwell, J., Martin, M., Azzapardi, W.B., Kosterewa-Tolman, D. and Hux, M. (2000) 'The Developing Nurse–Client Relationship: Nurses' Perspectives', *Journal of American Psychiatric Nurses Association* 6, 1, 3–10.

Geron, S.M. (2002) 'Cultural Competency: How is it Measured? Does it Make a Difference?' *Generations* 26, 3, 39–45, http://eric.ed.gov/ERICWebPortal/detail?accno=EJ658683, date accessed 13 August 2013.

Gezairy, H.A. 'The Role of Religion and Ethics in the Prevention and Control of AIDS', World Health Organisation Regional Office for the Eastern Mediterranean, World Health Organisation, www.emro.who.int/, date accessed 8 August 2013.

Giger, J. and Davidhizar, R. (2008) *Transcultural Nursing: Assessment and Intervention*, 5th edn (St Louis, MO: Mosby Yearbook).

Goode, T.D., Dunne, M.C. and Bronheim, S.M. (2006) *The Evidence Base for Cultural and Linguistic Competency in Health Care (Fund Report)*, The Commonwealth Fund, www.commonwealthfund.org, date accessed 8 August 2013.

Gulam, H. (2003) 'Care of the Muslim Patient', *ADF Health*, 4 September, www.defence.gov.au/health/infocentre/journals/adfhj_sep03/adfhealth_4_2_81-83.pdf, date accessed 8 August 2013.

Halligan, P. (2006) 'Caring for Patients of Islamic Denomination: Critical Care Nurses' Experiences in Saudi Arabia', *Journal of Clinical Nursing* 15, 12, 1565–73.

Hasnain, M. (2005) 'Patient-Centered Health Care for Muslim Women in the USA', *Medical News Today*, www.medicalnewstoday.com/releases/20788.php, date accessed 8 August 2013.

Hasnain, R., Shaikh, L.C. and Shanawani, H. (2008) *Disability and the Muslim Perspective: An Introduction for Rehabilitation and Health Care Providers* (New York: University at Buffalo, CIRRIE–Center for International Rehabilitation Research Information and Exchange, State University of New York) http://cirrie.buffalo.edu/culture/monographs/muslim.pdf, date accessed 9 August 2013.

Healthy People (2010) Centers for Disease Control and Prevention, www.cdc.gov/nchs/healthy_people/hp2010.htm, date accessed 8 August 2013.

Ibn Majah, cited in Zarabozo J. (2008) Hadith 32. *An-Nawawi Forty Hadith* (Denver, CO: Al-Basheer Company for Publications and Translations).

International Council of Nurses (ICN) (2006) *The ICN Code of Ethics for Nurses* (Geneva, (Switzerland: ICN).

ISPI (2006) Guidelines for Health Care Providers Interacting with Muslim Patients and their Families, www.ispi-usa.org/guidelines.htm, date accessed 10 August 2013.

Koenig, H.G. (2009) 'Research on Religion, Spirituality, and Mental Health: a Review', *Canadian Journal of Psychiatry* 54, 5, 283–91.

Leininger, M. and McFarland, M.R. (2006) *Culture Care Diversity and Universality: A World Wide Nursing Theory*, 2nd edn (Sudbury, MA: Jones and Bartlett).

Lopes, A.S. (2001) *Student National Medical Association, Cultural Competency Position Statement*. Prepared for: SNMA 36th House of Delegates, 12–15 April

2001, Annual Medical Education Conference, Atlanta, GA, www.snma.org/downloads/snma_cultural_competency.pdf, date accessed 9 August 2013.

Luna, L. (1989) 'Transcultural Nursing Care of Arab-Muslims', *Journal of Transcultural Nursing* 1, 22–7.

McKlindon, D. and Barnsteiner, J. (1999) 'Therapeutic Relationships: Evolution of the Children's Hospital of Philadelphia Model', *American Journal of Maternal Child Nursing* 24, 5, 237–43.

Merriam-Webster, www.merriam-webster.com/dictionary/acculturation, date accessed 8 August 2013.

Meyer, C.R. (1996) 'Medicine's Melting Pot', *Minnesota Medicine* 79, 5, 5.

Mosques and Imams National Advisory Board (MINAB) (2011) *Mosques and Youth Engagement: Guidelines and Toolkit* (Ealing, London: MINAB).

National Institutes of Health. 'What is Health Literacy?', www.nih.gov/clearcommunication/healthliteracy.htm, date accessed 8 August 2013.

Nooredin M. (2008) 'A Hermeneutic Phenomenological Inquiry into the Lived Experience of Muslim Patients in Australian Hospitals', PhD Thesis, University of Adelaide, School of Population Health and Clinical Practice, http://proxy.library.adelaide.edu.au/login?url=http://library.adelaide.edu.au/cgi-bin/Pwebrecon.cgi?BBID=1317115, date accessed 9 August 2013.

Okrentowich, A. (2007) 'Cultural Competence in Nursing', http://voices.yahoo.com/cultural-competence-nursing-190174.html?cat=4, date accessed 9 August 2013.

Padela, A., Gunter, K. and Killawi, A. (2011) *Needs of American Muslims: Challenges and Strategies for Healthcare Settings* (Washington, DC: Institute for Social Policy and Understanding).

Papadopoulos, I., Tilki, M. and Taylor, G. (1998) *Transcultural Care: A guide for Health Care Professionals* (Dinton, Wiltshire: Quay Books).

Pedersen, P.B. (1997) 'The Cultural Context of the American Counseling Association Code of Ethics', *Journal of Counseling and Development* 76, 23–8.

Rassool, G. Hussein (2006) 'Black and Ethnic Minority Communities: Substance Misuse and Mental Health: Whose Problems Anyway?' in G. Hussein Rassool (ed.), *Dual Diagnosis Nursing* (Oxford: Blackwell Publications).

Rassool, G. Hussein (2014) *Health Psychology from an Islamic Perspective: A Guide for Health Professionals* (Riyadh, Saudi Arabia: International Islamic Publication House) (Forthcoming).

Registered Nurses Association of Ontario (2002) *Establishing Therapeutic Relationships* (Toronto, Canada: Registered Nurses Association of Ontario), www.rnao.org, date accessed 8 August 2013.

Salman, K. and Zoucha, R. (2010) 'Considering Faith Within Culture When Caring for the Terminally Ill Muslim Patient and Family', *Journal of Hospice and Palliative Nursing* 12, 3, 156–63.

Seeleman, C., Suurmond, J. and Stronks, K. (2009) 'Cultural Competence: a Conceptual Framework for Teaching and Learning', *Medical Education* 43, 3, 229–37.

Stewart, M., Brown, J.B., Boon, H. et al. (1999) 'Evidence on Patient–Doctor Communication', Cancer Prevention Control 3, 1, 25–30.

Van Bommel, M. (2011) 'Expatriate Non-Muslim Nurses' Experiences of Working in a Cardiac Intensive Care Unit in Saudi Arabia', Master of Arts (Health Studies), University of South Africa.

van Ryn, M. and Burke, J. (2000) 'The Effect of Patient Race and Socioeconomic Status on Physicians' Perceptions of Patients', *Social Science and Medicine* 50, 6, 813–828.

Wehbe-Alamah, H. (2008) 'Bridging Generic and Professional Care Practices for Muslim Patients through Use of Leininger's Culture Care Modes', *Contemporary Nurse* 28: *Advances in Contemporary Transcultural Nursing* (2nd edn), pp. 83–97.

Woollett, A., Dosanjh, N., Nicolson, P., Marshall, H., Djhanbakhch, O. and Hadlow, J. (1995) 'The Ideas and Experiences of Pregnancy and Childbirth of Asian and Non-Asian Women in East London', *British Journal of Medical Psychology* 68 (Pt 1), 65–84.

World Health Organisation WHO) (2001) Fifty-fourth World Health Assembly, 30 March 2001, www.who.int/gb/EB_WHA/PDF/WHA54/ea548.pdf, date accessed 8 August 2013.

Worth, A., Irshad, T., Bhopal, R., Brown, D., Lawton, J., Grant, E., Murray, S., Kendall, M., Adam, J., Gardee, R. and Sheikh, A. (2009) 'Vulnerability and Access to Care for South Asian Sikh and Muslim Patients with Life Limiting Illness in Scotland: Prospective Longitudinal Qualitative Study', *British Medical Journal* 338: b183. Doi: 10.1136/bmj.b183.

Yosef, A.R. (2008) 'Health Beliefs, Practice, and Priorities for Health Care of Arab Muslims in the United States' [serial online], *Journal of Transcultural Nursing* 19, 3, 284–91. Doi: 10.1177/1043659608317450.

Appendix 1   Answers to Reflective Activities

Reflective Activity 1.1

1 True
2 False
3 True
4 False
5 True
6 False
7 False
8 True
9 False
11 True
12 False
13 True
14 False
15 False

Reflective Activity 2.1

1 True
2 False
3 True
4 True
5 False
6 False
7 False
8 True
9 True
10 False
11 True
12 False
13 True

Reflective Activity 3.1

1 True
2 False
3 True
4 False
5 True

6 False
7 True
8 True
9 True
10 False
11 True
12 True
13 False
14 True

Reflective Activity 4.1

1 False
2 True
3 False
4 True
5 True
6 False
7 True
8 False
9 False
10 True
11 True
12 False
13 True

Reflective Activity 5.1

1 True
2 False
3 False
4 True
5 True
6 False
7 True
8 False
9 True
10 False
11 True
12 True

13   False
14   True
15   False
16   True

Reflective Activity 6.1

1   True
2   False
3   True
4   False
5   True
6   True
7   True
8   False
9   True
10   False
11   True
12   False
13   True
14   True
15   False
16   True

Reflective Activity 7.1

1   True
2   False
3   True
4   False
5   True
6   True
7   True
8   False
9   False
10   False
11   True
12   True
13   False
14   True
15   False
16   True
17   False
18   True
19   False
20   True

Reflective Activity 8.1

1   False
2   True

3   False
4   False
5   True
6   False
7   True
8   False
9   True
10   False
11   True
12   True
13   True
14   True

Reflective Activity 9.1

1   True
2   False
3   True
4   True
5   False
6   True
7   True
8   False
9   True
10   True
11   True

Reflective Activity 10.1

1   True
2   False
3   True
4   True
5   False
6   False
7   True
8   True
9   False
10   False
11   True

Reflective Activity 11.1

1   True
2   False
3   True
4   False
5   False
6   True
7   True
8   True

9   False
10 True
11 True
12 False
13 True
14 True
15 False
16 False
17 True

3   False
4   False
5   True
6   False
7   True
8   False
9   True
10 True
11 True
12 False

Reflective Activity 12.1

1   True
2   False
3   False
4   True
5   False
6   True
7   False
8   True
9   False
10 True
11 False
12 True
13 True
14 False
15 True

Reflective Activity 13.1

1   True
2   False
3   False
4   True
5   False
6   False
7   True
8   False
9   True
10 True
11 False
12 True
13 True
14 True
15 False
16 False
17 True

Reflective Activity 14.1

1   True
2   True

Reflective Activity 15.1

1   True
2   False
3   False
4   True
5   True
6   False
7   True
8   True
9   False
10 True
11 True

Reflective Activity 16.1

1   False
2   False
3   True
4   False
5   True
6   False
7   False
8   True
9   False
10 True
11 False
12 False

Reflective Activity 16.2

1   False
2   False
3   True
4   False
5   True
6   True
7   True
8   False
9   True

Reflective Activity 17.1

1 True
2 False
3 False
4 True
5 False
6 False
7 True
8 True
9 False
10 True
11 True
12 False
13 True

Index